D0108467

WEIGHT BIAS

WEIGHT BIAS

■ ■ ■

Nature, Consequences, and Remedies

edited by

■ ■ ■

Kelly D. Brownell

Rebecca M. Puhl

Marlene B. Schwartz

Leslie Rudd

THE GUILFORD PRESS
New York London

A Division of Guilford Publications, Inc.
72 Spring Street, New York, NY 10012
www.guilford.com

Printed in the United States of America

This book is printed on acid-free paper.

Last digit is print number: 9 8 7 6 5 4 3 2 1

Library of Congress Cataloging-in-Publication Data

Weight bias : nature, consequences, and remedies / edited by Kelly D. Brownell ... [et al.].
p. cm.
Includes bibliographical references and index.
ISBN 1-59385-199-5 (hardcover : alk. paper)
1. Body image. 2. Body image—Social aspects. 3. Discrimination against overweight persons. 4. Physical-appearance-based bias. I. Brownell, Kelly D.
BF697.5.B63W43 2005
306.4′613—dc22

2005016816

About the Editors

Kelly D. Brownell, PhD, is Professor and Chair of the Department of Psychology at Yale University, where he also serves as Professor of Epidemiology and Public Health and as Director of the Rudd Center for Food Policy and Obesity. He has served as president of several national organizations, including the Society of Behavioral Medicine, the Association for Advancement of Behavior Therapy, and the Division of Health Psychology of the American Psychological Association. Dr. Brownell has received numerous awards and honors for his work, including the James McKeen Cattell Award from the New York Academy of Sciences, the award for Outstanding Contribution to Health Psychology from the American Psychological Association, and the Distinguished Alumni Award from Purdue University. He has published 14 books and more than 250 scientific articles and chapters. His book *Behavioral Medicine and Women* (coedited with Elaine A. Blechman) received the Choice Award for Outstanding Academic Book from the American Library Association, and his paper on "Understanding and Preventing Relapse" published in *American Psychologist* was listed as one of the most frequently cited papers in psychology.

Rebecca M. Puhl, PhD, is currently a researcher with the Rudd Center for Food Policy and Obesity at Yale University and a clinician at the Johns Hopkins Weight Management Center. Her research focuses on stigma against obese individuals, methods of reducing weight bias, and societal and behavioral contributors to obesity. Dr. Puhl's recent publications address the origins of weight stigma, stigma reduction interventions, coping with weight stigma, childhood food rules, and societal factors related to childhood obesity. She has presented on these topics to academic, professional, and community groups. Her clinical training at the Yale Center for Eating and Weight Disorders involved treating patients with anorexia nervosa, bulimia nervosa, binge-eating disorder, and obesity.

Marlene B. Schwartz, PhD, is Deputy Director of the Rudd Center for Food Policy and Obesity at Yale University and Co-chair of the Weight Bias Task Force of the North American Association for the Study of Obesity. Her research focuses on the stigma of obesity and environmental factors that contribute to poor nutrition for children. Dr. Schwartz has presented nationally on the treatment of eating disorders, parenting and food, and how to advocate for healthier food in schools. She is a coauthor of *Helping Your Child Overcome an Eating Disorder: What You Can Do at Home.*

Leslie Rudd established and funded the Rudd Foundation in December 1998, and is currently the owner and CEO of Leslie Rudd Investment Company, a privately held organization based in California. He is also the owner of Dean & DeLuca, the New York-based epicurean food store; Rudd Vineyards & Winery; PRESS restaurant in Napa Valley; and Distillery No. 209 in San Francisco. In 2005, Mr. Rudd funded the Rudd Center for Food Policy and Obesity at Yale University to continue and expand on the obesity-related work started by The Rudd Institute in 1999.

Contributors

Miriam Berg, BA, Council on Size and Weight Discrimination, Stowe, Pennsylvania

Steven N. Blair, PED, The Cooper Institute, Dallas, Texas

Diane Bliss, BS, Plus-Size Task Force of the Screen Actors Guild, Los Angeles, California

Kelly D. Brownell, PhD, Department of Psychology, Yale University, New Haven, Connecticut

Heather O. Chambliss, PhD, The Cooper Institute, Dallas, Texas

Christian S. Crandall, PhD, Department of Psychology, University of Kansas, Lawrence, Kansas

Jennifer Crocker, PhD, Department of Psychology, University of Michigan, Ann Arbor, Michigan

Morgan Downey, JD, American Obesity Association, Washington, DC

James L. Early, MD, Department of Preventive Medicine and Public Health, University of Kansas School of Medicine–Wichita, Wichita, Kansas

Marla Eisenberg, ScD, Department of Epidemiology and Community Health, School of Public Health, and Division of General Pediatrics and Adolescent Health, Department of Pediatrics, University of Minnesota, Minneapolis, Minnesota

Anthony N. Fabricatore, PhD, Department of Psychiatry, University of Pennsylvania School of Medicine, Philadelphia, Pennsylvania

Janna Fikkan, BA, Department of Psychology, University of Vermont, Burlington, Vermont

Gary D. Foster, PhD, Department of Psychiatry, University of Pennsylvania School of Medicine, Philadelphia, Pennsylvania

Julie A. Garcia, PhD, Department of Psychology, University of Michigan, Ann Arbor, Michigan

Bradley S. Greenberg, PhD, Departments of Communication and Telecommunication, Information Studies and Media, Michigan State University, East Lansing, Michigan

Todd F. Heatherton, PhD, Department of Psychology, Dartmouth College, Hanover, New Hampshire

Michelle R. Hebl, PhD, Department of Psychology, Rice University, Houston, Texas

Sylvia Herbozo, MA, Department of Psychology, University of South Florida, Tampa, Florida

Susan Himes, MA, Department of Psychology, University of South Florida, Tampa, Florida

Carol A. Johnson, MA, Planning Council for Health and Human Services, Milwaukee, Wisconsin

Judy A. Johnston, MS, RD/LD, Department of Preventive Medicine and Public Health, University of Kansas School of Medicine–Wichita, Wichita, Kansas

Eden B. King, MA, Department of Psychology, Rice University, Houston, Texas

Janet D. Latner, PhD, Department of Psychology, University of Canterbury, Christchurch, New Zealand

Robyn K. Mallett, PhD, Department of Psychology, University of Virginia, Charlottesville, Virginia

Lynn McAfee, Council on Size and Weight Discrimination, Stowe, Pennsylvania

Dianne Neumark-Sztainer, PhD, Division of Epidemiology and Community Health, School of Public Health, University of Minnesota, Minneapolis, Minnesota

Rebecca M. Puhl, PhD, Department of Psychology, Yale University, New Haven, Connecticut

April Horstman Reser, MA, Department of Psychology, University of Kansas, Lawrence, Kansas

Esther Rothblum, PhD, Department of Women's Studies, San Diego State University, San Diego, California

Marlene B. Schwartz, PhD, Department of Psychology, Yale University, New Haven, Connecticut

Gretchen B. Sechrist, PhD, Department of Psychology, University at Buffalo, The State University of New York, Buffalo, New York

Jeffery Sobal, PhD, Division of Nutritional Sciences, College of Human Ecology, Cornell University, Ithaca, New York

Sondra Solovay, JD, Law Office of Sondra Solovay, Oakland, California

Charles Stangor, PhD, Department of Psychology, University of Maryland, College Park, College Park, Maryland

Bethany A. Teachman, PhD, Department of Psychology, University of Virginia, Charlottesville, Virginia

Elizabeth E. Theran, JD, Office of General Counsel, U.S. Equal Employment Opportunity Commission, Washington, DC

J. Kevin Thompson, PhD, Department of Psychology, University of South Florida, Tampa, Florida

Thomas A. Wadden, PhD, Department of Psychiatry, University of Pennsylvania School of Medicine, Philadelphia, Pennsylvania

Christina C. Wee, MD, MPH, Division of General Medicine and Primary Care, Beth Israel Deaconess Medical Center and Harvard Medical School, Boston, Massachusetts

Michele Weston, BA, Curvy Media/Brand Consulting Firm, SellingStyle, Inc., New York, New York

Tracy R. Worrell, MA, Department of Communication, Michigan State University, East Lansing, Michigan

Yuko Yamamiya, MA, Department of Psychology, University of South Florida, Tampa, Florida

Susan Z. Yanovski, MD, Obesity and Eating Disorders Program, National Institute of Diabetes and Digestive and Kidney Diseases, National Institutes of Health, Bethesda, Maryland

Acknowledgments

We are grateful first and foremost to those individuals—clients, friends, colleagues, and others who contact us—for sharing their stories of living in a world that judges them for what they weigh. Their lives paint a picture of coping and strength, but also of great pain. The aim of this book is to understand these experiences, to document their impact, to understand how individuals react when confronted with bias and discrimination, and, above all, to stimulate the development and evaluation of efforts to ameliorate the injustice of weight bias.

We also thank the contributing authors for giving of their time, expertise, and creativity in helping us forge this book. Leading scholars, thinkers, and doers on the issue of weight bias have offered their thoughts in a way that not only advances knowledge but is also likely to have an important impact on the field.

One group of colleagues has worked with us from the outset and has been instrumental in advancing the field. This group includes Steven N. Blair and Heather O. Chambliss of The Cooper Institute, James L. Early at the University of Kansas School of Medicine, and James Hill at the University of Colorado Medical Center. Through their science, insight, and leadership, each has enriched us and the field overall. We thank also Ellen Hunt and John Olson for their support and guidance through their leadership roles in the Rudd Foundation. They have become good friends and colleagues.

We next thank our spouses and children for seeing us through the countless hours of work and for believing in us and in the importance of this book.

Finally, three of us (K. D. B., R. M. P., and M. B. S.) offer our heartfelt appreciation to Leslie Rudd who had the vision and courage to identify an area in need of attention, and through force of character created a foundation, assembled a fine group of scholars, and launched the most concerted effort ever on the topic of weight stigma. His objective was to make a difference. Let there be no doubt that he has.

Contents

Introduction

The Social, Scientific, and Human Context of Prejudice and Discrimination Based on Weight

KELLY D. BROWNELL

> The discovery of truth is prevented more effectively, not by the false appearance things present and which mislead into error, not directly by weakness of the reasoning powers, but by preconceived opinion, by prejudice.
>
> —ARTHUR SCHOPENHAUER (1851)

In free societies, bias, stigma, prejudice, and discrimination are considered inherently evil, seen as a threat to the health, happiness, and social status of those targeted, but also to a nation's fundamental values of inclusion and equality. The behaviors resulting from prejudice range from minor infractions of civility to genocide.

Prejudice and the discrimination it breeds are passed through generations, socialized through multiple channels, and often occur in people who believe themselves to be fair-minded. In areas such as race and gender bias, there is a rich tradition of research, advocacy, social action, and public policy designed to understand causes and to design methods for prevention. Bias based on race and gender has not been eliminated, but progress has been made. This is less the case with weight bias.

Research and social policy on weight bias and discrimination lag far behind, to the point where negative attitudes based on weight have been labeled the last acceptable form of discrimination (Puhl & Brownell,

2001). Because the prevalence of obesity is striking and because the consequences of weight stigma can be severe, the stakes are high.

This book aims to document those consequences, discuss the social and psychological origins of weight stigma, and propose what might be done at individual, institutional, and national levels to correct problems that may exist. This book is the first, we believe, to cover each of these areas and to combine what is known from scientific, legal, advocacy, and personal experience perspectives into a coherent picture of the problems and of potential solutions.

Why now? It is true that weight bias has existed for a very long time, but only in recent years has a critical mass of science accumulated to form the needed knowledge base. But there is more. Advocacy movements have more voice, legal challenges to weight discrimination are more common, employers are beginning to include prevention of weight bias as part of diversity training, and some legislators are considering policy as a means of preventing bias. Collecting this information from disparate sources may be one means for connecting the relevant parties and stimulating progress.

HUMAN AND SOCIAL CONTEXTS

A discussion of stigma and obesity might justifiably begin with consideration of the human toll. One might estimate the toll by inferring population consequences based on studies of depression, self-esteem, the impact of avoiding preventive medical care because of shame, and so on. But even then one emerges with only statistics, and the very real impact on the lives of human beings is easily overlooked.

Why care about individuals and their lives? Health professionals ply their trade to prevent and reduce human suffering, but physical suffering is only one target. Psychological torment and social discrimination are important in their own right, but may also affect health. Obese people suffer, plain and clear. They exist in a socially constructed world that determines what is right and wrong, what is pleasing and disgusting, how blame is assessed, and who deserves some version of a scarlet letter.

The depth of suffering can be profound. While anecdotes do not establish scientific fact, all professionals who have worked closely with obese individuals have heard wrenching stories. We offer a few to show why we believe the study of this problem is so important.

> When I was a child, I was sick and absent from school one day. The teacher taking attendance came across my name and said, "She must have stayed home to eat." The other kids told me about this the next day.
>
> —*Words from a person seeking treatment for obesity*

> I remember one incident when I was in the sixth grade and my teacher was looking at my latest handwriting assignment; she announced to the whole class that my handwriting was just like me—"fat and squatty." . . . The pain and humiliation aimed at you as an innocent child never leaves you!
>
> —*Words from a woman recalling stigma experiences*

> Gina Score, a 14-year-old girl in South Dakota, was sent in the summer of 1999 to a state juvenile detention camp. Gina was characterized as sensitive and intelligent, wrote poetry, and was planning to skip a grade when she returned to school. She was sent to the facility for petty theft—stealing money from her parents and from lockers at school "to buy food." She was said to have stolen "a few dollars here, a few dollars there," and paid most of the money back. The camp, run by a former Marine and modeled on the military, aimed, in the words of an instruction manual, to "overwhelm them with fear and anxiety." On July 21, a hot humid day, Gina was forced to begin a 2.7 mile run/walk. Gina was 5′4″ tall, weighed 224 lbs., and was unable to complete even simple physical exercises such as leg lifts. She fell behind early but was prodded and cajoled by instructors. A short time later, she collapsed, lay on the ground panting, with pale skin and purple lips. She was babbling incoherently and frothing from the mouth, with her eyes rolled back in her head. The drill instructors sat nearby drinking sodas, laughing and chatting, accusing Gina of faking, within 100 feet of an air-conditioned building. After 4 hours with Gina lying prostrate in the sun, a doctor came by and summoned an ambulance immediately. Gina's organs had failed and she died. (cited in Puhl & Brownell, 2001)

The chapters in this book help place these anecdotes in context by establishing the nature, frequency, and severity of prejudice and discrimination. Prejudice, when acted out in social interactions, generates stories like these. Educational and employment opportunities become constrained, interactions with health care providers are affected, and countless interactions in day-to-day life expose affected individuals to pain. Overweight people often report critical comments even from people they chose not to interact with (strangers in supermarkets, etc.).

Such stories have a purpose beyond the generation of hypotheses. They help keep us focused on what is most important—to improve health and well-being.

THE SCIENTIFIC CONTEXT

When parties disagree on how stigma develops, its consequences, and methods for prevention, science must be the referee. It must summon the parties to the center of the ring and establish the best way to proceed.

It is heartening, therefore, to see rapid changes in the quality and quantity of science on weight stigma. The chapters in this book represent the best of that science, but science alone is not sufficient to make change. Change may be possible through a variety of routes, including specific initiatives such as altering the portrayal of overweight people in the media, but also through broader means such as litigation and legislation. It is essential therefore that government agencies fund research on weight stigma, that a new generation of scientists be sensitized to its importance, that professional meetings and journals include work on the topic, and that connections remain open between scientists and those who might harness the science in the service of social change.

A number of key issues remain to be addressed. These are addressed in this book's chapters, but two issues are of special note: whether weight stigma affects health, and whether it has negative consequences, no impact, or even benefits for the overall well-being of affected individuals.

Weight Bias and Health

Excess weight is linked to ill health and mortality. Long lists of diseases associated with obesity have been constructed and include heart disease, cancer, hypertension, lipid dysregulation, and many more. Prominent on this list is Type 2 diabetes, whose prevalence tracks increasing obesity rates like a terribly unwanted companion.

Much work has been done to understand the mechanisms linking obesity to poor health. Without exception these have focused on biological mechanisms such as the impact of weight on blood pressure, lipids, and insulin resistance. Overlooked entirely is the impact obesity may have on health through its social consequences. To what extent does the impact of stigma, bias, and discrimination affect the health of obese individuals?

There is very good reason to study this issue. Mounting science on health disparities has shown clearly that disadvantaged groups suffer disproportionately, precisely because disadvantage creates conditions that in turn can compromise health. Stress, lack of access to medical care, exposure to environmental toxins, poor education about health, unsafe working conditions, lack of resources for preventive care, and of course poverty itself are examples.

Stated another way, quite apart from the direct effects of excess weight on physiology, being obese in an inhospitable, antagonistic environment may compromise health. A conceptual scheme for how this may take place is presented in Figure I.1.

Documenting the health consequences of weight bias may be extremely important. It could add an entire new dimension to efforts to reduce the medical impact of obesity to both individuals and society.

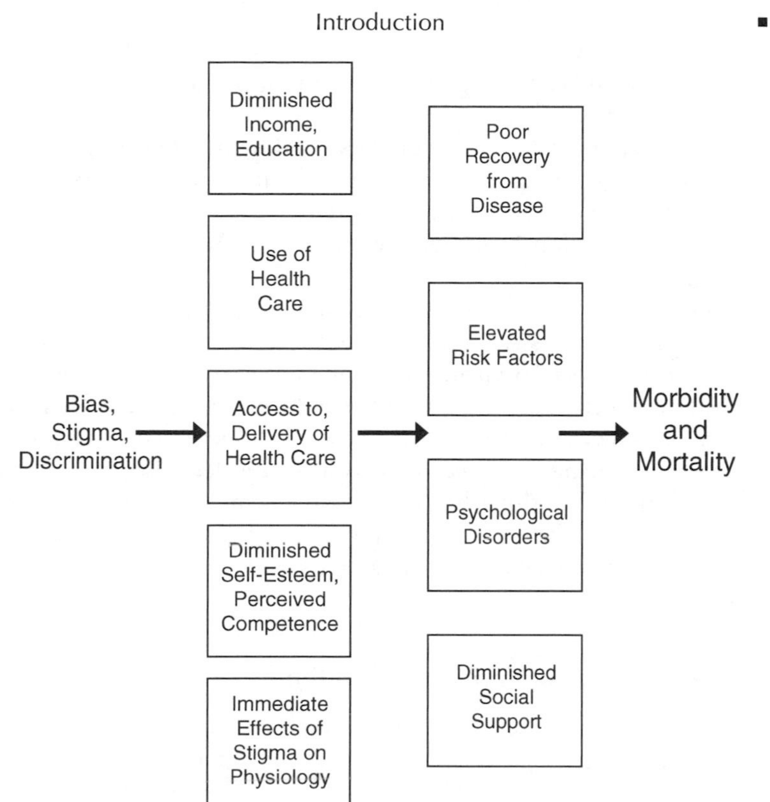

FIGURE I.1. A hypothetical scheme representing possible ways that the experience of bias and discrimination may be linked to important health outcomes.

One might eventually see, as an example, health insurance companies or large health maintenance organizations supporting bias reduction programs, not for reasons of social justice but to reduce health care costs.

Discrimination "for Their Own Good"

It is not uncommon to hear that stigma is beneficial because it serves as an incentive for people to avoid gaining weight and motivates overweight people to reduce. There are several corollaries of this stance:

1. Without bias there is insufficient motivation for people to lose weight.
2. The condition is under sufficient personal control that social contingencies will be sufficient to produce change.

3. Acts such as teasing, joking, and outright discrimination are acceptable.
4. The shame and humiliation produced by bias has positive effects.
5. Programs aimed at preventing bias may be counterproductive because motivation to be thin is reduced.
6. Discrimination "for their own good" is justifiable.

Those who work in the area of weight stigma bristle at such statements and classify this stance as a cynical attempt by those with biased attitudes to turn vice to virtue. It seems unlikely that being stigmatized has positive effects. Bias against overweight people has grown stronger at the same time the prevalence of obesity has increased. It is also hard to believe that being ridiculed, perceived to be defective, and discriminated against has anything but negative consequences. To be fair, however, these are testable and important questions. One reason to undertake the tests is to challenge arguments that the status quo should prevail.

Separating the Person from the Condition

Society sometimes attaches negative personal qualities to individuals with certain conditions, particularly when improper personal behavior is thought to be the cause. Alcoholism and AIDS are two examples. If the disease is bad, the person with the disease is bad as well.

It is important to uncouple the condition from the person. One can accept obesity as an undesirable and dangerous condition without despising the person with it. Having empathy for the obese person is not inconsistent with fighting obesity as a condition. This is an important conceptual point that must be made time and again if social progress is to be made. Questions of personal responsibility are central in this context and are key to framing the obesity issue in a constructive way.

A Brief History of Work on Weight Bias

Weight bias itself has been traced as far back as medieval times (Stunkard, LaFleur, & Wadden 1998), but Richardson, Goodman, Hastorf, and Dornbusch (1961) launched the science by asking children to rate line drawings of other children, one overweight and others with physical disabilities. The overweight child was rated as least likable. Other studies with children and adults in the 1960s came to similar conclusions (Goodman, Dornbusch, Richardson, & Hastorf, 1963; Maddox, Back, & Liederman, 1968). These were the predecessors to the social psychology research on weight stigma that began in earnest in the 1990s.

During the 1960s a field of obesity research began to take shape as researchers doing animal physiology studies of appetite and weight joined forces with physicians approaching obesity from a medical perspective. The great figures of this era, the ones who wrote the classic books, founded journals and associations, and made obesity a viable subject of research included George Bray, Theodore Van Itallie, Per Bjorntorp, Jules Hirsch, John Garrow, and Albert Stunkard. In 1976, Stunkard authored a book called *The Pain of Obesity*. This book contained a number of insights, among them recognition that obesity is highly stigmatized and has a very real impact on everyday life.

How did Stunkard come to these insights? He talked to people and he listened. Instead of seeing individuals as their weight or blood pressure, he attended to his patients as people. He heard them, understood them, and grasped what they were experiencing. In describing his own book, Stunkard said:

> This is a book about troubled people—those troubled by the modern American obsession with overweight and obesity. It tells something about the way they eat, how they feel about themselves and their bodies, and a good bit about how they cope with the preoccupation that dominates their lives—losing weight. (1976, p. 1)

Soon thereafter came feminist writers who emphasized social conditions that brought women into conflict with their bodies. Susie Orbach's *Fat Is a Feminist Issue* (1978) is perhaps the flagship publication. It spoke of the negative impact of dieting caused by fears of obesity and the impact of weight issues on the well-being of women. Other books appeared shortly thereafter and began to discuss the painful social and psychological consequences of being overweight. Marcia Millman's *Such a Pretty Face* (1980) is a key example.

The anti-dieting concept born from political and personal perspectives, exemplified by the Orbach and Millman books, had a basis in science as well. Susan Wooley was the pioneer who in the late 1970s began writing and speaking about compensatory metabolic reactions to weight loss, hunger during dieting, and other factors that would thwart weight loss and damage already weakened self-esteem (Wooley, Wooley & Dyrenforth, 1979). This work paved the path for what would follow; considerable research on the consequences of dieting, the arbitrary nature of weight and beauty standards, and the wisdom of the full-scale assault against overweight. Spanning three decades, Polivy and Herman's work (1983, 1985, 2002) is perhaps best known in this regard.

The study of weight stigma from a social psychology perspective also began around this time. A paper in 1979 by Natalie Allon presaged much of what would come. Allon argued that "the concept of stigma may be a viable analytical tool in studying overweight as: an exclusive focus in interaction, related to a negative body image, overwhelming others with mixed emotions, clashing with other attributes of the person, an equivocal predictor of activities, and related to one's sense of responsibility for one's overweight" (1979, p. 480). The social psychological study of weight bias, with figures like Christian Crandall and Jennifer Crocker leading the way, took firm hold in the 1990s.

Occurring in parallel to the science and feminist writings was the birth of an advocacy movement designed to expose bias and to fight injustice. The first group was founded in 1969 and was called the National Association to Aid Fat Americans (NAAFA), changed later to the National Association to Advance Fat Acceptance. For its small size, NAAFA generated considerable media attention, at first because it was considered an oddity, but with time because it addresses issues of social importance. More recent groups such as the Council on Size and Weight Discrimination also address issues of weight bias.

It was in the 1980s that the obesity field itself began to attend to the social consequences of obesity (Wadden & Stunkard, 1985). Personal experiences of obese individuals became important in understanding how to provide effective and compassionate care and studies began to appear on the way obese individuals were perceived by health care providers.

A key event occurred in 1998 when Leslie Rudd founded the Rudd Institute, "dedicated to identifying and ameliorating bias and stigma associated with obesity, and educating the public about obesity issues" (www.RuddInstitute.org). This organization has supported a great deal of research on weight stigma and has been a stimulus for organizing the efforts of scientists and others working on this issue.

This brings us to the turn of the century. More work than ever is occurring on weight stigma and discrimination, but has not been organized. The presence of this book is a sign that organization is beginning.

Another positive sign is action taken by the major professional obesity organization, The North American Association for the Study of Obesity (NAASO). At its annual meeting in 2001, President Charles Billington invited me to address the issue of weight bias in the opening session and to administer a measure of bias to those in the audience (Schwartz, Chambliss, Brownell, Blair, & Billington, 2003). NAASO then began to consider the issue of stigma and took two important steps. The first was to establish a NAASO Weight Discrimination Task Force. The second was to include organizational "values" in its 2005 strategic plan. Among these are the following:

- Compassion—For the lives and situations of those dealing with obesity both personally and professionally.
- Respect—For each other and all who are touched by obesity.

Much has been done but much remains to be done. The trajectory is positive.

DEFINITIONS AND TERMS

Terms Used to Describe Weight

Various terms are used by authors in this book to describe the condition of having excess weight, with *fat*, *obese*, and *overweight* being primary. Obesity and overweight have different technical meanings. *Overweight* is defined as body mass index between 25 and 29.9 kg/m^2 and *obesity* as body mass index 30 kg/m^2 and greater. The point at which overweight becomes obesity may have meaning in the context of health risk, but may be less important when considering social bias.

The term *fat* came into vogue because negative connotations attached to the word *obese* (as a condition) are applied to people who have the condition. It also attempts to remove the stigma from the word *fat* by using it in an open and forthright way. Several authors in this book prefer the word fat and offer a rationale for doing do.

Interchangeable use of these terms is unavoidable at this point. When science begins to identify breakpoints at which increasing weight confers elevated or very elevated social risk, more precise use of terms may be possible.

Bias, Stigma, Prejudice

Also used interchangeably are the terms *bias*, *stigma*, and *prejudice*. In general language, these refer to negative attitudes about individuals based on suppositions about a group they belong to. The Merriam-Webster Dictionary (www.m-w.com) offers the following definitions:

Bias: an inclination of temperament or outlook; *especially*: a personal and sometimes unreasoned judgment

Stigma: a mark of shame or discredit

Prejudice: preconceived judgment or opinion; an adverse opinion or leaning formed without just grounds or before sufficient knowledge; an instance of such judgment or opinion; an irrational attitude of hostility directed against an individual, a group, a race, or their supposed characteristics

Separating these terms might work as follows. *Bias* is the inclination to form unreasoned judgments, with *prejudice* (hostility) as a possible outcome. *Stigma* is the social sign or emblem carried by the individual who is the victim of *prejudice*. For some of the work represented in this book, precise definitions are important. This will be increasingly so as the field advances and work becomes more sophisticated.

THINKING AND ACTING BOTH LOCALLY AND GLOBALLY

> Where, after all, do universal human rights begin? In small places, close to home—so close and so small that they cannot be seen on any map of the world. Yet they are the world of the individual person: The neighborhood he lives in; the school or college he attends; the factory, farm or office where he works. Such are the places where every man, woman and child seeks equal justice, equal opportunity, equal dignity without discrimination. Unless these rights have meaning there, they have little meaning anywhere. Without concerted citizen action to uphold them close to home, we shall look in vain for progress in the larger world.
>
> —ELEANOR ROOSEVELT (1958 speech to the United Nations)

There is much that can be done to prevent weight stigma or to ameliorate its consequences. Actions by governments and institutions are possible, but so are actions individuals take as citizens. Children can be coached on attitudes regarding weight, schools can be encouraged to include weight as part of diversity issues, opinion pieces on the subject can be written for local newspapers, and local, regional, and national politicians can be approached regarding civil rights legislation.

One aim of this book is to open discussion on the optimal ways to proceed with eliminating prejudice and discrimination. Some of us will work on this by creating the needed science, others by attempting to create systemic change, and still others by working locally as individuals. All are important.

REFERENCES

Allon, N. (1979). Self-perceptions of the stigma of overweight in relationship to weight-losing patterns. *American Journal of Clinical Nutrition, 32*, 470–480.

Goodman, N., Dornbusch, S.M., Richardson, S.A., & Hastorf, A.H. (1963). Variant reactions of physical disabilities. *American Sociological Review, 28*, 429–435.

Maddox, G. L., Back, K. W., & Liederman, V. R. (1968). Overweight as social deviance and disability. *Journal of Health and Social Behavior, 9*, 287–298.

Millman, M. (1980). *Such a pretty face: Being fat in America*. New York: Norton.

Orbach, S. (1978). *Fat is a feminist issue: The anti-diet guide to permanent weight loss*. New York: Paddington.

Polivy, J., & Herman, C. P. (1983). *Breaking the diet habit: The natural weight alternative*. New York: Basic Books.

Polivy, J., & Herman, C. P. (1985). Dieting and binging: A causal analysis. *American Psychologist, 40*, 193–201.

Polivy, J., & Herman, C. P. (2002). If at first you don't succeed: False hopes of self-change. *American Psychologist, 57*, 677–689.

Puhl, R., & Brownell, K. D. (2001). Bias, discrimination, and obesity. *Obesity Research, 9*, 788–805.

Richardson, S. A., Goodman, N., Hastorf, A. H., & Dornbusch, S. M. (1961). Cultural uniformity in reaction to physical disabilities. *American Sociological Review, 26*, 241–247.

Roosevelt, E. (1958, March 27). Speech "In Your Hands," delivered to the United Nations. Retrieved March 22, 2005, from www.udhr.org/history/inyour.htm

Schopenhauer, A. (1851). *Parerga and paralipomena* (Vol. 2, ch. 1, sect. 17).

Schwartz, M. B., Chambliss, H. O., Brownell, K. D., Blair, S. N., & Billington, C. (2003). Weight bias among health professionals specializing in obesity. *Obesity Research, 11*, 1033–1039.

Stunkard, A. J. (1976). *The pain of obesity*. Palo Alto, CA: Bull.

Stunkard, A. J., LaFleur, W. R., & Wadden, T. A. (1998). Stigmatization of obesity in medieval times: Asia and Europe. *International Journal of Obesity, 22*, 1141–1144.

Wadden, T. A., & Stunkard, A. J. (1985). Social and psychological consequences of obesity. *Annals of Internal Medicine, 103*, 1062–1067.

Wooley, S. C., Wooley, O. W., & Dyrenforth, S. R. (1979). Theoretical, practical, and social issues in behavioral treatments of obesity. *Journal of Applied Behavior Analysis, 12*, 3–25.

PART I

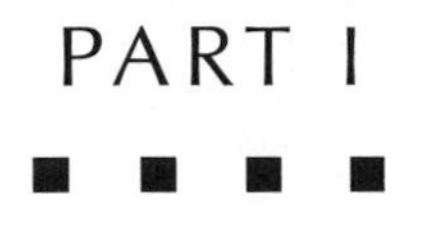

Nature and Extent of Weight Bias

CHAPTER 1

■ ■ ■

Weight Bias in Employment

JANNA FIKKAN
ESTHER ROTHBLUM

> Appearance, especially weight, has a lot to do with advancing. I have been normal size and have advanced. But since I have been heavy no one wants me. I have a high IQ and my productivity is extremely high. But, no one cares.
>
> —EMPLOYEE (quoted in Haskins & Ransford, 1999, p. 306).

> Under no circumstance . . . is it advisable to go on record as having turned someone down for reasons of size. Never write down in any note the fact that you didn't hire someone because they were overweight. Use code words and phrases, such as "presented poor image," or "poorly dressed," or "sloppy appearance."
>
> —LAWYER (quoted in Everett, 1990, p. 69)

In the past three decades, a growing body of literature has begun to document the marked discrimination that fat men and women face with regard to employment (Puhl & Brownell, 2001; Roehling, 1999, 2002; Solovay, 2000). This literature, which represents multiple disciplines, has reported both experimentally and anecdotally that fat people are less likely to be hired (Brink, 1988; Klesges et al., 1990; Larkin & Pines, 1979; Pingitore, Dugoni, Tindale, & Spring, 1994; Popovich et al., 1997), perceived as having numerous undesirable traits related to job performance (Jasper & Klassen, 1990a, 1990b; Klassen, Jasper & Harris, 1993; Rothblum, Miller, & Garbutt, 1988), more harshly disciplined on the job (Belizzi & Hasty, 1998, 2001; Belizzi & Norvell, 1991), assigned to inferior professional assignments (Belizzi & Hasty, 1998; Belizzi, Klassen, & Belonax, 1989), paid less than their nonfat coworkers (Averett & Korenman, 1993; Loh, 1996; Maranto & Stenoien, 2000; Pagán & Dávila, 1997; Register & Williams, 1990; Saporta & Halpern, 2002; Sargent & Blanchflower, 1994; Sarlio-Lähteenkarova & Lahelma, 1999; Sarlio-Lähteenkarova, Silventoinen, & Lahelma, 2004), and even terminated for failure to lose weight at the employer's request (cited in Berton, 2001). The self-report of fat men and women themselves has also revealed a high frequency of employment-related discrimination (Rothblum, Brand, Miller, & Oetjen, 1990). In addition to these barriers, fat people have been perceived by employers as a liability when it comes to providing health care insurance (Paul & Townsend, 1995; Roehling, 2002) and even penalized through some companies' benefits programs for their weight status (Reese, 2000).

Recent court cases brought to trial under the Rehabilitation Act and the Americans with Disabilities Act (ADA) have highlighted both the ways in which particular employees have been discriminated against because of their weight (see Ziolkowski, 1994, for a review) and the significant societal assumptions about fatness that persist in the general society. These assumptions address a range of issues from stereotypes of fat persons to the causes of fatness to the putative moral implications of being fat for men and women. Not only are these assumptions widespread at the societal level (Kolata, 1992), they also have impacted some court decisions and the legal interpretation of antidiscrimination laws that might protect fat persons from the negative treatment they face on the job (Maranto & Stenoien, 2000; Taussig, 1994; Ziolkowski, 1994).

EVIDENCE FOR WEIGHT-RELATED BIAS IN HIRING

Studies that have been designed to have raters evaluate both fat and nonfat hypothetical job applicants on suitability for a job have consistently found that fat applicants are chosen less often, despite having similar or identical credentials to nonfat applicants. One recent study even showed that *nonfat* male job applicants who were shown in close proximity with fat women were evaluated more harshly than men in the presence of nonfat women (Hebl & Mannix, 2003), evidencing the magnitude of anti-fat bias in employment settings.

In one of the earliest and most often cited experimental studies in this area, Larkin and Pines (1979) showed that there was a strong negative stereotype of fat people. When assessed on work-related personality traits, fat applicants were rated as significantly less neat, active, productive, likely to take initiative, energetic, ambitious, attractive, and healthy than "normal weight" applicants. They were also seen as significantly more likely to need prompting, lack self-discipline, and give up easily (Larkin & Pines, 1979).

Brink (1988) asked college students to evaluate hypothetical candidates' suitability for a position as a professor of psychology using sex, age, race, marital status, number of children and weight as independent variables. No discrimination was reported for any of the categories except weight; when the candidate was described as a man weighing 425 lbs. his suitability rating was significantly lower than when he was described as weighing 165 lbs. A separate group of students rated a worker described as weighing 365 lbs. as much less likely to be promoted than a worker described as weighing 165 lbs., despite the fact that, in this study, there were no differences between weight status in the ascription of *positive* personality traits to the workers, such as "hardworking," "intelligent," and "persistent" (Brink, 1988).

Jasper and Klassen (1990a) also asked students to rate hypothetical job applicants who varied by "body type" on (1) their desire to work with the person, (2) how effective they thought the person would be in selling them a product, and (3) how the target person's size affected their decision. Results showed that students were significantly less likely to report a desire to work with a fat person than a nonfat person. Students also reported that the nonfat target would be significantly more effective in selling them a product. Interestingly, male students reported significantly less desire to work with a fat woman, whereas there was no gender difference on desire in working with a fat man (Jasper & Klassen, 1990a). When asked about their decisions, students reported that body size had negatively impacted their impression of the target, their desire to work with the person, and how effective they estimated the target to be as a salesperson. Additionally, Popovich et al. (1997) reported from their studies that fat job applicants were specifically less likely to be hired for jobs perceived as being more active, especially by raters who scored higher on negative attitudes toward fat persons in general.

Studies that have utilized simulated job interviews to assess discrimination against fat persons have found similar results. Klesges et al. (1990) reported that, when levels of qualifications between applicants viewed on brief videotape clips were described as being equal, raters preferred "normal weight" applicants to fat applicants. Moreover, fat applicants were viewed as having poorer work habits; being less able to get along with others; having less self-control and discipline; being lonely, depressed, and anxious; and having an offensive appearance, regardless of their level of qualification. Whereas applicants described as being diabetic were viewed as more likely to have medically related absences, fat applicants were viewed as having more nonmedically related absences (e.g., being late for work) and as being less conscientious (e.g., more likely to abuse company privileges).

Pingitore et al. (1994) found that applicants' body weight explained about 35% of the variance in the hiring decision, after controlling for facial attractiveness and qualifications. Fat applicants, especially women, were less likely to be recommended for hiring, especially by raters who were satisfied with their own bodies and for whom this was central to their self-concept. Polinko and Popovich (2001) also controlled for facial attractiveness, and although raters in this study did perceive applicants in the "overweight" condition as having more negative work-related attributes than those in the "average-weight" condition, this did not result in the fat applicants being less likely to be recommended to be hired (Polinko & Popovich, 2001).

Rothblum et al. (1988) asked college students to rate résumés of female job applicants. When résumés were accompanied by written information about the applicants' appearance (clothing, hair, height, and weight), fat applicants were rated more negatively than nonfat applicants on supervisory potential, self-discipline, professional appearance, personal hygiene, and ability to perform a physically strenuous job. However, when photos that had been matched for level of attractiveness were attached to the résumé, raters exhibited little negative stereotyping of the fat applicants, leading the authors to speculate that negative reactions to fat women may be attributable to the effects of obesity on perceived attractiveness.

NEGATIVE PERCEPTIONS OF FAT EMPLOYEES AND DISPARATE DISCIPLINARY TREATMENT

A number of studies have dealt with the question of how fat employees, once hired, are perceived and evaluated in comparison with their nonfat counterparts. Results from a study by Klassen et al. (1993) showed that fat targets who displayed behavior that was consistent with the fat stereotype (e.g., "lazy") were judged more negatively then their nonfat counterparts. Specifically, harsher discipline was recommended, their behavior was seen as more likely to recur, and raters expressed the least desire to work with them. Although the presence of a discounting cue (explanation for behavior) did result in less harsh disciplinary recommendations and less of a tendency to believe the behavior would recur, it did not increase raters' desire to work with the fat employee.

Jasper and Klassen (1990b) also found that raters were significantly more eager to work with a person described as "normal weight" than an employee who was described as "obese." Moreover, raters who read a description about a fat female employee were much less eager to work with her than those who read about a fat male employee. Fat employees were more likely to be rated as lazy and lacking in self-discipline. Additionally, fat men were most frequently cited as being "unkempt" and fat women as being "insecure."

Bellizzi and colleagues (Bellizzi & Hasty, 1998, 2001; Bellizzi et al., 1989; Bellizzi & Norvell, 1991) have used samples of actual sales managers recruited through mass mailings to assess treatment of hypothetical employees in "role play" scenarios. Bellizzi et al. (1989) showed that employees described as "extremely overweight" were more likely to be assigned by sales managers to undesirable sales territories or *no* territory within the manager's region and less likely to be assigned an important or desirable region. This discrimination was stronger than that exhibited against employees who were described as heavy smokers and was stronger for fat women than fat men. Bellizzi and Hasty (1998) likewise found that fat sales recruits were found to be significantly less fit for a more challenging sales assignment than nonfat recruits. Additionally, whereas only 24% of the managers indicated a preference for not placing the new recruit in *any* assignment, 40% of the fat recruits fell into this category while only 10% of the nonfat recruits did.

Finally, in three separate studies (Bellizzi & Hasty, 1998, 2001; Bellizzi & Norvell, 1991), this same group of researchers found disparate treatment of fat employees in response to unethical selling behavior. In two of these studies (Bellizzi & Hasty, 1998; Bellizzi & Norvell, 1991), both male and female employees who were described as "extremely overweight" or "obese" were disciplined more harshly for unethical conduct than their nonfat counterparts. Specifically, sales managers were more willing to endorse as appropriate responses termination and issuing written and verbal reprimands, and less willing to suggest counseling for fat sales employees. Managers also rated the fat salesperson as significantly less self-disciplined, ambitious, clean-cut, healthy, and serious, and more lazy, insecure, and untidy than the "normal weight" salesperson (Bellizzi & Norvell, 1991).

Interestingly, though Bellizzi and colleagues report that a general finding in the sales and marketing literature has been that saleswomen are less harshly disciplined than salesmen for unethical sales behavior, this effect seems to disappear when the saleswoman is fat (Bellizzi & Hasty, 2001). In the third and most recent study by Bellizzi and colleagues (Bellizzi & Hasty, 2001), the finding that salesmen are recommended harsher forms of reprimand is qualified by size. As the authors state, "the lenient treatment of women disappears in the case of obesity. Obese women were disciplined at about the same severity level as both obese and non-obese men" (p. 195).

EVIDENCE FOR INEQUITY IN PAY

In addition to having less chance of getting hired and facing more on-the-job discrimination, fat people have also been found in many studies to earn less than their nonfat counterparts, even after controlling for other relevant variables such as education and family socioeconomic status. Numerous studies using data from the United States' National Longitudinal Survey of Youth (NLSY) and Britain's National Child Development Study (NCDS) have found a significant impact of weight on employees' earnings (Averett & Korenman, 1996; Cawley, 2000; Loh, 1993; Maranto & Stenoien, 2000; Pagán & Dávila, 1997; Register & Williams, 1990; Sargent & Blanchflower, 1994).

While controlling for conventional variables associated with disparity in income (e.g., years of education, ethnicity, geographic region) Register and Williams (1990) found that fat women (those in excess of 20% of standard weight for height) in their NLSY sample earned an average of 12% less than nonfat women, whereas this finding did not extend to fat men. Pagán and Dávila (1997) also reported an income disparity for fat women but not fat men.

Cawley (2000) estimated that white women who are "significantly overweight" (defined as being two standard deviations above the mean) are paid on average 7% less than women of mean weight. He proposes this wage difference is equal to that associated with roughly 3 years of prior work experience, 2 years of job tenure, or 1 year of education. This effect was not found for Hispanic or black women. Maranto and Stenoien (2000) also found the negative effect of weight on salaries to be highly significant for white women and only marginally significant for black women. White and black men, on the other hand, only experience wage penalties at the very highest weight levels (100% above standard for their height), with white men suffering a much larger penalty (19.6% lower wages) than black men (3.5% lower wages). In fact, white women in this sample were found to suffer a greater wage penalty for "mild obesity" (20% over standard weight for their height) than black men do for weight that is 100% over standard weight.

Sargent and Blanchflower (1994), found an inverse relationship between obesity at age 16 and earnings at age 23 for British women, using longitudinal data from the NCDS. The magnitude of weight was similar to that of other determinants of earnings, such as gender, job training, and union membership, and increased for women as weight increased. Even fatness at age 11 was associated with earning approximately 3.5% less at age 23 for females. What is perhaps most intriguing about this study's findings is that, even while controlling for non-weight-related variables, young women who were fat at age 16 suffered a wage penalty at age 23 *whether or not they maintained their fatness during that time.* Averett and Korenman (1996) used data from the 1988 NLSY and controlled for family background. Women who were "obese" or "overweight" between ages 16 and 25 had, at ages 23–31, a lower family income, lower hourly wages (30+ age category only), a lower likelihood of being married, and lower spousal income (if married) than women in the recommended weight range.

Sarlio-Lähteenkarova and colleagues (Sarlio-Lähteenkarova & Lahelma, 1999; Sarlio-Lähteenkarova et al., 2004) have also found income differences by body weight in a large, representative sample of Finnish men and women. For women, "overweight" was associated with current unemployment and "obesity" with long-term unemployment as well as low household disposable income and individual incomes (Sarlio-Lähteenkarova & Lahelma, 1999). In contrast, among men only thinness was associated with unemployment and low income, whereas high body mass index (BMI) was not associated with adverse economic outcomes at all.

In more recent analyses of these data, Sarlio-Lähteenkarova et al. (2004) found that the income penalty for fat women was most apparent among more highly educated women, who were found to have income levels about 30% lower than their nonfat counterparts. Women in the lowest educational group did not differ in income according to body weight, and self-employed women showed a *positive* association between their body weight and income. This led the authors to suggest that highly qualified fat women might find better job options being self-employed instead of taking a salaried job.

Haskins and Ransford (1999) also found that the income penalties for fatness in women varied by occupational level. Their study surveyed the female employees of a large industrial organization in the aerospace industry and found that, whereas weight was an important and significant predictor of occupational attainment in the entire sample, it only significantly impacted wages for those women in entry-level professional and managerial strata. The authors speculated that this finding could reflect the fact that women may undergo the most intense "screening" at this occupational level, when they are, in theory, moving from lower-paying blue-collar positions into upper-level professional and managerial positions. This reasoning is further supported by the finding that thinness or ideal weight was especially related to high occupational status in the male-dominated cluster of professions (e.g., research scientist, senior engineer, physicist, etc.). "Perhaps," the authors conclude, "for women in positions typically dominated by males, there is a more careful screening of the 'rational' qualifications criteria as well as attractiveness characteristics such as weight" (Haskins & Ransford, 1999, p. 311).

Findings for the impact of being fat on men's wages have been inconsistent. Some studies found no effects for men, or even a wage *premium* associated with fatness in men (Maranto & Stenoien, 2000; McLean & Moon, 1980; Register & Williams, 1990). Others, however, have found a significant negative impact of fatness on men's wages. Loh (1993) found that fatness did not affect the wage levels of full-time workers, but did lower the rate of wage *growth* for men, but not women. Melamed (1994) also found a correlation between BMI and salaries for men, but not for women. Of interest here is that this correlation was curvilinear, so that, for men, wages were negatively impacted by being too fat *or too thin* (Melamed, 1994). Saporta and Halpern (2002) likewise found in a survey of lawyers that male lawyers were penalized for deviating in either direction from the "ideal" physique. Not surprisingly, women were only penalized for being *above* the "ideal" weight. Though the pay difference between fat and nonfat female lawyers did not reach statistical significance in this particular study, the authors speculated that this may be an artifact due to the fact that there were so few fat female lawyers in this sample.

THEORETICAL EXPLANATIONS AND SOCIOCULTURAL CONTEXTS

These findings document a significant impact on the work experiences of fat persons, especially women, due to anti-fat discrimination. Certainly, the fact that this discrimination is embedded in a much broader societal denigration of fatness is important to recognize. Fatness as a "social deviance" (Maddox, Back, & Leiderman, 1968) has been the focus of a large body of literature that has shown this negative bias to be pervasive (Puhl & Brownell, 2001); exhibited in children as young as preschool age (Cramer & Steinwert, 1998); reproduced in mass media (Greenberg, Eastin, Hofschire, Lachlan, & Brownell, 2003); deeply rooted in, connected to, and justified by conservative American values (Crandall, 1994; Crandall & Martinez, 1996; Crocker, Cornwell, & Major, 1993) and of long-standing origin as represented in widely read cultural texts (Stunkard, LaFleur, & Wadden, 1998).

Despite the large amount of empirical evidence that fat people are discriminated against, much of the research on the well-established relationship between fatness and poverty in Western culture has hesitated to conclude that fat people become poor *because* of this level of discrimination (Sobal, 1991; Sobal & Stunkard, 1989). Instead, a popular hypothesis is that men and women become fat because they are poor and do not have access to nutritious food, safe ways of exercising, education about energy exchange, and the like. However, as the literature reviewed here and elsewhere shows, the obverse is more likely true: people are fat and, because of multiple sources of discrimination, become poor. This argument seems especially compelling in the case of women, who have already been shown to suffer greater social and emotional consequences for fatness than men (Rothblum, 1992; Stake & Lauer, 1987), especially in the United States (Tiggemann & Rothblum, 1988).

A well-cited study by Gortmaker, Must, Perrin, Sobol, and Dietz (1993) showed that women who had been fat in adolescence (unlike those with other chronic conditions) completed fewer years of schooling, were less likely to be married, had lower household incomes, and higher rates of household poverty than women who had not been fat, regardless of their baseline socioeconomic status and aptitude-test scores. Furthermore, although fatness has not been shown to negatively impact the performance of high school students (Canning & Mayer, 1967), it *has* been shown to have a negative impact on rates of college acceptance and attendance (again, more so for females than for males; Canning & Mayer, 1966) and even on the willingness of parents to pay for their children's educational expenses (more so for fat daughters than for fat sons; Crandall, 1991, 1995). Interestingly, although all of these factors negatively impact the earning potential of fat women, Averett and Korenman (1996) found that between 50 and 95% of fat women's lower economic status can be explained by differences in marriage probabilities. That is, not only do fat women earn less money themselves but, in comparison with women whose weight falls within the recommended range, they are much more likely to marry men who earn less in their respective occupations.

LEGAL RECOURSE AND INTERVENTIONS FOR DISCRIMINATION

The question remains whether there are reasonable options for fat persons to redress the discrimination they face in the job market. Reviews of relevant case law have shown that discrimination suits brought under the Rehabilitation Act or the ADA have met with mixed results (Solovay, 2000; Taussig, 1994; Ziolkowski, 1994). Most of those who have won have only been able to do so by showing that they were "morbidly obese" (defined as being in excess of 100 lbs. or 100% over maximum recommended weight) and that this qualifies them as "disabled." A recent example was the case of Bonnie Cook, whose employment discrimination suit against the Rhode Island Department of Mental Health, Retardation and Hospitals was eventually heard before the First Circuit

U.S. Court of Appeals. In the first federal court decision to acknowledge obesity as a disability under federal law, the First Circuit awarded Ms. Cook monetary compensation and reinstatement in a job that she was deemed unsuitable for by the staff of the hospital. Legal scholars who have reviewed this case, however, have stated that the case was unique in that Ms. Cook met medical criteria for "morbid obesity," and was able to provide clear evidence that her denial of employment was based solely on her weight (Taussig, 1994; Ziolkowski, 1994). Furthermore, there is heated controversy within the community of fat individuals about the ramifications of considering fatness a "disability" under any circumstances (Solovoy, 2000).

Neither judiciary nor legislative action at the federal level has yet provided protection to the vast majority of fat persons who do not qualify as "morbidly obese" but who still face marked discrimination in the job market (Solovay, 2000). One state (Michigan) and a few municipalities (like San Francisco and Washington, DC) have specifically passed legislation that makes it illegal to discriminate against persons based on weight or physical appearance (Solovay, 2000). Some have argued that a promising avenue for litigation is bringing a "disparate impact" suit under Title VII of the Civil Rights Act, since it has been shown that certain protected populations (e.g., women, the elderly, and ethnic minorities) have higher rates of fatness and therefore would suffer disproportionately from anti-fat discrimination (Paul & Townsend, 1995). Otherwise, the legal recourse available to people who face discrimination based on their weight remains limited, lengthy, and costly.

The other domain in which state and federal law will perhaps come into play is providing protection for fat persons whose employers coerce them into losing weight through built-in "incentives" in their health insurance plans and/or company wellness programs (Grossman, 2004; Reese, 2000; Zablocki, 1998). The passage of the Health Insurance Portability and Accountability Act (HIPAA) in 1996 restricts employers from using health status as a basis for incentive or disincentive qualification but does not prohibit them from encouraging participants to enroll in wellness programs aimed at increasing "healthy lifestyle" changes (Reese, 2000). Prior to this, a team of researchers at Emory University who were evaluating the effectiveness of an employee program that gave monetary rewards for meeting certain health-related criteria reported that "the major place where people could lose points was in the things that were tough to change . . . measures such as achieving an ideal body fat ratio" (cited in Reese, 2000). Furthermore, after 3 years of following participants in this program, the researchers found no impact on behavior (Reese, 2000).

CONCLUSIONS

Clearly there is ample evidence of differential treatment in employment settings for fat people, especially fat women. That such discrimination continues to exist, despite legislation such as Title VII of the Civil Rights Act and the ADA designed to eradicate discrimination in the workplace, is cause for concern. Research on the stigma of weight has only begun to examine the psychosocial origins of weight-related stigma and how this information may serve to inform interventions (Puhl & Brownell, 2003). However, until such interventions are developed, empirically tested, and utilized, the real and present economic hardship faced by fat men and women needs to be addressed. Currently, it appears that creating laws and policies at a more local level may be most effective in combating weight discrimination. In addition, there is some evidence that the introduction of a company policy can have an impact on the disparate treatment of employees based on personal characteristics such as weight (Bellizzi & Hasty, 2001). More research examining the benefits of such small-scale interventions should continue until, on a broader level, federal policies can be developed and passed to protect all workers.

AUTHOR NOTE

This chapter was written while Esther Rothblum was on sabbatical at the Lesbian Health Research Center of the University of California at San Francisco, the Women's Leadership Institute at Mills College, and the Beatrice M. Bain Center for Research on Women at the University of California at Berkeley.

REFERENCES

Averett, S., & Korenman, S. (1996). The economic reality of the beauty myth. *Journal of Human Resources, 31*, 304–330.

Bellizzi, J. A., & Hasty, R. W. (1998). Territory assignment decisions and supervising unethical selling behavior: The effects of obesity and gender as moderated by job-related factors. *Journal of Personal Selling and Sales Management, 18(2)*, 35–49.

Bellizzi, J. A., & Hasty, R. W. (2001). The effects of a stated organizational policy on inconsistent disciplinary action based on salesperson gender and weight. *Journal of Personal Selling and Sales Management, 21*(3), 189–198.

Bellizzi, J. A., Klassen, M. L., & Belonax, J. J. (1989). Stereotypical beliefs about overweight and smoking and decision-making in assignments to sales territories. *Perceptual and Motor Skills, 69*, 419–429.

Bellizzi, J. A., & Norvell, D. W. (1991). Personal characteristics and salesperson's justifications as moderators of supervisory discipline in cases involving unethical salesforce behavior. *Journal of the Academy of Marketing Science, 19*(1), 11–16.

Berton, L. (2001). Discrimination suit may have "heavy" implications for profession. *Accounting Today, 15*(11), 6.

Brink, T. L. (1988). Obesity and job discrimination: Mediation via personality stereotypes? *Perceptual and Motor Skills, 66*, 494.

Canning, H., & Mayer, J. (1966). Obesity—its possible effect on college acceptance. *New England Journal of Medicine, 275*, 1172–1174.

Canning, H., & Mayer, J. (1967) Obesity: An influence on high school performance? *American Journal of Clinical Nutrition, 20*(4), 352–354.

Cawley, J. (2000, August). Body weight and women's labor market outcomes. NBER Working Paper No. W7841. Available at ssrn.com/abstract=239096

Cramer, P., & Steinwert, T. (1998). Thin is good, fat is bad: How early does it begin? *Journal of Applied Developmental Psychology, 19*(3), 429–451.

Crandall, C. S. (1991). Do heavy-weight students have more difficulty paying for college? *Personality and Social Psychology Bulletin, 17*(6), 606–611.

Crandall, C. S. (1994). Prejudice against fat people: Ideology and self-interest. *Journal of Personality and Social Psychology, 66*(5), 882–894.

Crandall, C. S. (1995). Do parents discriminate against their heavy-weight daughters? *Personality and Social Psychology Bulletin, 21*(7), 724–735.

Crandall, C. S., & Martinez, R. (1996). Culture, ideology, and antifat attitudes. *Personality and Social Psychology Bulletin, 22*(11), 1165–1176.

Crocker, J., Cornwell, B., & Major, B. (1993). The stigma of overweight: Affective consequences of attributional ambiguity. *Journal of Personality and Social Psychology, 64*(1), 60–70.

Everett, M. (1990). Let an overweight person call on your best customers? Fat chance. *Sales and Marketing Management, 142*, 66–70.

Gortmaker, S. L., Must, A., Perrin, J. M., Sobol, A. M., & Dietz, W. H. (1993). Social and economic consequences of overweight in adolescence and young adulthood. *New England Journal of Medicine, 329*(14), 1008–1012.

Greenberg, B. S., Eastin, M., Hofschire, L., Lachlan, K., & Brownell, K. D. (2003). Portrayals of overweight and obese individuals on commercial television. *American Journal of Public Health, 93*(8), 1342–1348.

Grossman, R. J. (2004). Weight in the workplace. *HRMagazine, 49*(3), 43–51.

Haskins, K. M., & Ransford, H. E. (1999) The relationship between weight and career payoffs among women. *Sociological Forum, 14*(2), 295–318.

Hebl, M. R., & Mannix, L. M. (2003). The weight of obesity in evaluating others: A mere proximity effect. *Personality and Social Psychology Bulletin, 29*(1), 28–38.

Jasper, C. R., & Klassen, M. L. (1990a). Perceptions of salespersons' appearance and evaluation of job performance. *Perceptual and Motor Skills, 71*, 563–566.

Jasper, C. R., & Klassen, M. L. (1990b). Stereotypical beliefs about appearance: Implications for retailing and consumer issues. *Perceptual and Motor Skills, 71*, 519–528.

Klassen, M. L., Jasper, C. R., & Harris, R. J. (1993). The role of physical appearance in managerial decisions. *Journal of Business and Psychology, 8*(2), 181–198.

Klesges, R. C., Klem, M. L., Hanson, C. L., Eck, L. H., Ernst, J., O'Laughlin, D., et al. (1990). The effects of applicants health status and qualifications on simulated hiring decisions. *International Journal of Obesity, 14*, 527–535.

Kolata, G. (1992, November 22). The burdens of being overweight: Mistreatment and misconceptions. *New York Times*, pp. 1, 38.

Larkin, J. C., & Pines, H. A. (1979). No fat persons need apply: Experimental studies of the overweight stereotype and hiring preference. *Sociology of Work and Occupations, 6*(3), 312–327.

Loh, E. S. (1993). The economic effects of physical appearance. *Social Science Quarterly, 74*(2), 421–438.

Maddox, G. L., Back, K. W., & Liederman, V. R. (1968). Overweight as social deviance and disability. *Journal of Health and Social Behavior, 9*(4), 287–298.

Maranto, C. L., & Stenoien, A. F. (2000). Weight discrimination: A multidisciplinary analysis. *Employee Responsibilities and Rights Journal, 12*(1), 9–24.

McLean, R. A., & Moon, M. (1980). Health, obesity and earnings. *American Journal of Public Health, 70*(9), 1006–1009.

Melamed, T. (1994). Correlates of physical features: some gender differences. *Personality and Individual Differences, 17*(5), 689–691.

Pagán, J. A., & Dávila, A. (1997). Obesity, occupational attainment and earnings. *Social Science Quarterly, 78*(3), 757–770.

Paul, R. J., & Townsend, J. B. (1995). Shape up or ship out? Employment discrimination against the overweight. *Employee Responsibilities and Rights Journal, 8*(2), 133–145.

Pingitore, R., Dugoni, B. L., Tindale, R. S., & Spring, B. (1994). Bias against overweight job applicants in a simulated employment interview. *Journal of Applied Psychology, 74*(6), 909–917.

Polinko, N. K., & Popovich, P. M. (2001). Evil thoughts but angelic actions: Responses to overweight job applicants. *Journal of Applied Social Psychology, 31*(5), 905–924.

Popovich, P. M., Everton, W. J., Campbell, K. L., Godinho, R. M., Kramer, K. M., & Mangan, M. R. (1997). Criteria used to judge obese persons in the workplace. *Perceptual and Motor Skills, 85*, 859–866.

Puhl, R., & Brownell, K. D. (2001). Bias, discrimination, and obesity. *Obesity Research, 9*(12), 788–805.

Puhl, R., & Brownell, K. D. (2003). Psychosocial origins of obesity stigma: Toward changing a powerful and pervasive bias. *Obesity Reviews, 4*, 213–227.

Reese, S. (2000). New concepts in health benefits: Employee incentives. *Business and Health, 18*(5), 21.

Register, C. A., & Williams, D. R. (1990). Wage effects of obesity among young workers. *Social Science Quarterly, 71*(1), 131–141.

Roehling, M. V. (1999). Weight-based discrimination in employment: Psychological and legal aspects. *Personnel Psychology, 52*(4), 969–1016.

Roehling, M. V. (2002). Weight discrimination in the American workplace: Ethical issues and analysis. *Journal of Business Ethics, 40*, 177–189.

Rothblum, E. D. (1992). The stigma of women's weight: Social and economic realities. *Feminism and Psychology, 2*(1), 61–73.
Rothblum, E. D., Brand, P. A., Miller, C. T., & Oetjen, H. A. (1990). The relationship between obesity, employment discrimination, and employment-related victimization. *Journal of Vocational Behavior, 37*, 251–266.
Rothblum, E. D., Miller, C. T., & Garbutt, B. (1988). Stereotypes of obese female job applicants. *International Journal of Eating Disorders, 7*(2), 277–283.
Saporta, I., & Halpern, J. J. (2002). Being different can hurt: Effects of deviation from physical norms on lawyers' salaries. *Industrial Relations, 41*(3), 442–466.
Sargent, J. D., & Blanchflower, D. G. (1994). Obesity and stature in adolescence and earnings in young adulthood: Analysis of a British birth cohort. *Archives of Pediatric Medicine, 148*, 681–687.
Sarlio-Lähteenkarova, S., & Lahelma, E. (1999). The association of body mass index with social and economic disadvantage in women and men. *International Journal of Epidemiology, 28*, 445–449.
Sarlio-Lähteenkarova, S., Silventoinen, K., & Lahelma, E. (2004). Relative weight and income at different levels of socioeconomic status. *American Journal of Public Health, 94*(3), 468–472.
Sobal, J. (1991). Obesity and socioeconomic status: A framework for examining relationships between physical and social variables. *Medical Anthropology, 13*, 231–247.
Sobal, J., & Stunkard, A. J. (1989). Socioeconomic status and obesity: A review of the literature. *Psychological Bulletin, 105*(2), 260–275.
Solovay, S. (2000). *Tipping the scales of justice: Fighting weight-based discrimination*. Amherst, NY: Prometheus Books.
Stake, J., & Lauer, M. L. (1987). The consequences of being overweight: A controlled study of gender differences. *Sex Roles, 17*(1/2), 31–47.
Stunkard, A. J., LaFleur, W. R., & Wadden, T. A. (1998). Stigmatization of obesity in medieval times: Asia and Europe. *International Journal of Obesity, 22*, 1141–1144.
Taussig, W. C. (1994). Weighing in against discrimination: *Cook v. Rhode Island, Department of Mental Health, Retardation, and Hospitals* and the recognition of obesity as a disability under the Rehabilitation Act and the Americans with Disabilities Act. *Boston College Law Review, 35*, 927–963.
Tiggemann, M., & Rothblum E. D. (1988). Gender differences in social consequences of perceived overweight in the United States and Australia. *Sex Roles, 18*(1/2), 75–86.
Zablocki, E. (1998). Weight and work. *Business and Health, 16*(8, Suppl. A), 20–24.
Ziolkowski, S. M. (1994). Case comment: The status of weight based-employment discrimination under the Americans with Disabilities Act after *Cook v. Rhode Island Department of Mental Health, Retardation, and Hospitals. Boston University Law Review, 74*, 667–686.

CHAPTER 2

■ ■ ■

Bias in Health Care Settings

ANTHONY N. FABRICATORE
THOMAS A. WADDEN
GARY D. FOSTER

> Whatever houses I may visit, I will come for the benefit of the sick, remaining free of all intentional injustice. . . .
>
> —FROM THE HIPPOCRATIC OATH (Edelstein, 1943, p. 3)

The Hippocratic Oath, still taken by many medical students upon their graduation, is frequently summarized as, "First, do no harm." This statement does not explicitly appear in the oath, but captures the essence of the pledge. The present chapter investigates whether physicians and other health care providers are free of injustice in caring for obese individuals, intentional or not. We first examine the attitudes of health care providers toward obese persons and then describe obese patients' perceptions of their providers' attitudes and practices. Next, we review objective findings that show that health care utilization, and possibly assessment and treatment practices, are related to patients' body weight. The chapter closes with recommendations for creating a health care environment that will provide optimal weight-related care for obese individuals.

ATTITUDES OF HEALTH CARE PROVIDERS TOWARD OBESE INDIVIDUALS

The first logical method of studying negative attitudes is simply to ask about them. In much of the research on this topic, respondents have rated their agreement or disagreement with statements about individuals with obesity. This method, however, is subject to the effects of social desirability. People are often reluctant to endorse attitudes they believe are inconsistent with values they feel they "should" hold. Thus, researchers have developed methods of assessing implicit negative attitudes and beliefs. These methods typically reveal greater bias than respondents are willing to admit and are thought to provide a more accurate assessment than direct, explicit measures of attitudes. Results of these two types of studies are reviewed separately.

Explicit Attitudes

A survey conducted over 35 years ago found that physicians had very negative attitudes toward obese patients, describing them as unintelligent, unsuccessful, inactive, and weak-willed (Maddox & Liederman, 1969). This sample of doctors also stated that they preferred not to treat patients for their obesity and that they did not expect successful outcomes when they did provide such care. Klein and colleagues (Klein, Najman, Kohrman, & Munro, 1982) surveyed 400 doctors, who associated obesity with poor hygiene and adherence, as well as dishonesty and hostility. Only drug addiction, alcoholism, and mental illness aroused more negative feelings than obesity.

These findings suggest that obese patients are at risk not only of developing adverse medical conditions but also negative interactions with their physicians. Physicians' negative attitudes could reduce the quality of care they provide to obese individuals, thus, potentially increasing the patients' risk of developing health complications and then reinforcing the original negative attitudes (see Figure 2.1).

Physicians in the 1980s were not alone in their negative attitudes toward obese individuals. In a sample of 107 nurses, nearly 1 in 4 reported that they were repulsed by caring for their obese patients and 1 in 8 indicated that they would prefer to avoid touching those individuals (Bagley, Conklin, Isherwood, Pechiulis, & Watson, 1989). It is possible that nurses who disliked touching severely overweight patients might dress wounds less frequently or make transfers less carefully with their heavier patients. Additionally, they might be more reluctant to assist with toileting, thus, increasing the likelihood patients would further "repulse" the nurse. (It should be noted that the two previous scenarios are hypothetical. Empirical data to support or refute them are not available.)

A study of nutrition professionals found that most respondents attributed obesity to emotional problems (70%) and believed that obesity was a form of compensation for lack of love or attention (88%) (Maiman, Wang, Becker, Finlay, & Simonson, 1979). Such misconcep-

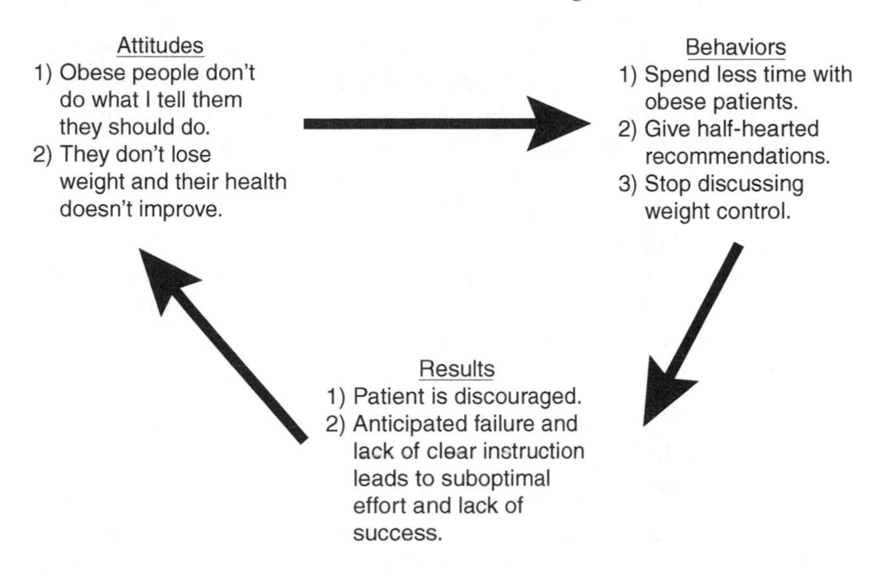

FIGURE 2.1. A hypothetical example of how negative attitudes of health care providers have the potential to become self-perpetuating.

tions about the causes of obesity may lead nutritionists and dietitians to the inappropriate conclusion that their obese patients need psychotherapy rather than nutritional counseling, thus lowering their expectations for success and, possibly, their efforts in treating obesity. A study of medical students similarly found that they linked obesity with a number of derogatory adjectives including worthless, unpleasant, bad, ugly, awkward, unsuccessful, and lacking self-control (Blumberg & Mellis, 1980).

Recent investigations indicate that today's practitioners still hold negative attitudes and beliefs about obese persons. Foster et al. (2003) surveyed 5,000 primary care physicians about their attitudes toward obese patients as well as the causes and treatment of obesity. Of the 620 persons who responded, at least 50% endorsed statements that obese individuals are awkward, unattractive, ugly, and noncompliant. Approximately 30% reported that obese individuals are lazy and sloppy. Beliefs that obese persons are unpleasant and dishonest were less common, endorsed by fewer than 10% of respondents.

Whereas a sample of obesity experts rated genetic factors as the most important cause of obesity (Bray, York, & DeLany, 1992), Foster and colleagues' (2003) general practitioners rated physical inactivity as the most important contributor. Psychological problems were rated as important in the development of obesity as genetic factors. Similarly, Harvey and Hill (2001) reported that primary care physicians and clinical psychologists believed that physical inactivity was the leading cause of overweight and obesity, with psychological factors (e.g., depression, "food addiction") viewed as more important than genetic factors.

Over 90% of Foster et al.'s (2003) respondents agreed that obesity is a chronic disease. However, over 40% agreed or strongly agreed that medications for obesity should only be used short-term (< 3 months). The same proportion also agreed that obese patients can reach "normal weight" if they are motivated. While this latter finding could be interpreted as physicians' optimism that patients can be successful, it implicitly suggests that physicians attribute the inability to lose weight to lack of motivation.

Implicit Attitudes

Rather than asking physicians directly how they feel about obese individuals, studies of implicit attitudes take a more subtle approach. Two methodologies have been employed: (1) experimental designs in which some physicians respond to a description of obese patients and others respond to vignettes of otherwise identical normal-weight patients, and (2) designs that compare performance when respondents attempt to pair obesity with positive versus negative attributes.

Using the first of these methodologies, Hebl and Xu (2001) sent one of six vignettes to 122 primary care physicians. Each vignette depicted an otherwise healthy patient who presented with two migraine headaches per week over the past 2 years. The sex (male or female) and body mass index (BMI; 23, 30, or 36 kg/m^2) of the hypothetical patient were manipulated by the experimenters. Respondents were asked to indicate (1) the tests, procedures, and referrals they would recommend; (2) how much time they would spend with the patient; and (3) their emotional and behavioral reactions to the patient.

Differences in the tests and procedures that physicians recommended were mostly weight-related (e.g., test for cholesterol and triglycerides, consult on nutrition and exercise) and, thus, not surprising. One difference, however, revealed a negative stereotype about obese persons. A referral to a psychologist was recommended by a significantly greater percentage of physicians when they were told the patient was mildly (15%) or moderately obese (23%) instead of average weight (3%). In addition, the physicians' desire to help the patient differed significantly based on BMI, as did beliefs about whether the patient was self-disciplined or annoying, or whether seeing the individual would be a waste of time. In each case, beliefs and expectations about the obese patients were less favorable than those about the average-weight patient. Given their negative judgments and expectations, it is not surprising that the amount of time respondents said they would spend with the patient also varied significantly by patient BMI. As compared with the average-weight patient (31.1 ± 9.4 minutes), respondents reported they would spend 20% and nearly 30% less time, respectively, with patients with mild and moderate obesity.

Health care professionals who specialize in obesity treatment might be expected to be immune to implicit negative attitudes toward obese persons. Two studies, however, showed that they are not. In the first, Teachman and Brownell (2001) assessed both explicit and implicit anti-obesity bias among 84 health care providers (72% physicians, 71% male) who were attending a continuing education meeting on obesity. Explicitly, "thin people" were seen as more motivated than "fat people," but there were no differences in the extent to which thin and fat people were rated as good or bad. The evidence of anti-obesity attitudes and beliefs was much stronger on the implicit measures.

The Implicit Association Test (IAT) requires subjects to correctly categorize stimulus words based on different response keys. In one key, "fat people" might be paired with "bad" and "thin people" with "good." In an opposite key, "fat people" and "good" would comprise one pairing, and "thin people" and "bad" would comprise the other. The difference in the time it takes to associate obesity with a list of positive qualities, rather than negative ones, is considered a measure of implicit bias. Teachman and Brownell's (2001) sample of obesity specialists were much more successful in classifying words when "fat people" was paired with "bad" or "lazy" than with "good" or "motivated," thus providing evidence of implicit negative attitudes toward obese persons. The implicit biases among those specialists, though strong, were weaker than the implicit attitudes found in the general population.

A second study also employed the IAT with obesity specialists (Schwartz, Chambliss, Brownell, Blair, & Billington, 2003). Participants in this study were 389 health professionals who attended an international obesity conference. As in Teachman and Brownell's (2001) study, reports of explicit anti-fat attitudes were modest, while implicit negative attitudes were robust (Schwartz et al., 2003). Figure 2.2 shows that more stimulus words were correctly categorized when "fat people" was paired with negative attributes, such as "bad," "lazy," "stupid," and "worthless," than with positive attributes, including "good," "motivated," "smart," and "valuable." Implicit anti-fat attitudes were found to be related to sex, age, BMI, and professional experience. Women, younger respondents, lighter respondents, and those who did not work directly with obese patients held stronger negative implicit attitudes (Schwartz et al., 2003).

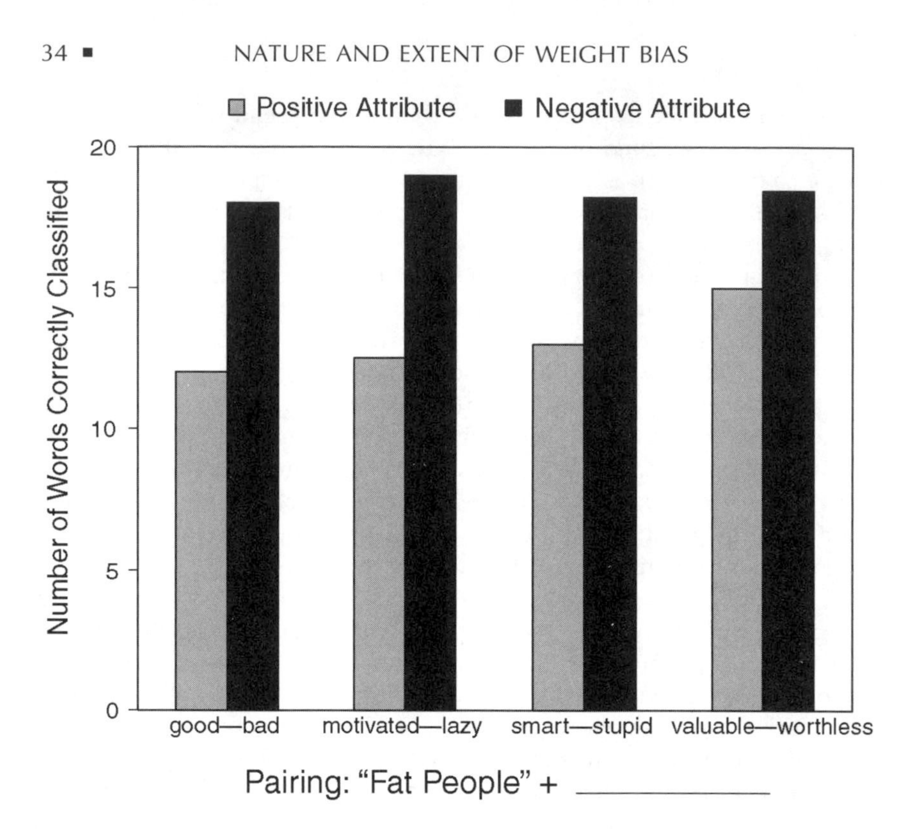

FIGURE 2.2. Results of implicit attitude testing in obesity specialists. Subjects categorized more words correctly when "fat people" was paired with negative, versus positive, attributes. This discrepancy suggests implicit negative attitudes toward obese individuals. Adapted from Schwartz, Chambliss, Brownell, Blair, and Billington (2003). Copyright 2003 by the North American Association for the Study of Obesity. Adapted by permission.

OBESE PATIENTS' EXPERIENCE OF WEIGHT-RELATED BIAS

The research reviewed earlier indicates that anti-obesity attitudes are common in health care professionals. This section examines the extent to which patients perceive weight-related bias in their interactions with doctors. In the first study of this issue, Rand and MacGregor (1990) asked 57 extremely obese individuals who presented for bariatric surgery to report on their experiences of having been treated unfairly. Discrimination in the health care setting was acutely felt. Nearly 80% of respondents indicated that they were "usually" or "always" treated disrespectfully by medical professionals.

Anderson and Wadden (2004) recently sought to replicate Rand and MacGregor's (1990) findings in a larger sample of bariatric surgery patients and to compare the experiences of these individuals with those of more moderately obese patients who sought behavioral and pharmacological treatment. Their sample of surgery patients included 79 women and 26 men with a mean age of 41.5 ± 9.7 years and BMI of 54.8 ± 12.5 kg/m^2. Nonsurgery patients were 176 women and 38 men with a mean age of 43.6 ± 10.2 years and BMI of 37.8 ± 4.2 kg/m^2. Participants completed questionnaires pertaining to medical visits, perceived mistreatment, and satisfaction with medical care.

These authors found substantially less perceived disrespect than did Rand and MacGregor (1990). Only 13.5% of their sample of surgery patients reported that they were usually or always treated disrespectfully by the medical profession because of their weight, compared with 78% of Rand and MacGregor's respondents. Among nonsurgery patients in Anderson and Wadden's (2004) study, only 6.6% said that they were treated disrespectfully by medical professionals. Scare tactics, however, were commonly reported by both surgery and nonsurgery patients. Nearly two-thirds of the surgery candidates and one-third of the nonsurgery patients indicated that their physicians had tried to scare them into losing weight by warning about the health risks associated with excess weight.

In another study, 259 obese women (BMI 35.2 ± 4.5 kg/m^2) who sought professional weight loss responded to several questions about their satisfaction with their physicians' treatment of their health in general and their weight in particular (Wadden et al., 2000). Respondents indicated that they were moderately satisfied, on average, with the care they received for their overall health, but either neutral or slightly satisfied with the care their physicians provided for their weight. Two-thirds of the sample said their doctors discussed weight only once in a while or never, and three-quarters said they looked to their doctors only a slight amount or not at all for help with weight control.

The women in Wadden et al.'s (2000) study reported few negative interactions with their doctors concerning weight: 90% said their physicians never or rarely criticized them when they lost and regained weight, and 87% said their doctors were rarely or never critical or insulting about weight. Thus, their reluctance to seek weight-related help from their physicians did not appear to be due to perceived hostility. Perhaps the participants did not turn to their physicians because of a perceived lack of empathy. Over 60% of participants reported feeling that most doctors do not understand how difficult it is to be overweight. Alternatively, they may not seek help from their physicians because they receive little guidance when they do. Despite 60% of participants reporting that their doctors tell them they need to lose weight (even if the patient did not ask), nearly 45% indicated that their physicians did not prescribe any of the 10 weight control methods that the authors listed, including diet plans, commercial programs, medication, and calorie-controlled diets.

WEIGHT-RELATED DIFFERENCES IN HEALTH CARE UTILIZATION

It is well known that obesity is associated with several adverse medical consequences, including hypertension, type 2 diabetes, osteoarthritis, sleep apnea, and even some forms of cancer (National Task Force on the Prevention and Treatment of Obesity, 2000). Not surprisingly, several studies have found positive relationships between BMI and various indicators of health care utilization, such as number of prescription medications, frequency of outpatient visits and inpatient stays, and total medical costs (see Fontaine & Bartlett, 2000). Thus, obese individuals do see physicians more frequently than do persons of average weight, probably because of their greater number of health complications (associated with their obesity). One study also found that obese persons sought mental health services more frequently than nonobese persons (Trakas, Lawrence, & Shear, 1999). Fontaine and Bartlett noted that the relationship between BMI and health care utilization holds when controlling for age, sex, physical activity, and smoking, but "becomes weaker, if not eliminated completely, when obesity-related comorbidities are added to the statistical models" (p. 405).

Findings of a study by Sansone and colleagues (Sansone, Sansone, & Wiederman, 1998) support this conclusion. These researchers reviewed 12 months of medical records for 88 overweight/obese women (BMI = 35 ± 6 kg/m^2) and 111 nonobese women (BMI = 21.9 ± 2.3 kg/m^2) who received services in a primary care clinic. The heavier group had a mean of 3.2 diagnoses, compared to 2.6 for the lighter group. When controlling for that difference, BMI was unrelated to number of prescriptions and number of contacts with the clinic. However, BMI remained positively related to the number of physicians seen at the clinic, even after controlling for the number of diagnoses. The authors suggested that embarrassment about body shape and weight may increase heavier patients' reluctance to continue contact with a single physician. Alternatively, shame over a lack of weight loss may lead heavier patients to schedule future appointments with another physician, particularly if the previous physician recommended weight loss.

A study of a nationally representative sample of nearly 7,000 women also found a positive relationship between BMI and physician visits (Fontaine, Faith, Allison, & Cheskin, 1998). Obesity, however, appeared to be negatively related to receiving preventive health care services. Controlling for age, race, socioeconomic status, smoking, and health insurance, women with a BMI of 35 kg/m^2 were 26–39% more likely than those with a BMI of 25 kg/m^2 to delay gynecological examinations, clinical breast examinations, and Papanicolaou smear tests for more than 3 years. Whether the delays can be explained by obese patients' reluctance to undergo those procedures or by physicians' reluctance to recommend or perform those services is unknown. Regardless, the authors suggested that the reduction in preventive health services may contribute to the increased health risks associated with obesity.

Access to health care is a separate issue from service utilization. Data on the link between obesity and health care access could not be found. There is clear evidence, however, that minorities and individuals of low socioeconomic status have reduced access to health care. Both of these subgroups have disproportionately high rates of obesity for which they are unlikely to receive care.

CREATING A MORE "WEIGHT-FRIENDLY" HEALTH CARE ENVIRONMENT

Trips to the physician may be uncomfortable or awkward for obese persons for a variety of reasons. Like airplanes, sports arenas, and movie theaters, doctors' offices may require larger patients to squeeze into chairs that are too narrow. Thus, we recommend that waiting and examination rooms be equipped with sturdy armless chairs. Examination gowns, blood pressure cuffs, and examination tables should likewise be size-appropriate. Given the increasing prevalence of extreme obesity in the United States—5% of adults according to most recent data (Hedley et al., 2004)—physicians' offices also must have scales that will measure individuals who weigh more than 300 pounds.

Health care providers can also incorporate subtler, less expensive changes to make their practices more weight-friendly. For instance, scales should be moved out of the public view so that only the patient and the staff member measuring the weight can see the result. Additionally, the staff member can write the number in the chart and show it to the patient rather than announcing it.

All health care professionals (including physicians, nurses, nutritionists, and psychologists) who work with obese individuals can practice two methods of increasing patients' satisfaction with weight-related care. First, educate patients about weight control. Discussion should include available treatment options, the safety and efficacy of various approaches, the role of genetic and environmental factors in determining weight, and how to induce negative energy balance (see National Heart, Lung, and Blood Association & North American Association for the Study of Obesity, 2000). In Anderson and Wadden's (2004) survey, mentioned earlier, the degree to which physicians described the causes and consequences of overweight accounted for 82% of the variance in patients' satisfaction with weight-related care. It was also important for the physician to communicate empathy regarding the difficulties of being overweight and attempting to lose weight.

In explaining the importance of weight control to patients, it is preferable to list the benefits of modest weight loss (e.g., control diabetes, reduce cardiovascular risk factors, improve mobility) than to attempt to induce fear by enumerating the drastic health consequences of obesity. While a certain degree of anxiety can increase motivation, we believe that the "lose-weight-or-else" approach is more likely to be paralyzing than motivating, especially for patients with a history of repeated weight loss and regain.

Second, practitioners should use acceptable terms when discussing the issue of weight control with patients. A study by Wadden and Didie (2003) found that "weight" was clearly preferred by obese men (BMI = 35.1 ± 4.1 kg/m^2) and two samples of obese women (BMIs = 35.3 ± 5.1 and 52.7 ± 10.4 kg/m^2). Terms that elicited a neutral reaction included "excess weight" and "BMI." "Fatness," "excess fat," and even the clinical term "obesity" evoked strong negative reactions from patients. These descriptors frequently are used in a pejorative manner by the public and may be offensive or hurtful to overweight individuals.

CONCLUSIONS

Health care professionals' anti-obesity attitudes, originally reported nearly 40 years ago, appear to persist today. Beliefs that obese persons are lazy, unintelligent, or worthless are less likely, however, to be explicitly endorsed. Instead, many providers appear to hold implicit negative attitudes toward obese individuals. Experimental and descriptive studies have shown that physicians often expect that they will be annoyed by obese patients and that treatment efforts will be unsuccessful. Whether those expectations impact treatment decisions and practices is not yet clear. What is clear, however, is that obese patients report experiencing less discrimination in medical settings than would be expected based on the literature on negative attitudes. Possible explanations include the following: (1) Practitioners may not discuss weight so as to avoid offending obese patients; (2) negative attitudes may be suppressed or expressed so subtly that obese patients do not perceive them in their providers; or (3) implicit attitude tests may overestimate the degree of anti-obesity bias held by health care professionals. Further research clearly is needed to determine if negative weight-related attitudes, whether explicit or implicit, result in obese individuals receiving suboptimal care from health professionals. There currently are not adequate data to answer this question.

The research described in this chapter has several limitations. For example, the surveys of health care providers had very low response rates (Foster et al., 2003; Harvey & Hill, 2001). It is possible that those who responded differed in important ways from those who did not. Studies that included patient reports of unfair treatment (Anderson & Wadden, 2004; Rand & MacGregor, 1990) and their doctors' practices (Wadden et al., 2000) should be interpreted with caution. The participants in those studies were seeking specialized weight loss therapies and thus may have been primed to remember previous failures and negative experiences surrounding weight control. In addition, most studies examined small convenience samples. Randomly selected nationally representative samples are needed to examine responses of both overweight individuals and health care providers.

In the meantime, health professionals can reduce bias and increase patient satisfaction by considering and communicating knowledge of the genetic and environmental forces that influence obesity. While psychological factors may interact with weight, it is inappropriate and inaccurate to assume that obese individuals must also have some form of psychopathology (Fabricatore & Wadden, 2004). Care must be taken when discussing weight with patients, so as not to induce defensiveness or otherwise reduce the likelihood that the message of healthy weight control will be received and acted upon. The value of warm and empathetic communication should not be underestimated. As Stunkard (1993) has noted, health care providers have

> a golden opportunity. As with chronic illness, we rarely have the opportunity to cure. But we do have the opportunity to treat the patient with respect. Such an experience may be the greatest gift that a doctor can give an obese patient; it compares favorably with the modest benefits of our programs of weight reduction. (pp. 355–356)

ACKNOWLEDGMENTS

Completion of this chapter was supported in part by Grant No. K24-DK065018 from the National Institutes of Health and by an unrestricted educational grant from Abbott Laboratories.

REFERENCES

Anderson, D. A., & Wadden, T. A. (2004). Bariatric surgery patients' views of their physicians' weight-related attitudes and practices. *Obesity Research, 12,* 1587–1595.

Bagley, C. R., Conklin, D. N., Isherwood, R. T., Pechiulis, D. R., & Watson, L. A. (1989). Attitudes of nurses toward obesity and obese patients. *Perceptual and Motor Skills, 68,* 954.

Blumberg, P., & Mellis, L. P. (1980). Medical students' attitudes toward the obese and morbidly obese. *International Journal of Eating Disorders, 4,* 169–175.

Bray, G. A., York B., & DeLany, J. (1992). A survey of the opinions of obesity experts on the causes and treatment of obesity. *American Journal of Clinical Nutrition, 55,* 151–154.

Edelstein, L. (1943). *The Hippocratic Oath: Text, translation, and interpretation.* Baltimore, MD: Johns Hopkins University Press.

Fabricatore, A. N., & Wadden, T. A. (2004). Psychological aspects of obesity. *Clinics in Dermatology, 22,* 332–337.

Fontaine, K. R., & Bartlett, S. J. (2000). Access and use of medical care among obese persons. *Obesity Research, 8,* 403–406.

Fontaine, K. R., Faith, M. S., Allison, D. B., & Cheskin, L. J. (1998). Body weight and health care among women in the general population. *Archives of Family Medicine, 7,* 381–384.

Foster, G. D., Wadden, T. A., Makris, A. P., Davidson, D., Sanderson R. S., Allison, D. B., et al. (2003). Primary care physicians' attitudes about obesity and its treatment. *Obesity Research, 11,* 1168–1177.

Harvey, E. L., & Hill, A. J. (2001). Health professionals' views of overweight people and smokers. *International Journal of Obesity, 25,* 1253–1261.

Hebl, M. R., & Xu, J. (2001). Weighing the care: Physicians' reactions to the size of a patient. *International Journal of Obesity, 25,* 1246–1252.

Hedley, A. A., Ogden, C. L., Johnson, C. L., Carroll, M. D., Curtin, L. R., & Flegal, K. M. (2004). Prevalence of overweight and obesity among U.S. children, adolescents, and adults, 1999–2002. *Journal of the American Medical Association, 291,* 2847–2850.

Klein, D., Najman, J., Kohrman, A. F., & Munro, C. (1982). Patient characteristics that elicit negative responses from family physicians. *Journal of Family Practice, 14,* 881–888.

Maddox, G. L., & Liederman, V. (1969). Overweight as a social disability with medical implications. *Journal of Medical Education, 44,* 214–220.

Maiman, L. A., Wang, V. L., Becker, M. H., Finlay, J., & Simonson, M. (1979).

Attitudes toward obesity and the obese among professionals. *Journal of the American Dietetic Association, 74,* 331–336.

National Heart, Lung, and Blood Institute and North American Association for the Study of Obesity. (2000). *Practical guide to the identification, evaluation, and treatment of overweight and obesity in adults.* Bethesda, MD: National Institutes of Health.

National Task Force on the Prevention and Treatment of Obesity. (2000). Overweight, obesity, and health risk. *Archives of Internal Medicine, 160,* 898–904.

Rand, C. S. W., & MacGregor, A. M. C. (1990). Morbidly obese patients' perceptions of social discrimination before and after surgery for obesity. *Southern Medical Journal, 83,* 1390–1395.

Sansone, R. A., Sansone, L. A., & Wiederman, M. W. (1998). The relationship between obesity and medical utilization among women in a primary care setting. *International Journal of Eating Disorders, 23,* 161–167.

Schwartz, M. B., Chambliss, H. O., Brownell, K. D., Blair, S. N., & Billington, C. (2003). Weight bias among health professionals specializing in obesity. *Obesity Research, 11,* 1033–1039.

Stunkard, A. J. (1993). Talking with patients. In A. J. Stunkard & T. A. Wadden (Eds.), *Obesity: Theory and therapy* (pp. 355–363). New York: Raven Press.

Teachman, B. A., & Brownell, K. D. (2001). Implicit anti-fat bias among health professionals: Is anyone immune? *International Journal of Obesity, 25,* 1525–1531.

Trakas, K., Lawrence, K., & Shear, N. H. (1999). Utilization of health care resources by obese Canadians. *Canadian Medical Association Journal, 160,* 1457–1462.

Wadden, T. A., Anderson, D. A., Foster, G. D., Bennett, A., Steinberg, C., & Sarwer, D. B. (2000). Obese women's perceptions of their physicians' weight management attitudes and practices. *Archives of Family Medicine, 9,* 854–860.

Wadden, T. A., & Didie, E. (2003). What's in a name? Patients' preferred terms for describing obesity. *Obesity Research, 11,* 1140–1146.

CHAPTER 3

■ ■ ■

The Portrayal of Weight in the Media and Its Social Impact

BRADLEY S. GREENBERG
TRACY R. WORRELL

In the field of media studies, identifying the impact of the potential influence of any mass medium and its influence on consumers follows a systematic approach. First, researchers do qualitative and quantitative assessments of the message content. For example, in the beginning of the study of media violence in the 1950s, researchers enumerated the frequency of violence on television, the characteristics of the combatants, and the form of violence (e.g., hitting, shooting, stabbing). Second, researchers elaborate on the frequency data by identifying the context of the messages. In the study of violence, research assessed the motives, rewards, and justification for violence, and these content analyses established trends, themes, and topics. Finally, researchers use this information to design laboratory experiments and field surveys. In the violence field, lab studies manipulated variables to see if there was an enhancement or diminishment of mediated violence, and cross-sectional and longitudinal surveys tested the link between measures of exposure to potential or actual consequences. To date, the academic literature on the issue of mediated violence numbers in the hundreds (see Anderson & Bushman, 2002).

Research addressing weight and body imagery in the media is far less developed than research on violence, but the research approach is the same. In this chapter, we first review the research identifying how body image is portrayed in the media and the context surrounding these images. Second, we review the field studies that test the relationship between exposure to media images of particular body sizes and one's own body image and eating behaviors. Third, we review the laboratory experiments that manipulate media exposure and measure impact on body image and eating behaviors. Finally, we outline directions for future research.

WHAT DO THE MEDIA PORTRAY?

Bodies from magazines and beauty pageants provided early opportunities to examine media portrayals of body images (e.g., Garner, Garfinkel, Schwartz, & Thompson, 1980; Silverstein, Perdue, Peterson, & Kelly, 1986; Wiseman, Gray, Mosimann, & Ahrens, 1992). These studies focused on an anticipated trend that women portrayed were becoming thinner. Garner et al. (1980) found that the busts and hips of *Playboy* centerfolds had decreased whereas waist and height both increased over the two decades examined. They also found that Miss America contestants had become thinner, with a significant decrease in weight during the same time period that the average weight of U.S. women under the age of 30 had been increasing (Garner et al., 1980).

The articles and advertisements in 12 issues each of four highly read female-targeted (e.g., *Family Circle* and *Ladies Home Journal*) and male-targeted (e.g., *Rolling Stone* and *Sports Illustrated*) magazines from 1980 were analyzed for body shape and size, as well as dieting, food, drink, and cooking (Silverstein et al., 1986). There were large discrepancies on most topics: 96 ads and articles that were body-related for the women compared to 10 for the men; 63 ads for diet foods in the women's issues versus 1 in the men's; 228 articles on food in the women's magazines and 10 in the men's; 1,179 food ads for the women and 15 for the men. Only in ads for alcohol did the men's magazines surpass the women's, by a count of 624 to 19.

Examining the top 10 magazines most read by 18- to 24-year-old males (e.g., *Sports Illustrated* and *Playboy*) and 10 different ones most read by females (e.g., *Cosmopolitan* and *Glamour*) in 1987, Anderson and DiDomenico (1992) reported that the number of diet articles and advertisements in female-targeted magazines was greater by a 10 to 1 margin over male-targeted magazines. In a longer time frame, Garner et al. (1980) identified 467 articles in six popular women's magazines (e.g., *Vogue* and *Ladies Home Journal*) from 1959 to 1978 that dealt with dieting and/or weight loss. The trend across the 20-year period inclined significantly from an average of 17 articles per year to 30 ($p < .001$).

Wiseman et al. (1992) also cited an increase from 1959 to 1988 in the number of articles on diet and exercise in the same six magazines examined by Garner et al. (1980). They also noted that the number of articles aimed at exercise continued to increase while articles specific to dieting decreased during the 1980s.

All these studies, which do not go beyond the 1980s, suggest that the substantive and commercial focus of magazine content for women is aimed at the body, and methods designed to change it. Even then, the question arose as to the comparison between this ideal woman and her real-life counterpart. For example, Garner et al. (1980) found that *Playboy* centerfolds weighed significantly less than the average U.S. woman. A study of the next decade of *Playboy* centerfolds (1979–1988) and Miss America contestants (1979–1985) found that 69% of centerfolds and 60% of Miss America contestants weighed an average of 15% below the expected weight for their age and height (Wiseman et al., 1992).

A smaller number of studies of body types on television programs have been done. In one early study, Kaufman (1980) examined body types on 10 TV series from 1977. She found these body types: obese, 5%, overweight, 15%, average, 42%, and thin, 38%. Two decades later, from a 1997 sample of situation comedies, Fouts and Burggraf (2000) indicated that 76% of their major female characters were below average in weight, contrasted with 24% in the general population. Greenberg, Eastin, Hofschire, Lachlan, and Brownell (2003) examined 275 episodes from 56 different TV series during the 1999–2000 season. They reported that 1 in 3 women portrayed on television were underweight, whereas only 5% of all women in reality are underweight, according to the National Institutes of Health. Only 3 in 100 women were shown as obese, while 1 in 4 real women are classified as overweight. The body shape distribution for men also was skewed significantly in the same direction, but to a lesser extent.

The visibility, attractiveness, interactions, and treatment of TV characters have also been analyzed in relation to body type. Overall, few overweight or obese persons are seen on TV; only 24% of males and 13% of females were classified in these weight categories (Greenberg et al., 2003). Heavier characters are typically found in minor TV roles, while thinner characters are disproportionately more likely to be in major roles (Greenberg et al., 2003; Hofschire, 2001). Younger characters are thinner than older ones, and thinner characters are perceived as more attractive than larger ones (Greenberg et al., 2003; Hofschire, 2001; Silverstein et al., 1986).

An examination of TV character interactions showed that heavier characters are less likely to be involved in friendships, have fewer romantic relationships and have fewer positive interactions with others, compared with thinner characters. In addition, larger female characters were more often the objects of humor than thinner females (Greenberg et al., 2003). In the Fouts and Burggraf (2000) study, the frequency of negative comments was positively related to the weight of the comments' recipients; heavier female characters received more negative comments and thinner women received more positive comments from males. This study also found that the audience laughter responses (both live and canned) were stronger to the negative comments directed at heavier women.

WHAT DO THE FIELD STUDIES SHOW?

Research suggests that exposure to "distorted" body images for women and men is related to negative self-perceptions and negative social behaviors. For women, the distortion is in the direction of the excessively thin body; for men, the distortion is in the direction of the overly muscular body, as identified in the media content analyses. These findings emerge consistently across a variety of measures of media exposure (as predictor variables) and across an even larger variety of body image and body satisfaction measures (as dependent variables). Here we summarize key studies, moving from work done with adults to those with younger age groups.

An early substantial work is that of Harrison and Cantor (1997), based on data gathered from 232 female and 190 male undergraduates in 1994. They assessed exposure to TV programs that featured thin, average, and heavy bodies, and to beauty, fashion, and entertainment magazines. The full set of media exposure variables significantly predicted tendencies for disordered eating, anorexia, bulimia, body dissatisfaction, and drive for thinness among the women. The strongest correlate of disordered eating was reading fitness magazines, followed by fashion magazines. The women's drive for thinness was best predicted by the degree to which they viewed shows featuring thin characters and read fashion magazines. For the adolescent males in this study, overall magazine reading and viewing of TV shows featuring thin characters related to their own drive for thinness and dieting.

Harrison (2003) followed up this work with another college student sample of 149 women and 82 men. Exposure to the ideal body image on TV was measured by how frequently people watched certain shows and the prevalence of thin characters on those shows. Exposure was positively related to the female participants' desire for a smaller waist and hips, but not a smaller bust. Degree of exposure did not influence men's estimate of the ideal female figure; however, it was positively related to approval of breast surgery and liposuction. For women, there was a relationship between media exposure to the thin-ideal and approval for breast surgery, liposuction, and wearing a special bra to change bust appearance or size.

At the same time, Botta (2003) surveyed 400 high school and college students and their reading of fashion, sports, and health/fitness magazines. For the adolescent girls, frequent fashion magazine reading related to higher rates of bulimic behaviors; greater reading of health/fitness magazines related to increased bulimic and anorexic behaviors; greater reading of sports magazines related to increased muscularity. Among the boys in the study, fashion magazine reading related to decreased body satisfaction, whereas health/fitness magazine reading related to increased muscularity. This study also assessed the importance of social comparisons made by the readers between themselves and the magazine images they saw. Increased social comparisons enhanced the magazines' effects for both boys and girls, in terms of decreased body satisfaction, increased drive to be thin, and increased bulimic *and* anorexic behaviors. Botta's earlier work (1999) with adolescent girls failed to find relationships between exposure to thin TV characters and body dissatisfaction, the thin-ideal, and a drive for thinness; what did make a difference in these dispositions was the extent to which the girls made comparisons between the TV models and themselves.

Having demonstrated a positive relationship between young adults' thin-ideal media exposure and eating disorders (Harrison & Cantor, 1997), Harrison (2000) turned to studying 366 adolescents from 6th-, 9th-, and 12th-grade classes. She obtained measures of exposure to TV shows featuring thin *and* fat characters and to thin-ideal magazines (there were no fat-ideals). Exposure to the magazines predicted anorexic tendencies for all the females, and bulimia activities for the 9th- and 12th-grade females. For both sexes, interest in these magazines predicted their drive for thinness. With TV, exposure to fat characters was a positive predictor of bulimia for females. Although exposure to thin-ideal characters did not predict disordered eating among the females when controlling for the influence of overall TV exposure, that exposure was positively related to bulimia, and interest in thin-ideal TV was positively associated with anorexia and the drive for thinness for both boys and girls. Overall, Harrison concludes that the media images, including interest in them, were stronger influences on disordered eating for the adolescent girls than boys.

In a cross-sectional survey with 548 5th–12th-grade girls in public schools, 69% reported that magazine pictures influenced their image of the ideal body and 47% wanted to lose weight because of those pictures (Field et al., 1999). More impressively, their multivariate analysis demonstrated that "frequent readers of fashion magazines were two to three times more likely than infrequent readers to diet to lose weight [and] to exercise to lose weight because of a magazine article" (p. e36).

A second cross-sectional survey examined the same grade groups, but from private religious schools (Polce-Lynch, Myers, Kliewer, & Kilmartin, 2001). The researchers assessed the Rosenberg Self-Esteem Inventory in terms of a group of predictor variables that included a "Media Influence Scale" containing items that asked the youngsters their thoughts and feelings about how their physical appearance may have been influenced by advertisements, movies, or TV (e.g., "When I compare myself to movie stars on TV or in the movies, I feel disappointed with how I look"). They did not ask directly about media exposure. Also included was a personal body-image scale. Their chief finding was that acceptance of media messages about the importance of body image was negatively related to their measure of self-esteem for all the girls and boys in each age group, except the youngest boys. This replicates findings obtained by Henderson-King and Henderson-King (1997). In addition, Polce-Lynch et al. (2001) report from a path analysis that perceived media influence was by far the strongest single correlate of youngsters' own body image, which in turn was strongly related to their self-esteem.

In considering young people's responses to content elements of television shows, parents can opt to actively mediate that activity. They can offer positive, negative, or neutral comments about the content, and they can direct those comments toward the central content of the show, (e.g., the plot, the nature of the conflict), or toward "incidental" content (e.g., the physical appearance of the characters, their body size, eating behaviors). Nathanson and Botta (2003) surveyed 149 parent–adolescent pairs to determine the role of such mediation in shaping the effects of television on adolescent body-image disturbance. The focus was on body dissatisfaction, drive for thinness, and symptoms of anorexia and bulimia, as well as negative emotions while viewing and social comparisons with television characters. There was no obtained relationship between parental mediation of central content and these disturbances. It was the mediation of incidental content that was critical. First, the valence of the mediation was unimportant; regardless of valence, parental mediation of body-image and character appearance content on television makes the adolescent more vulnerable to various body-image disturbances. Talking about it positively, negatively, or neutrally upgraded the salience of body characteristics and led to a stronger drive for thinness or symptoms of anorexia, for example.

WHAT DO THE EXPERIMENTAL STUDIES SHOW?

Sufficient laboratory research on the issue of the media's impact on body satisfaction has been completed to warrant an initial meta-analysis. Groesz, Levine, and Murnen (2002) identified 25 studies, all with females, in which experimental stimuli depicted the entire body of thin media-type models, control groups received stimuli, and effect sizes could be computed. In all studies, body/weight dissatisfaction or physical attractiveness was the dependent variable. There were 43 effect sizes, of which 38 demonstrated a negative impact on body satisfaction. In addition to greater body dissatisfaction ($p < .0001$), the effects were stronger among those with a history of eating disorders or higher preexperimental body dissatisfaction ($p < .01$), and those not yet in college ($p < .05$). However, greater amounts of exposure did not lead to greater dissatisfaction; in fact, the trend was for stronger effects in experiments that presented fewer thin models.

In addition, studies that did not meet the specific criteria for this meta-analysis yield parallel findings. Laboratory research using exposure to the media's thin-ideal portrayal increased body dissatisfaction (Meyers & Biocca, 1992), increased body-size distortion (Waller, Hamilton, & Shaw, 1992), and increased mood disturbance (Pinhas, Toner, Alia, Garfinkel, & Stuckless, 1999).

Clearly, these findings for studies published through 1999 set expectations for more recent work. Here, we can update the experimental literature for females and determine what evidence there is among males, but focus more on the increasing introduction of variables that may moderate or mediate the impact of media models.

Recently, objectification theory (Fredrickson & Roberts, 1997) has been offered to explain women's body-image disturbance problems. It proposes that Western women are socialized to consider themselves based on how they appear physically rather than on their physical competence. In one test of these ideas, Hofschire (2003) manipulated magazine articles that emphasized physical appearance and/or physical competence with 219 undergraduate women. She predicted that exposure to the physical appearance content would enhance self-definition based on self-objectification and would increase body shame, while exposure to the physical efficacy content would enhance self-definition in terms of physical competence. Results supported the self-appraisal expectations for each kind of content, without an increase in body shame.

Three experiments by Mills, Polivy, Herman, and Tiggemann (2002) used thin models in each, but paired them alternatively with heavy models or magazine articles that argued dieting worked or did not work. Participants seeing the thin model ads felt worse and had higher depression scores. However, those who read prodieting articles and then saw thin body ads were less anxious, less upset, and less depressed, and had higher appearance-state self-esteem. If the diet articles can be considered an attempt at intervention, then Irving and Berel's (2001) work is relevant. Their three different media literacy interventions surpassed their control group in increasing skepticism about media images that depict the thin-ideal, reduced perceptions of the realism of those images, and decreased the similarity of those images to the study subjects.

Tiggemann and McGill (2004) chose to see if a focus on body parts, such as a pair of female legs in shoe advertisements or a flat stomach to advertise breakfast cereal, in magazine ads differed from presentation of the full bodies of thin models. Both produced more negative moods and more social comparisons, but body dissatisfaction and state weight anxiety were highest in the body parts condition. Using clever software to "stretch" thin models into average-size models, Halliwell and Dittmar (2004) split subjects into high and low levels of internalization of the thin-ideal. The former experienced greater anxiety from the thin models, with the latter showing no change.

Three studies emerged recently that examined male responses or compared males with females. Girls and boys, ages 6–12, were shown four pictures of objectified images of their own sex (e.g., Britney Spears, a male model) and asked for their response (Murnen, Smolak, Mills, & Good, 2003). There was no sex difference in positive responses, but girls were more consistent in their responses of acceptance or rejection, and those who consistently rejected them had higher body esteem. In Australia, boys ages 13–15 viewed or did not view 20 commercials with the female thin ideal (Hargreaves & Tiggemann, 2003). Exposure did not impact on attractiveness of the models, but those in the midlevel on a preexposure measure of importance of appearance rated slimness and attractiveness as more important attributes. For older males, Agliata and Tantleff-Dunn (2004) exposed 158 undergraduates to TV ads with an ideal male image or neutral ads within the context of a TV show. Regardless of their initial body-image disposition or attitude toward appearance, exposure increased depression and dissatisfaction with their own body parts, such as muscles.

DISCUSSION AND A RESEARCH AGENDA

Clearly the content analytic literature is sparse and dated in several dimensions. Although magazines have been the primary benefactors of these analyses, little if any data reflect the past decade, during which eating disorders and obesity have come to the forefront of academic and national interests. The National Eating Disorders Association states that the media are one factor that contributes to the prevalence of eating disorders (10 million females and 1 million males) and to the 80% of women who are dissatisfied with their appearance (Smolak, 1996).

TV studies have been rare, no trend studies have been completed, and only fictional series and advertising have been examined. For example, body images have not been analyzed on children's television programs, yet according to the National Eating Disorders Association 42% of first- to third-grade girls want to be thinner (as cited in Collins, 1991). Other media have been ignored completely. How do children's books depict the human body and what do they have to say about diet and exercise? Which of any of several romantic book series read by millions of teenage girls impact body-image perceptions?

Video games are now a staple of the American media environment. They are highly visual and strongly male-oriented. Adolescents and preadolescent boys spend as much time with videogames as with TV, and girls are creeping ever higher in play time. Are the games likely to influence young male images about one's self and others, and are they more likely to do so than other mass media that may be less involving? That content has yet to be analyzed.

Furthermore, what attributes may be considered critical in addition to body thinness? Do the media character's personality, interrelationships, and interpersonal behaviors make a difference? For example, an oft-cited emaciated TV character (in a now-cancelled show) was Ally McBeal. Was she admired and emulated for her body, given her interpersonal problems and continuous self-absorption and self-deprecation? By whom?

The studies reported pay little attention to heavy models, although there are relatively few in media presentations. Do they function as opposites to the thin-ideal, by reminding audiences that "fat is bad"? We may suggest that if the presence of the thin-ideal is so common, then the more rare appearance of a heavy model may receive greater attention. This would argue for increasing attention to the potential influence of media models who do not fit the ideal standard. There is more variability in the body image of male than female role models in the media. Does this account for greater variability in what males consider acceptable for themselves?

The survey findings reviewed here suffer singularly from the lack of longitudinal work. Cross-sectional evidence is highly suggestive but not conclusive. It would be opportune to follow preadolescent young men and women for some period of time, document a broad range of their media experiences and media preferences (as well as their eating, exercise, and diet regimens) and examine body-image disturbances and change over that time frame.

Throughout the experimental evidence runs the theme that there are moderating or mediating variables that influence the relationship between media exposure and body-image attributes and behaviors. In their efforts to account for more variance in their dependent measures, researchers have discussed the possibility that the media's impact may be indirect, based on self-definition (Hofschire, 2003), social comparisons (Tiggemann & McGill, 2004), upward comparisons (Han, 2003), drive for thinness (Hausenblas, Janelle, Gardner, & Focht, 2004), and high levels of internalization of the thin-ideal (Halliwell & Dittmar, 2004), among others. There is considerable conceptual (and measurement) overlap here that requires clarification and parsimony.

However, there seems little reason to argue with the basic finding supported with great consistency in all bodies of research reviewed. The media present far more thin women than otherwise, and the men tend in that direction as well—with bulges in different body areas. Regular exposure or immediate exposure to these images is related to personal attitudes, moods, and behaviors that have been linked to eating disorders. Although we may continue to monitor this linkage and demonstrate it with different groups under different circumstances, a companion approach would begin to conceive how that linkage might be reduced or broken. Among such approaches are intervention strategies, identifying moderating variables that can be manipulated to diminish the media's influence, galvanizing parental mediation efforts, enhancing healthy exercise options, and so on.

We have no basis for prioritizing such research stratagems, but there is clearly a basis for continuing interest in the mass media's content related to these issues. Here is the conundrum: While characters on television are thinner than in real life, diet or exercising behaviors are almost invisible. Hofschire (2001) found that only 2% of the men and women exercised, and another 2% of the women talked about it. She found considerable evidence of eating and drinking, however, among characters of all shapes and sizes. Thus, television portrays in programs and commercials that you can eat and drink a lot of just about everything and be thin, but does not show or tell viewers how that can be accomplished.

REFERENCES

Agliata, D., & Tantleff-Dunn, S. (2004). The impact of media exposure on males' body image. *Journal of Social and Clinical Psychology, 23*(1), 7–22.

Anderson, A. E., & DiDomenico, L. (1992). Diet vs. shape content in popular male and female magazines: A dose-response relationship to the incidence of eating disorders? *International Journal of Eating Disorders, 11*, 283–287.

Anderson, C. A., & Bushman, B. J. (2002). The effects of media violence on society. *Science, 295*(5564), 2377–2379.

Botta, R. A. (1999). Television images and adolescent girls' body image disturbance. *Journal of Communication*, *49*, 22–41.

Botta, R. A. (2003). For your health?: The relationship between magazine reading and adolescents' body image and eating disturbances. *Sex Roles*, *48*(9/10), 389.

Collins, M. E. (1991). Body figure perceptions and preferences among preadolescent children. *International Journal of Eating Disorders*, *10*(1), 199–208.

Field, A. E., Cheung, L., Wolf, A. M., Herzog, D. B., Gortmaker, S. L., & Colditz, G. A. (1999). Exposure to the mass media and weight concerns among girls. *Pediatrics*, *103*(3), e36.

Fouts, G., & Burggraf, K. (2000). Television situation comedies: Female weight, male negative comments, and audience reactions. *Sex Roles*, *42*(9/10), 925–932.

Fredrickson, B. L., & Roberts, T. A. (1997). Objectification theory: Toward understanding women's lived experiences and mental health risks. *Psychology of Women Quarterly*, *21*, 173–206.

Garner, D. M., Garfinkel, P. E., Schwartz, D., & Thompson, M. (1980). Cultural expectations of thinness in women. *Psychological Reports*, *47*, 483–491.

Greenberg, B. S., Eastin, M., Hofschire, L., Lachlan, K., & Brownell, K. (2003). Portrayals of overweight and obese individuals on commercial television. *American Journal of Public Health*, *93*(8), 1342–1348.

Groesz, L. M., Levine, M. P., & Murnen, S. K. (2002). The effect of experimental presentation of thin media images on body satisfaction: A meta-analytic review. *International Journal of Eating Disorders*, *31*(1), 1–16.

Halliwell, E., & Dittmar, H. (2004). Does size matter? The impact of model's body size on women's body-focused anxiety and advertising effectiveness. *Journal of Social and Clinical Psychology*, *23*(1), 104–122.

Han, M. (2003). Body image dissatisfaction and eating disturbance among Korean college female students: Relationship to media exposure, upward comparison, and perceived reality. *Communication Studies*, *54*(1), 65–78.

Hargreaves, D. A., & Tiggemann, M. (2003). Female "thin ideal" media images and boys' attitudes toward girls. *Sex Roles*, *49*(9/10), 539–544.

Harrison, K. (2000). The body electric: Thin-ideal media and eating disorders in adolescents. *Journal of Communication*, *50*(3), 119–146.

Harrison, K. (2003). Television viewers' ideal body proportions: The case of the curvaceously thin woman. *Sex Roles*, *48*(5/6), 255–264.

Harrison, K., & Cantor, J. (1997). The relationship between media consumption and eating disorders. *Journal of Communication*, *47*(1), 40–67.

Hausenblas, H. A., Janelle, C. M., Gardner, R. E., & Focht, B. C. (2004). Viewing physique slides: Affective responses of women at high and low drive for thinness. *Journal of Social and Clinical Psychology*, *23*(1), 45–60.

Henderson-King, E., & Henderson-King, D. (1997). Media effects on women's body esteem: Social and individual difference factors. *Journal of Applied Social Psychology*, *27*, 399–417.

Hofschire, L. (2001). *Body type portrayals on prime time television*. Paper presented at the 51st meeting of the International Communication Association, Washington, DC.

Hofschire, L. (2003). *The role of entertainment media in promoting self-objectification, body shame, and physical competence*. Unpublished doctoral dissertation, Michigan State University.

Irving, L. M., & Berel, S. R. (2001). Comparison of media-literacy programs to strengthen college women's resistance to media images. *Psychology of Women Quarterly, 25*(2), 103–111.

Kaufman, L. (1980). Prime-time nutrition. *Journal of Communication, 30*(3), 37–46.

Meyers, P., & Biocca, F. (1992). The elastic body image: An experiment on the effect of advertising and programming on body image distortions in young women. *Journal of Communication, 42*(3), 108–133.

Mills, J. S., Polivy, J., Herman, C. P., & Tiggemann, M. (2002). Effects of exposure to thin media images: Evidence of self-enhancement among restrained eaters. *Personality and Social Psychology Bulletin, 28*(12), 1687–1699.

Murnen, S. K., Smolak, L., Mills, J. A., & Good, L. (2003). Thin, sexy women and strong, muscular men: Grade-school children's responses to objectified images of women and men. *Sex Roles, 49*(9/10), 427–438.

Nathanson, A. I., & Botta, R. A. (2003). Shaping the effects of television on adolescents' body image disturbance: The role of parental mediation. *Communication Research, 30*(3), 304–331.

Pinhas, L., Toner, B. B., Ali, A., Garfinkel, P. E., & Stuckless, N. (1999). The effects of the ideal of female beauty on mood and body satisfaction. *International Journal of Eating Disorders, 25*, 223–226.

Polce-Lynch, M., Myers, B. J., Kliewer, W., & Kilmartin, C. (2001) Adolescent self-esteem and gender: Exploring relations to sexual harassment, body image, media influence, and emotional expression. *Journal of Youth and Adolescence, 20*(2), 225–244.

Silverstein, B., Perdue, L., Peterson, B., & Kelly, E. (1986). The role of the mass media in promoting a thin standard of attractiveness for women. *Sex Roles, 14*(9/10), 519–532.

Smolak, L. (1996). *Next Door Neighbors Eating disorders awareness and prevention puppet guide book*. Seattle, WA: National Eating Disorders Association.

Tiggemann, M., & McGill, B. (2004). The role of social comparison in the effect of magazine advertisements on women's mood and body dissatisfaction. *Journal of Social and Clinical Psychology, 23*(1), 23–44.

Waller, G., Hamilton, K., & Shaw, J. (1992). Media influences on body size estimation in eating disordered and comparison subjects. *British Review of Bulimia and Anorexia Nervosa, 6*, 81–87.

Wiseman, C. V., Gray, J. J., Mosimann, J. E., & Ahrens, A. H. (1992). Cultural expectations of thinness in women: An update. *International Journal of Eating Disorders, 11*, 85–89.

CHAPTER 4

■ ■ ■

Weight Bias in a Child's World

JANET D. LATNER
MARLENE B. SCHWARTZ

One of the most compelling reasons to fight weight stigma is to protect overweight children. The argument that bias is deserved because it results from controllable behaviors (see Crandall & Reser, Chapter 6, this volume) is especially damaging when one considers children. Bias is also rationalized by blaming parents for doing a poor job of child rearing; several legal cases (see Solovay, Chapter 15, this volume) imply that simply having an obese child is evidence of neglect or abuse.

Obese children can face bias from multiple sources, including peers, family members, health professionals, and educators. The most common place where children experience bias is at school (see Neumark-Sztainer & Eisenberg, Chapter 5, this volume). According to the National Education Association (1994), "For fat students, the school experience is one of ongoing prejudice, unnoticed discrimination, and almost constant harassment. . . . From nursery school through college, fat students experience ostracism, discouragement, and sometimes violence."

In the present chapter, we first review the literature on the nature and extent of childhood weight bias. Second, we present research on the consequences of weight bias for children in the areas of interpersonal difficulties, victimization, psychological effects, impact on quality of life, and academic and occupational consequences. Third, we address the question of how small children learn to feel negatively toward their overweight peers, with particular focus on the portrayal of overweight people in children's popular culture.

NATURE AND EXTENT OF CHILDHOOD WEIGHT BIAS

Early Studies

Bias against overweight children was first investigated in the early 1960s and used two principal methods. The first method had children rate their liking of a series of figures that differed in key characteristics. In a classic study, 640 participants, ages 10–11 years old, viewed six drawings of children, four with various disabilities, an average-weight child with no disabilities, and an overweight child (Richardson, Goodman, Hastorf, & Dornbusch, 1961). By an overwhelming margin, children of various cultural backgrounds rated the overweight child as least likable.

Subsequent studies used similar methods with additional cultural groups (Goodman, Dornbusch, Richardson, & Hastorf, 1963), additional stimulus materials (Richardson & Royce, 1968), and adult participants as well as children (Maddox, Back, & Liederman, 1968). Similar stigmatizing attitudes were held across a broad spectrum of populations, including individuals who worked with disabled children, medical patients, and elderly adults.

In a recent replication of the Richardson et al. (1961) study, the bias appears to have worsened. A sample of 458 fifth- and sixth-grade children ranked the six drawings used in the original study in order of how well they liked each child. Not only were overweight boys and girls again consistently liked the least, but they were ranked significantly lower than in 1961. The distance between the child ranked the highest (the thin child) and the lowest (the overweight child) increased by 41% since 1961 (Latner & Stunkard, 2003).

The second method had participants assign adjectives to silhouettes depicting children of different body sizes, typically a "mesomorph" (healthy child), an "ectomorph" (skinny child), and an "endomorph" (overweight child). When asked to assign positive and negative adjectives to these three silhouettes, both boys and girls ages 6–11 ascribed unfavorable characteristics to the overweight child, such as *lazy, sloppy, dirty, naughty, cheats, lies, argues, mean, ugly,* and *stupid* (Staffieri, 1967, 1972). Children were asked who they would prefer to look like, and both boys and girls preferred not to look like the overweight child. Lerner and Gellert (1969) replicated these findings; 86% of 5- to 6-year-old boys and girls said they did not want to look like a chubby child. Recent studies demonstrate continued weight bias using variants of the adjective checklist method, such as showing videos of a child wearing or not wearing a "fat suit" to appear overweight and asking participants to ascribe adjectives to the child (Bell & Morgan, 2000).

Girls and Boys

Several studies have demonstrated greater weight bias among girls than boys. Richardson et al. (1961) found that girls liked overweight peers significantly less than boys did. These investigators attributed this finding to boys' greater bias against functional disabilities, such as being in a wheelchair, compared to girls' dislike for appearance-related difficulties, such as facial disfigurement or overweight. Girls were also more likely than boys to rank the drawings of overweight children last, indicating they were liked the least (Richardson & Royce, 1968). Whereas 7- to 9-year-old boys assigned more negative adjectives to a chubby child than to an average-weight or thin child, girls rated both chubby and average-weight children less favorably than a thin child (Kraig & Keel, 2001). These findings suggest that among young girls, the preference for thinness is so strong that even average weight is unacceptable.

Children of Different Ethnic and Cultural Backgrounds

Richardson and Royce (1968) included two sets of the drawings used by Richardson et al. (1961), one each of white and black children. Children's rankings of the most disliked drawing were not altered by the additional variable of skin color; indeed, "the least liked was the obese child regardless of the color of the drawing" (p. 476). This finding held across groups of white, black, and Hispanic participants. The authors concluded by predicting that weight prejudice would be more difficult to counter than race bias.

A study of 50 overweight adolescent girls found that stigmatizing experiences were frequent (96%) and were equally common in black and white girls (Neumark-Sztainer, Story, & Faibisch, 1998). Black girls reported that they had experienced both weight-based and racial discrimination, but that the discrimination related to their weight felt more personal and thus more hurtful than racial discrimination.

Although the victims of weight bias might be distributed equally across ethnic groups, it is possible that the degree to which people endorse negative stereotypes and negative attitudes toward overweight people varies by ethnic group. For example, black girls have lower vulnerability to the influence of the thin-body ideal (Wildes, Emery, & Simons, 2001) and lower body dissatisfaction than white girls (Striegel-Moore et al., 2000), suggesting that black girls may show greater acceptance of overweight peers. In fact, limited evidence among young adult women suggests that black women stigmatize obesity less than white women do (Hebl & Heatherton, 1998; Latner, Stunkard, & Wilson, in press). Further, 13- to 14-year-old overweight black girls have similar levels of self-esteem to average-weight girls. In contrast, self-esteem is significantly lower in overweight white and Hispanic girls than in average-weight white or Hispanic girls (Strauss, 2000). Considering that self-esteem in overweight children may be mediated by the critical reactions of others and internalized weight concerns (as discussed later), this finding suggests that the negative effects of the stigmatization of obesity among black girls may be mediated by a more weight-tolerant attitude in their social network. Future research is needed to address this question.

Children of Different Age Groups

Goodman and colleagues (1963) proposed that weight stigma stems from the assimilation of cultural norms. At what age does this learning begin and is there sufficient information to define its developmental trajectory? Children as young as 3 years have demonstrated bias against chubby children; when read a story about a mean child and asked to select the picture of this child, a heavy child was chosen most often (Cramer & Steinwert, 1998). By age 4, children were able to articulate that the reason for their selection was the child's size. An adjective assignment task showed that stigmatizing attitudes increased through age 5 among boys and girls (Cramer & Steinwert, 1998), as it also did in 4- to 11-year-old children (Wardle, Volz, & Golding, 1995). Two studies of boys showed increases in negative stereotypes about overweight children across second, fourth, and sixth grades (Lawson, 1980), and across the ages of 5–6, 14–15, and 19–20 years (Lerner & Korn, 1972). Among kindergarten through fourth-grade children, a significantly stronger bias against chubby children first manifested itself between the first and second grade (Brylinsky & Moore, 1994). Moreover, increased negative evaluations of an overweight child emerged at the second-grade level in a study of nursery to third grade children (Sigelman, Miller, & Whitworth, 1986).

On the other hand, there is also evidence of increasing tolerance of excess weight in adulthood. Compared to elementary school children, adolescents and adults viewed a wider range of body sizes as acceptable (Rand & Wright, 2000). College students ranked drawings of overweight peers more highly than fifth- and sixth-grade children did (Latner et al., in press). It is possible that weight bias increases during early childhood, when cultural norms might first be understood and internalized, followed by a leveling off or decrease in young and middle adulthood. Prior studies have been cross-sectional in design; prospective research is needed to test this hypothesis.

CONSEQUENCES OF CHILDHOOD WEIGHT BIAS

Interpersonal Consequences

Self-report studies have documented that children dislike and harshly judge their overweight peers, suggesting that weight bias may severely undermine friendship formation. Staffieri (1967) first addressed this issue by asking 6- to 10-year-old boys to list their five closest friends. Overweight boys were least likely to receive nominations as best or second-best friends by their schoolmates. Other researchers have found no difference in peer-rated popularity between 313 overweight and average-weight 9-year-old girls, despite peer ratings that overweight girls were less attractive (Phillips & Hill, 1998). However, a recent investigation examined friendship networks among 90,118 adolescents ages 13–18 using a sophisticated social network analysis (Strauss & Pollack, 2003). Participants designated their five best friends of both sexes. Overweight adolescents were more isolated and peripheral to social networks. They were less often selected as friends or best friends and more likely to receive zero friendship nominations from peers. Their own friends were less popular, and the more overweight adolescents were, the fewer friendship nominations they received. Non-Hispanic white girls faced the strongest social penalties for their overweight.

Obese 9th- to 12th-grade girls are also less likely to have dated than their average-weight counterparts (Pearce, Boergers, & Prinstein, 2002). Half of obese girls reported never having dated, compared to 17% of overweight girls and 20% of average-weight girls. This was not by choice: Obese girls and boys were significantly less satisfied with their dating status than nonobese girls and boys.

Victimization

In addition to being teased, criticized, and less often selected as friends and romantic partners, overweight children are vulnerable to harsher forms of victimization. In a study of 434 children ages 12–16 in Finland, investigators examined the phenomenon of "mobbing": repeated ganging up on and tormenting the same victim (Lagerspetz, Kjorkqvist, Berts, & King, 1982). Based on ratings by their classmates, 4% of children were rated by their peers as being victims. Nearly a third of the victims were overweight, while only 2% of nonvictims were overweight.

An investigation with 416 adolescents in the United States measured two types of victimization: overt victimization such as teasing and physical aggression, and "relational victimization," exclusionary and hurtful treatment occurring in the context of purported friendships (Pearce et al., 2002). As predicted, obese girls experienced more relational victimization, and obese boys more overt victimization, than their nonobese peers. The findings suggest that obese girls may have to cope with less supportive and more antagonistic friendships.

A more recent Canadian study found a significant correlation between body mass index (BMI) and the likelihood of peer victimization within a large sample (n = 5,749) of preadolescent and adolescent boys and girls (Janssen, Craig, Boyce, & Pickett, 2004). With the exception of 15- to 16-year old boys, overweight and obese boys and girls of all ages were more likely than normal-weight children to experience overt and relational victimization. Among 15- and 16-year-old boys, there was a greater likelihood of being the perpetrator of bullying behavior as BMI increased. Among 15- to 16-year old girls, there was an increase in both victimization and bullying behavior associated with higher BMI levels. Clearly, the experience of victimization and later bullying behavior might impair the social development of overweight and obese children.

Psychological Consequences

Numerous studies have addressed the question of whether overweight has adverse psychological consequences such as low self-esteem. In a prospective study of 1,520 girls ages 9–10, overweight girls did not differ from nonoverweight girls in global self-esteem (Strauss, 2000). However, 4 years later, the overweight Hispanic and white girls showed significantly lower self-esteem than their nonoverweight counterparts. Decreased self-esteem was associated with greater sadness, loneliness, and nervousness, and overweight children with poor self-esteem were more likely to smoke and drink alcohol.

Other studies have shown an association between overweight and specific domains of self-esteem. Compared with their thin peers, overweight 9-year-old girls had lower self-esteem with respect to physical appearance and athletic competence (Phillips & Hill, 1998), and overweight 5-year-old girls had lower body esteem and perceived cognitive ability (Davison & Birch, 2001). Overweight girls from this sample later had lower self-concept at age 7 than their average-weight peers (Davison & Birch, 2002). Among children presenting for treatment at a weight management clinic, 31% were diagnosed with depression and 22% had borderline depression (Sheslow, Hassink, Wallace, & DeLancey, 1993). It seems appropriate that 74–100% of health care providers for overweight adolescents routinely address issues of self-acceptance during treatment (Neumark-Sztainer, Story, Evans, & Ireland, 1999).

These findings suggest a link between childhood obesity and psychological problems, a position supported by studies with obese adults showing that earlier onset of obesity in childhood is related to greater psychopathology (Mills & Andrianopoulous, 1993) and body dissatisfaction (Grilo, Wilfley, Brownell, & Rodin, 1994) in adulthood. However, a modest association between BMI and depressive symptoms found in 439 third-grade girls disappeared when controlling for concerns with overweight (Erickson, Robinson, Haydel, & Killen, 2000). Weight concerns, on the other hand, were associated with depressive symptoms independent of BMI. Similarly, 4,746 boys and girls in 7th- to 12th-grade were assessed on five outcome measures of emotional well-being (Eisenberg, Neumark-Sztainer, & Story, 2003). Once the history of being teased (by peers and/or family members) was included in the regression model, weight was no longer significantly associated with most outcomes. However, all five measures were elevated in adolescents who had been teased.

In the prospective study of 7-year-old girls described earlier (Davison & Birch, 2002), the presence of weight-related peer teasing and parental criticism about weight mediated the relationship between higher BMI and lower self-concept. In a retrospective study with adults, a history of childhood teasing about body weight and shape was correlated with negative evaluation of appearance and body dissatisfaction in adulthood, which in turn correlated with lower self-esteem (Grilo et al., 1994). Finally, weight-related criticism during physical activity has also been shown to specifically reduce enjoyment of sports and perceived amounts of activity performed, among 576 fifth- to eighth-grade children (Faith, Leone, Ayers, Heo, & Pietrobelli, 2002). This form of criticism was more common among girls and heavier children.

Overall, these findings suggest that the negative psychological outcomes that have at times been connected with heavier body weight may be primarily the consequence of the negative reactions of others to excess weight. When statistically controlling for these negative reactions, the psychological outcomes often disappear. The findings suggest that if these negative reactions were substantially limited, then the numerous adverse psychological consequences associated with childhood obesity would be greatly reduced.

Quality of Life

Considering the widespread weight bias against them, it is not surprising that overweight children have a severely impaired quality of life (QOL). One hundred and six obese children and adolescents presenting for weight loss treatment had significantly lower health-related QOL than nonobese comparison children (Schwimmer, Burwinkle, & Varni, 2003). QOL among the obese group was lower across all domains: physical health, psychosocial health, emotional functioning, social functioning, and school functioning. The most striking finding was that obese children had QOL scores similar to those of children with cancer. Another study assessed QOL as reported by parents in a nonclinical sample of 371 8- to 11-year-old children. Relative to average-weight children, overweight children had lower psychosocial health summary scores and lower subscale scores for self-esteem, emotional well-being, physical functioning, behavior, and global general health (Friedlander, Larkin, Rosen, Palermo, & Redline, 2003).

Academic and Occupational Consequences

As described earlier, girls of higher weight at age 5 have a lower perception of their own cognitive ability (Davison & Birch, 2001). Is there any validity to this perception? A case-controlled study of 102 obese and average-weight children ages 6–13 in China found significantly lower full-scale IQ scores (11 points lower) and performance IQ scores (14 points lower) in obese children (Li, 1995). School records revealed that examination grades were also lower in obese children. A more recent study showed that among 11,192 children, overweight children had lower math and reading test scores in kindergarten and at the end of first grade (Datar, Sturm, & Magnabosco, 2004). However, when controlling for socioeconomic status (SES) and background variables such as mother's education and ethnicity, these differences became nonsignificant. The authors concluded that obesity is a marker, not a cause, of poor academic achievement.

Although the results from the Datar et al. (2004) study support the position that obesity is only a marker for the actual correlates of poorer academic performance, the apparent link between weight and achievement might contribute to weight stigma. Indeed, a significant proportion of 115 school teachers, nurses, and social workers endorsed stigmatizing views about obesity (Neumark-Sztainer, Story, & Harris, 1999). Over half believed that obesity is caused primarily by one's own behaviors and 20–25% believed that obese persons are more emotional, less tidy, and less likely to succeed at work, and have different personalities and more family problems.

It is also possible that the perception of poorer performance serves to reinforce preexisting biases about obesity, which in turn may adversely affect children's actual potential for achievement in school and occupational settings. Results from an early study suggest that obese girls and boys are less likely to be accepted for admission to high-ranking colleges despite comparable academic performance (Canning & Mayer, 1966). Once enrolled in college, heavier females receive less financial support from their parents, even when controlling for income, ethnicity, and family size (Crandall, 1991).

This disadvantage continues to haunt overweight girls throughout their subsequent professional and personal lives, regardless of whether they continue to be overweight. Sixteen-year-old girls in the top 10% of the BMI range in the United Kingdom earned 7.4% less income than nonoverweight girls 7 years later (Sargent & Blanchflower, 1994). This occurred whether or not the young women were still overweight. The degree of obesity at age 16 was inversely correlated with earnings at age 23, controlling for parental social class and academic test scores. Another prospective study of overweight 16- to 24-year-olds in the United States found that 7 years later, controlling for baseline SES and aptitude test scores, overweight males and females were less likely to have married and had lower household income. Females also completed fewer years of education and had higher rates of poverty (Gortmaker, Must, Perrin, Sobol, & Dietz, 1993). The authors suggested that weight-related discrimination could explain these findings. This research indicates that there may be a strong causal relationship between childhood / adolescent obesity and low SES in later life. How great a role weight-based discrimination plays in the etiology of poor educational and occupational outcomes is an important topic for future research.

HOW IS WEIGHT BIAS LEARNED BY CHILDREN?

The research reviewed here on weight bias among very young children suggests that by age 3, children have learned that an overweight child is an undesirable playmate, and these attitudes strengthen through adolescence. How weight bias is transmitted to children remains unclear and is an important area for future research. A better understanding of how children acquire biased beliefs could be helpful in reversing the situation.

Parental Transmission

Only one study provides information on how parents may transmit negative associations with obese individuals to their children. Adams, Hicken, and Salehi (1988) asked parents to tell a story to their preschool child about an overweight, average-weight, or handicapped child. During stories about the overweight child, more negative descriptions were used, and peer reactions to the overweight child were presented as deeply disapproving. Parents may thus communicate and model stereotypical expectations to their children directly, without being aware of their own behaviors.

If parents transmit negative attitudes about obesity directly to their children, then there should be a correlation between parental and child levels of bias. A recent study, however, did not find a significant relationship between negative stereotypes about overweight people held by 9-year-old girls and their parents (Davison & Birch, 2004). Instead, the factors reflecting endorsement of the thin-ideal were significantly related to the girls' level of stereotyping, specifically, parental encouragement to lose weight, peer interactions focused on body shape and weight, and girls' maladaptive eating attitudes and weight concerns. These findings suggest that weight-based stereotypes may be transmitted indirectly via the idealization of being thin, rather than directly by teaching stereotypes about obese people.

Transmission through the Media

There is evidence that overweight individuals are portrayed in negative stereotypical roles in adult-oriented television shows (see Greenberg & Worrell, Chapter 3, this volume). We know of no similar empirical examination of children's literature or movies; however, a few salient characters from popular children's culture stand out as examples of how children may acquire negative views of overweight people.

In the beginning of the bestselling novel *Harry Potter and the Sorcerer's Stone* (Rowling, 1997), the hero, Harry, lives with his Aunt Marge, Uncle Vernon, and their son Dudley. Dudley is portrayed as a selfish, mean, fat boy. He is introduced in the second chapter, and the scene is his birthday:

> The table was almost hidden beneath all Dudley's birthday presents. It looked as though Dudley had gotten the new computer he wanted, not to mention the second television and the racing bike. Exactly why Dudley wanted a racing bike was a mystery to Harry, as Dudley was very fat and hated to exercise—unless of course it involved punching somebody. Dudley's favorite punching bag was Harry, but he couldn't often catch him. (pp. 19–20)

Later, Dudley is punished by Hagrid, and it is described: "Dudley was dancing on the spot with his hands clasped over his fat bottom, howling in pain. When he turned his back on them, Harry saw a curly pig's tail poking through a hole in his trousers." Afterwards, Hagrid said he "meant to turn him into a pig, but . . . . he was so much like a pig anyway there wasn't much left [to] do" (p. 59).

Even books directed at younger children contain the idea that being fat is synonymous with being selfish. The message that overweight people sneak and cheat in order to eat more is clearly conveyed in the book *The Hungry Pig* (Fun Works, 1998):

> The hungry pig's so hungry that he eats his breakfast slop.
> And when the farmer's good and gone, he finds a doughnut shop.
> The hungry pig's so hungry that he gobbles up his lunch.
> He sets his watch an hour back and sneaks out for some brunch.

Another example is found in a book series designed to teach very small children about particular characteristics. *Mr. Greedy* (Hargreaves, 1998) is about being greedy. The book begins, "Mr. Greedy, liked to eat! In fact, Mr. Greedy loved to eat, and the more he ate the fatter he became. . . . " As the book goes on, Mr. Greedy learns not to be so greedy, and therefore eats less and loses weight. It is interesting that the author chose overeating and body weight as the salient behaviors and physical characteristics of someone who is greedy.

Once sensitized to this issue, examples in children's movies are easy to find as well. In the classic *Willy Wonka and the Chocolate Factory* (Marguilies & Stuart, 1971), one of the primary themes is the punishment of greedy children. The first child to vanish from the factory is the only overweight child, who falls into the chocolate creek while trying to eat from it, after explicitly being told not to do so. In *A Little Princess* (Cuaron, 1995), there is a scene of a math lesson where a child is humiliated for not knowing the answer; she is the only overweight child in the class. Clearly, there are also examples of evil or selfish people who are not overweight, and overweight people who are loved (consider Scrooge and Santa Claus). The challenge facing researchers, however, is to identify and change the cultural messages directed at children that reinforce weight stigma.

CONCLUSION

In sum, the bias against overweight children is pervasive and powerful. The impact of this stigma is felt throughout a child's life and the damage can be significant. Relatively little is known about how this stigma develops, how to prevent it, and how to help children cope more effectively with it. It is logical to experiment with antibullying programs in schools and education of adults on how to approach situations where weight discrimination is observed. Parents of overweight children likely need help in methods to assist their children in coping with bias and discrimination. Finally, children need adults to advocate for them and fight against the stigma of obesity. Innovation in designing and evaluating stigma-prevention programs is necessary for this field to move forward.

REFERENCES

Adams, G. R., Hicken, M., & Salehi, M. (1988). Socialization of the physical attractiveness stereotype: Parental expectations and verbal behaviors. *International Journal of Psychology, 23,* 137–149.

Bell, S. K., & Morgan, S. B. (2000). Children's attitudes and behavioral intentions toward a peer presented as obese: Does a medical explanation for the obesity make a difference? *Journal of Pediatric Psychology, 25,* 137–145.

Brylinsky, J. A., & Moore, J. C. (1994). The identification of body build stereotypes in young children. *Journal of Research in Personality, 28,* 170–181.

Canning, H., & Mayer, J. (1966). Obesity—its possible effect on college acceptance. *New England Journal of Medicine,* 275, 1172–1174.

Cramer, P., & Steinwert, T. (1998). Thin is good, fat is bad: How early does it begin? *Journal of Applied Developmental Psychology, 19,* 429–451.

Crandall, C. S. (1991). Do parents discriminate against their heavyweight daughters? *Personality and Social Psychology Bulletin, 21,* 724–735.

Cuaron, A. (Director). (1995). *A little princess* [Film]. United States: Warner Home Video.

Datar, A., Sturm, R., & Magnabosco, J. L. (2004). Childhood overweight and academic performance: National study of kindergartners and first-graders. *Obesity Research, 12,* 58–68.

Davison, K. K., & Birch, L. L. (2001). Weight status, parent reaction, and self-concept in five-year-old girls. *Pediatrics, 107,* 46–52.

Davison, K. K., & Birch, L. L. (2002). Processes linking weight status and self-concept among girls from ages 5 to 7 years. *Developmental Psychology, 38,* 735–748.

Davison, K. K., & Birch, L. L. (2004). Predictors of fat stereotypes among 9-year-old girls and their parents. *Obesity Research, 12,* 86–94.

Eisenberg, M. E., Newmark-Sztainer, D., & Story, M. (2003). Associations of weight-based teasing and emotional well-being among adolescents. *Archives of Pediatric and Adolescent Medicine, 157,* 733–738.

Erickson, S. J., Robinson, T. N., Haydel, F., & Killen, J. D. (2000). Are overweight children unhappy? Body mass index, depressive symptoms, and overweight concerns in elementary school children. *Archives of Pediatric and Adolescent Medicine, 154,* 931–935.

Faith, M. S., Leone, M. A., Ayers, T. S., Heo, M., & Pietrobelli, A. (2002). Weight criticism during physical activity, coping skills, and reported physical activity in children. *Pediatrics, 110,* 23.

Friedlander, S. L., Larkin, E. K., Rosen, C. L., Palermo, T. M., & Redline, S. (2003). Decreased quality of life associated with obesity in school-aged children. *Archives of Pediatric and Adolescent Medicine, 157,* 1206–1211.

Fun Works. (1998). *The hungry pig.* New York: Mouse Works.

Goodman, N., Dornbusch, S. M., Richardson, S. A., & Hastorf, A. H. (1963). Variant reactions of physical disabilities. *American Sociological Review, 28,* 429–435.

Gortmaker, S. L., Must, A., Perrin, J. M., Sobol, A. M., & Dietz, W. H. (1993). Social and economic consequences of overweight in adolescence and young adulthood. *New England Journal of Medicine, 329,* 1008–1012.

Grilo, C. M., Wilfley, D. E., Brownell, K. D., & Rodin, J. (1994). Teasing, body image, and self-esteem in a clinical sample of obese women. *Addictive Behaviors, 19,* 443–450.

Hargreaves, R. (1998). *Mr. Greedy.* New York: Price Stern Sloan.

Hebl, M. R., & Heatherton, T. F. (1998). The stigma of obesity in women: The difference is black and white. *Personality and Social Psychology Bulletin, 24,* 417–426.

Janssen, I., Craig, W. M., Boyce, W. F., & Pickett, W. (2004). Associations between overweight and obesity with bullying behaviors in school-aged children. *Pediatrics, 113,* 1187–1194.

Kraig, K. A., & Keel, P. K. (2001). Weight-based stigmatization in children. *International Journal of Obesity, 25,* 1661–1666.

Lagerspetz, K. M. J., Kjorkqvist, K. A. J., Berts, M., & King, E. (1982). Group aggression among school children in three schools. *Scandinavian Journal of Psychology, 23,* 45–52.

Latner, J. D., & Stunkard, A. J. (2003). Getting worse: The stigmatization of obese children. *Obesity Research, 11,* 452–456.

Latner, J. D., Stunkard, A. J., & Wilson, G. T. (in press). Stigmatized students: Age, sex, and ethnicity effects in the stigmatization of obesity. *Obesity Research.*

Lawson, M. C. (1980). Development of body build stereotypes, peer ratings, and self-esteem in Australian children. *Journal of Psychology, 104,* 111–118.

Lerner, R. M., & Gellert, E. (1969). Body build identification, preference, and aversion in children. *Developmental Psychology, 1,* 456–462.

Lerner, R. M., & Korn, S. J. (1972). The development of body-build stereotypes in males. *Child Development, 43,* 908–920.

Li, X. (1995). A study of intelligence and personality in children with simple obesity. *International Journal of Obesity, 19,* 355–357.

Maddox, G. L., Back, K. W., & Liederman, V. R. (1968). Overweight as social deviance and disability. *Journal of Health and Social Behavior, 9,* 287–298.

Marguilies, S. (Producer), & Stuart, M. (Director). (1971). *Willy Wonka and the chocolate factory* [Film]. United States: Warner Home Video.

Mills, J. K., & Andrianopoulos, G. D. (1993). The relationship between childhood onset obesity and psychopathology in adulthood. *Journal of Psychology, 127,* 547–550.

National Education Association (1994). Report on Size Discrimination. Available: www.lectlaw.com/file/con28.htm. Accessed December 4, 2004.

Neumark-Sztainer, D., Story, M., Evans, T., & Ireland, M. (1999). Weight-related issues among overweight adolescents: What are health care providers doing? *Topics in Clinical Nutrition, 14,* 62–68.

Neumark-Sztainer, D., Story, M., & Faibisch, L. (1998). Perceived stigmatization among overweight African-American and Caucasian adolescent girls. *Journal of Adolescent Health, 23,* 264–270.

Neumark-Sztainer, D., Story, M., & Harris, T. (1999). Beliefs and attitudes about obesity among teachers and school health care providers working with adolescents. *Journal of Nutrition Education, 31,* 3–9.

Pearce, M. J., Boergers, J., & Prinstein, M. J. (2002). Adolescent obesity, overt and

relational peer victimization, and romantic relationships. *Obesity Research 10,* 386–393.
Phillips, R. G., & Hill, A. J. (1998). Fat, plain, but not friendless: Self-esteem and peer acceptance of obese pre-adolescent girls. *International Journal of Obesity, 22,* 287–293.
Rand, C. S. W., & Wright, B. A. (2000). Continuity and change in the evaluation of ideal and acceptable body sizes across a wide age span. *International Journal of Eating Disorders, 28,* 90–100.
Richardson, S. A., Goodman, N., Hastorf, A. H., & Dornbusch, S. M. (1961). Cultural uniformity in reaction to physical disabilities. *American Sociological Review, 26,* 241–247.
Richardson, S. A., & Royce, J. (1968). Race and physical handicap in children's preference for other children. *Child Development, 39,* 467–480.
Rowling, J. K. (1997). *Harry Potter and the sorcerer's stone.* New York: Scholastic.
Sargent, J. D., & Blanchflower, D. G. (1994). Obesity and stature in adolescence and earnings in young adulthood. *Archives of Pediatric and Adolescent Medicine, 148,* 681–687.
Schwimmer, J. B., Burwinkle, T. M., & Varni, J. W. (2003). Health-related quality of life of severely obese children and adolescents. *Journal of the American Medical Association, 289,* 1813–1819.
Sheslow, D., Hassink, S., Wallace, W., & DeLancey, E. (1993). The relationship between self-esteem and depression in obese children. *Annals of the New York Academy of Science, 699,* 289–291.
Sigelman, C. K., Miller, T. E., & Whitworth, K. A. (1986). The early development of stigmatizing reactions to physical differences. *Journal of Applied Developmental Psychology, 7,* 17–32.
Staffieri, J. R. (1967). A study of social stereotype of body image in children. *Journal of Personality and Social Psychology, 7,* 101–104.
Staffieri, J. R. (1972). Body build and behavioral expectancies in young females. *Developmental Psychology, 6,* 125–127.
Strauss, R. S. (2000). Childhood obesity and self-esteem. *Pediatrics. 105,* 1–5.
Strauss, R. S., & Pollack, H. A. (2003). Social marginalization of overweight children. *Archives of Pediatric and Adolescent Medicine, 157,* 746–752.
Striegel-Moore, R. H., Schreiber, G. B., Lo, A., Crawford, P., Obarzanek, E., & Rodin, J. (2000). Eating disorder symptoms in a cohort of 11 to 16–year-old black and white girls: The NHLBI growth and health study. *International Journal of Eating Disorders, 27,* 29–66.
Wardle, J., Volz, C., & Golding, C. (1995). Social variation in attitudes to obesity in children. *International Journal of Obesity, 19,* 562–569.
Wildes, J. E., Emery, R. E., & Simons, A. D. (2001). The roles of ethnicity and culture in the development of eating disturbance and body dissatisfaction: A meta-analytic review. *Clinical Psychology Review, 21,* 521–551.

CHAPTER 5

■ ■ ■

Weight Bias in a Teen's World

DIANNE NEUMARK-SZTAINER
MARLA EISENBERG

Adolescence is characterized as a period of transition from childhood to adulthood, during which there are many physical, psychological, and social changes. Because of the many physical changes that adolescents experience and their increased attention to their physical appearance, and because they are in the stage of developing their self-identity, body image and self-esteem tend to be very intertwined during adolescence. Although adolescents are striving to be independent and find their own identity, they are still reliant on input from significant others to do so. Pressures on adolescents to conform to social norms regarding an ideal body shape and size can be particularly strong. For these and other related reasons, weight bias—particularly in the form of weight teasing—has the potential to be extremely detrimental to adolescents in terms of their body image, self-esteem, eating behaviors, and emotional well-being.

In this chapter we examine the experience of weight bias in a teen's world by addressing three major questions. First, how prevalent is weight teasing as an expression of weight bias? We discuss who is being teased about weight, who is doing the teasing, and where the teasing occurs. Second, because teens spend so much of their time at school, we examine factors in the school environment that may affect teasing and weight attitudes among teens. We look in particular at school staff working in middle schools and high schools, and their attitudes toward obesity. Finally, we address the question: Does weight teasing really matter? We discuss the extent to which teens are bothered by weight teasing and the impact of teasing on body image, disordered eating behavior, and psychosocial well-being.

THE PREVALENCE OF WEIGHT STIGMATIZATION

Our research team conducted in-depth individual interviews with 50 overweight adolescent girls to learn more about the experience of being fat in a thin-oriented society (Neumark-Sztainer, Story, & Faibisch, 1998; Neumark-Sztainer, Story, Faibisch, Ohlson, & Adamiak, 1999). Virtually all (*n* = 48) of the girls described hurtful comments and/or differential treatment or rejection owing to being overweight. Three-fourths of the girls described intentionally hurtful comments including weight teasing, jokes, and derogatory names. Many discussed being teased in elementary and middle schools and indicated that the situation had either improved in high school or that they had learned how to better cope with hurtful situations.

While these interviews helped us understand the experience of being overweight, we were interested in learning more about the prevalence of weight stigmatization in a larger adolescent population and seeing whether there were differences across gender and weight status. In Project EAT (Eating Among Teens), a study of eating, activity, and weight-related issues in 4,746 middle school and high school adolescents, we examined the prevalence of weight teasing (Neumark-Sztainer et al., 2002). Nearly a quarter of the adolescents reported being teased about their weight at least a few times a year (25.5% of girls and 22.2% of boys). Weight teasing by peers (ever) was reported by 30.0% of the girls and 24.6% of the boys. Weight teasing by family members was slightly lower and was reported by 28.7% of the girls and 16.1% of the boys. Table 5.1 shows the prevalence of weight teasing for girls and boys by weight status. Teens in all weight categories reported being teased about their weight, but the prevalence was much higher among teens whose weight deviated from the norm and who were either underweight or overweight. Teens with body mass index (BMI) values ≥ 95th percentile (labeled as overweight in Table 5.1) reported the highest prevalence of weight teasing by peers; 63.2% of these overweight girls and 58.3% of these overweight boys reported that they had been teased about their weight by their peers.

These numbers are high, and based upon our experiences in the individual interviews, we expect that experiences of weight bias are even higher. Early on in the interviews, the overweight girls were reluctant to admit, or did not recognize, that they had been teased or treated poorly

TABLE 5.1. Weight Teasing (≥ Few Times/Year) by Weight Status in Adolescent Girls and Boys

	n	%
Girls		
Underweight (*n* = 95)	40	44.0
Average weight (*n* = 1,267)	236	18.7
Moderately overweight (*n* = 406)	115	28.5
Overweight (*n* = 250)	112	45.3
Boys		
Underweight (*n* = 116)	41	36.6
Average weight (*n* = 1,300)	168	13.0
Moderately overweight (*n* = 297)	66	22.3
Overweight (*n* = 333)	167	50.2

Note. From Neumark-Sztainer et al. (2002). Adapted by permission.

because of their weight. Often, only after talking about their experiences did they realize that they had been treated unfairly. Furthermore, in the Project EAT survey, we only asked about weight teasing and not about more subtle forms of weight bias such as being excluded from school activities or social groups or being treated differently because of one's weight. For example, Sobal and his colleagues found that overweight high school students, especially girls, were stigmatized regarding dating activities (Sobal, Nicolopoulos, & Lee, 1995). Only 12% of the students had dated someone who was overweight, with girls (16%) more often dating overweight peers than boys did (8%). Adolescents, in particular boys, expressed low comfort levels in dating overweight peers, and comfort levels were low for dating a very overweight individual.

Both in the interviews that we conducted with overweight teens, and in the survey that was done on a population-based sample, peers were most frequently mentioned as the instigators of hurtful weight-related experiences, followed by family members. In the interviews, girls were more likely to describe hurtful situations with boys, rather than with other girls. Not surprisingly, the school was the most commonly mentioned place in which weight stigmatization took place.

WEIGHT BIAS IN THE SCHOOL ENVIRONMENT

Adolescents report that they get teased about their weight, or experience other forms of weight stigmatization, at school more than any other place. The school is a central place in the lives of most teens because of the amount of time spent at school, the numerous social interactions that go on at school, and the school's role in formally and informally educating teens.

Interestingly, in a study aimed at identifying factors within the school social and physical environments that support or interfere with efforts to promote physical activity and healthful nutrition, weight teasing and other forms of teasing/bullying arose as obstacles to both. Bauer and her colleagues conducted focus groups and interviews with middle school students and school staff (Bauer, Yang, & Austin, 2004). Students and staff indicated that teasing and bullying were among the predominant barriers to students fully participating in physical education class. The findings indicated that being female, having fewer athletic abilities, and being overweight cause many students to feel uncomfortable. While most of their comments suggested that they were teased by their peers, students also reported that the staff, on occasion, makes negative comments regarding students' athletic abilities. They noted that this type of criticism could be so upsetting that it leads them to feel self-conscious and to avoid participating. They also talked about overweight peers being targeted for teasing during lunch. While students acknowledged that teasing and harassment are in violation of school policy, many felt there was no enforcement of those rules. Both students and staff felt that teasing and bullying occur so frequently that it would be impossible monitor and discipline everyone.

School faculty and school health care providers have an important role to play in either decreasing or perpetuating negative weight-related attitudes. They are well educated and care about the well-being of their students; in our experience, most school staff members are interested in protecting their students from any form of teasing, and are highly unlikely to intentionally mistreat students because of their weight. However, school staff members are not immune to social pressures stigmatizing overweight persons, and could unintentionally perpetuate misconceptions about overweight individuals or treat overweight students differently than their nonoverweight peers. Thus, our research team conducted a study to assess beliefs and attitudes regarding obesity among school staff most likely to discuss health-related issues with students (Neumark-Sztainer, Story, & Harris, 1999).

Mailed surveys were completed by 115 science, health, home economics, and physical education teachers, school nurses, and school social workers from 17 middle schools and high schools in a large urban school district. We assessed beliefs about causes of obesity (Table 5.2) and attitudes toward obese persons (Table 5.3) using scales developed by Allison and his colleagues (Allison, Basile, & Yuker, 1991).

School faculty and health care providers were aware that multiple factors contribute to obesity (Table 5.2). Nevertheless, it was interesting that overall belief scores (mean = 14.0; *SD* = 5.4) were lower, and more indicative of beliefs that obesity is caused by individual factors, than scores found in other studies among undergraduate psychology students (mean = 19.4; *SD* = 8.7), graduate psychology students (mean = 20.8; *SD* = 7.0), and members of the National Association to Advance Fat Acceptance (mean = 31.7; *SD* = 10.5) (Allison et al., 1991). Similarly, Price and his colleagues found that physical education teachers working in elementary schools tend toward the belief that obesity is largely caused by individual behaviors; 92% indicated that peer eating behaviors play a major role in causing obesity, while 58% indicated that heredity plays a major role, and only 23% indicated that cultural factors

TABLE 5.2. Beliefs about Obese Persons among School Staff

	Strongly agree/agree[a]		Strongly disagree/ disagree[b]		Mean score[c]	
	n	%	*n*	%	*M*	*SD*
Obesity often occurs when eating is used as a form of compensation for lack of love or attention.	63	54.8	14	12.2	1.2	1.7
In many cases, obesity is the result of a biological disorder.	62	54.4	13	11.4	1.0	1.7
Obesity is caused by overeating.	60	52.2	8	7.0	1.2	1.5
Most obese people cause their problem by not getting enough exercise.	56	48.7	14	12.1	0.9	1.7
Most obese people eat more than nonobese people.	36	31.3	25	21.8	0.4	1.8
The majority of obese people have poor eating habits, which lead to their obesity.	64	55.6	8	6.9	1.2	1.5
Obesity is rarely caused by a lack of willpower.	28	24.6	25	21.9	0.2	1.7
People can become addicted to food, just as others are addicted to drugs, and these people usually become obese.	71	61.8	8	7.0	1.5	1.5

Note. *n* = 115. From Neumark-Sztainer, Story, and Harris (1999). Copyright 1999 by the Society for Nutrition Education. Reprinted by permission.

[a]Responses 1 or 2 on a 6-point scale (1 = strongly agree; 6 = strongly disagree).

[b]Responses 5 or 6 on a 6-point scale (1 = strongly agree; 6 = strongly disagree).

[c]Responses were recoded with values ranging from +3 (strongly agree) to –3 (strongly disagree) in order to calculate mean scores for each item.

play a major role (Price, Desmond, & Ruppert, 1990). It may be that by nature of their profession, school staff, who are involved in the education of youth, believe more in people's ability to control their behaviors and resultant health outcomes such as weight status. This type of thinking appears to have positive implications in terms of supporting school efforts addressing obesity; in our study, school staff holding stronger beliefs that obesity is under individual control were more likely to support school-based activities aimed decreasing obesity. However, this type of thinking could possibly have negative implications in terms of blaming overweight adolescents for their condition.

In examining the attitudes of school staff toward overweight people, it was encouraging to find that the vast majority did *not* associate obesity with characteristics unrelated to weight such as personality, tidiness, and work success (Table 5.3). Two-thirds of the respondents disagreed with statements such as "Obese workers cannot be as successful as other workers" or "Obese people should not expect to lead normal lives." Nevertheless, school staff are not immune to weight stigmatization and the tendency to assign nonpersonality characteristics to obesity. Approximately one-fifth of the respondents viewed obese persons as more emotional, less tidy, less likely to succeed at work, and as having different personalities than nonobese persons. About one-fourth viewed obese persons as having more family problems than nonobese individuals and agreed with the statement that "one of the worst things that could happen to a person would be for him/her to become obese."

Because of the ongoing contact that school faculty and health care providers have with youth, these findings suggest a need for staff training. Even if school staff are not contributing to the weight stigmatization that many teens experience at school, they need to know how to be effective in preventing and intervening when kids are victims of weight stigmatization from their peers. Staff training should include activities aimed at increasing knowledge about weight problems and their etiology, skills for addressing and minimizing weight teasing, skills in meeting the needs of overweight teens, and sensitivity toward their own weight biases. Our research team has recently been involved in implementing a school-based program to decrease weight teasing in an elementary school (Haines, Neumark-Sztainer, & Thiel, 2004). The staff training began with an activity aimed at increasing teachers' sensitivity to their own biases about overweight people (Greenwald, McGhee, & Schwartz, 1998; Teachman, Gapinski, Brownell, Rawlins, & Jeyaram, 2003). This type of exercise can be very effective, as long as participants are not made to feel bad about their attitudes, but rather made aware of how ingrained weight-related biases can be in all of us.

TABLE 5.3. Attitudes toward Obese Persons among School Staff

	Strongly agree/agree[a]		Strongly disagree/ disagree[b]		Mean score[c]	
	n	%	*n*	%	*M*	*SD*
Obese people are as happy as nonobese people.	44	38.6	37	32.4	0.1	2.2
Most obese people feel that they are not as good as other people.	65	57.0	13	11.4	1.1	1.9
Most obese persons are more self-conscious than other people.	75	65.8	7	6.2	1.5	1.5
Obese workers cannot be as successful as other workers.	20	17.5	78	68.5	–1.4	2.0
Most nonobese people would not want to marry anyone who is obese.	53	46.5	25	21.9	0.5	2.1
Severely obese people are usually untidy.	23	20.2	77	67.5	–1.3	2.2
Obese persons are just as confident as other people.	42	36.9	33	29.0	0.2	2.1
Most people feel uncomfortable when they associate with obese people.	49	42.9	41	36.0	0.2	2.4
Obese people are often less aggressive than nonobese people.	38	33.3	38	33.3	–0.2	2.2
Most obese people have different personalities than nonobese people.	24	20.9	67	58.2	–1.0	2.1
Obese people are more emotional than other people.	22	19.3	69	60.5	–1.1	2.0
Obese people should not expect to lead normal lives.	19	16.5	79	68.7	–1.4	2.1
Obese people are just as healthy as nonobese people.	20	17.4	68	59.1	–1.3	1.9
Obese people are just as sexually attractive as nonobese people.	35	30.4	48	41.8	–0.4	2.2
Obese people tend to have family problems.	31	27.5	47	41.6	–0.5	2.2
One of the worst things that could happen to a person would be for him or her to become obese.	32	27.9	62	53.9	–0.7	2.3

Note. n = 115. From Neumark-Sztainer, Story, and Harris (1999). Copyright 1999 by the Society for Nutrition Education. Reprinted by permission.

[a]Responses 1 or 2 on a 6-point scale (1 = strongly agree; 6 = strongly disagree).

[b]Responses 5 or 6 on a 6-point scale (1 = strongly agree; 6 = strongly disagree).

[c]Responses were recoded with values ranging from +3 (strongly agree) to –3 (strongly disagree) in order to calculate mean scores for each item.

DOES WEIGHT TEASING REALLY MATTER?

How do teens feel when they are teased, or otherwise treated differently because of their weight? In interviews with overweight girls, they talked about how painful it was and how damaging it could be for one's self-esteem (Neumark-Sztainer, Story, Faibisch, et al., 1999). In Project EAT, many of the teens who were teased by peers or family reported that it bothered them "somewhat" or "very much." Girls were more likely to be bothered than boys, and overweight teens were more likely to be bothered than nonoverweight teens. Two-thirds of the overweight girls who were teased by peers or family members reported that they were bothered by the teasing (Neumark-Sztainer et al., 2002).

Beyond feeling upset or hurt, research has demonstrated a number of other psychosocial and behavioral problems related to being teased about weight. In the Project EAT study, we found that teens who were teased by peers or family members were more likely to use unhealthy weight control behaviors, including taking diet pills, using laxatives, skipping meals, and binge eating (Neumark-Sztainer et al., 2002). While the teen may be attempting to lose weight and avoid further teasing, behaviors such as these rarely result in sustained weight loss, and may even lead to weight gain (Field et al., 2003; Stice, Cameron, Killen, Hayward, & Taylor, 1999). Comments from significant others do not always come in the form of hurtful teasing; parents, for example, may simply encourage their teens to diet. This type of feedback about weight and body shape can also be harmful, however. Project EAT findings showed that boys in particular were more likely to binge eat and use other weight control behaviors if their mothers encouraged them to diet (Fulkerson et al., 2002). Interestingly, almost half of teens who were encouraged to diet were not considered overweight according to federal guidelines.

These associations of weight teasing with body dissatisfaction and disordered eating have been replicated in several countries. Similar studies with adolescents in the United States, Canada, Australia, Sweden, and India have shown repeatedly that being teased about one's weight is associated with body dissatisfaction and eating pathology (Lieberman, Gauvin, Bukowski, & White, 2001; Lunner et al., 2000; Shroff & Thompson, 2004; Thompson, Coovert, Richards, Johnson, & Cattarin, 1995; van den Berg, Wertheim, Thompson, & Paxton, 2002). Specifically, these studies suggest that teasing may be a more important factor than BMI in predicting body dissatisfaction, which in turn predicts eating disturbance. Such consistent cross-cultural findings point to the importance of teasing as a modifiable risk factor in a variety of social contexts.

The experience of being teased about weight may influence teens' well-being beyond their weight control behaviors and beliefs (Eisenberg, Neumark-Sztainer, & Story, 2003; Fabian & Thompson, 1989; Jackson, Grilo, & Masheb, 2000). Using data from Project EAT, we found that teens were 2–3 times more likely to report high depressive symptoms, suicidal ideation, and suicide attempts if they were teased by peers and/or family members, compared to those who were not teased. For example, 51% of girls who had been teased about weight by both peers and family members had ever thought about committing suicide, compared to 25% of those who had not been teased. Similarly, 13% of boys who had been teased by family members reported a suicide attempt, compared to only 4% of boys who were not teased. Again, teasing was a more important factor than BMI in relation to these emotional health problems (Eisenberg et al., 2003).

A significant limitation of the work described is that most studies are cross-sectional and do not speak to the causal relationship between teasing and related attitudes and behaviors. Two longitudinal studies, however, have found that teasing and other pressures to be thin may contribute to subsequent body dissatisfaction in girls (Cattarin & Thompson, 1994; Stice & Whitenton, 2002). In one study, being teased about weight and size predicted appearance dissatisfaction 3 years later (Cattarin & Thompson, 1994). In a second study, pressure to be thin that participants felt from family, friends, dating partners, and the media predicted body dissatisfaction after 1 year, although teasing per se was not a significant predictor when considered alongside pressure to be thin (Stice & Whitenton, 2002).

NEXT STEPS IN RESEARCH AND PRACTICE

Research on the causal relationship of teasing and teens' behaviors and psychosocial well-being has just begun. New prospective studies are needed to examine the effect of teasing on weight-control behaviors and additional outcomes such as self-esteem, depression, and suicide involvement. Longitudinal research must also include boys, for whom teasing and other weight-related pressure have been associated with eating and emotional disturbances in cross-sectional studies. More qualitative research is also needed to disentangle some of the experiences captured in quantitative research as "teasing," compared to "encouraged to diet" and "pressured to be thin." Qualitative feedback from teens would also be useful in unpacking the subjective meaning of weight teasing and how it relates to well-being. Finally, programs aimed at reducing weight teasing and ameliorating its effects in clinical, family, and community settings will need to be developed and evaluated in order to identify promising avenues for intervening on this health issue.

Far from being a rare or harmless social interaction, weight teasing is extremely common and can be very hurtful, contributing to both weight-specific and general disturbances. We need to take teasing seriously and take steps to increase awareness of the problem and its consequences. Training for adults who interact with young people—including school staff, health care providers, and parents—should include general discussions about the prevalence and seriousness of weight teasing, as well as strategies for preventing teasing or other types of weight bias. Education about healthful ways to address a teen's overweight status (for example, adopting healthier eating and physical activity practices for the whole family) may allow parents an alternative to teasing or pressuring their kids, which may result in less healthy behaviors.

At many schools across the country, recent decades have seen increased attention and sensitivity given to prejudices such as racism and sexism. Weight bias, however, has rarely received such attention. Explicitly articulating the parallels in these various forms of discrimination may help students and staff to recognize the similarities and come to view weight bias as an equally unacceptable attitude. In addition, schools—and society in general—have recently begun addressing the problem of bullying among youth. The time is right to capitalize on this development and incorporate a focus on weight teasing into school-based and communitywide bullying prevention programs.

REFERENCES

Allison, D. B., Basile, V. C., & Yuker, H. E. (1991). The measurement of attitudes toward and beliefs about obese persons. *International Journal of Eating Disorders, 10*(5), 599–607.

Bauer, K. W., Yang, Y. W., & Austin, S. B. (2004). "How can we stay healthy when you're throwing all of this in front of us?" Findings from focus groups and interviews in middle schools on environmental influences on nutrition and physical activity. *Health Education and Behavior, 31*(1), 34–46.

Cattarin, J., & Thompson, J. K. (1994). A three year longitudinal study of body image and eating disturbance in adolescent females. *Eating Disorders: The Journal of Prevention and Treatment, 2*(2), 114–125.

Eisenberg, M. E., Neumark-Sztainer, D., & Story, M. (2003). Associations of weight-based teasing and emotional well-being among adolescents. *Archives of Pediatrics and Adolescent Medicine, 157*(8), 733–738.

Fabian, L. J., & Thompson, J. K. (1989). Body image and eating disturbance in young females. *International Journal of Eating Disorders, 8*(1), 63–74.

Field, A. E., Austin, S. B., Taylor, C. B., Malspeis, S., Rosner, B., Rockett, H. R., et al. (2003). Relation between dieting and weight change among preadolescents and adolescents. *Pediatrics, 112*(4), 900–906.

Fulkerson, J. A., McGuire, M. T., Neumark-Sztainer, D., Story, M., French, S. A., & Perry, C. L. (2002). Weight-related attitudes and behaviors of adolescent boys and girls who are encouraged to diet by their mothers. *International Journal of Obesity, 26*, 1579–1587.

Greenwald, A. G., McGhee, D. E., & Schwartz, J. L. K. (1998). Measuring individual differences in implicit cognition: The Implicit Association Test. *Journal of Personality and Social Psychology, 74*(6), 1464–1480.

Haines, J., Neumark-Sztainer, D., & Thiel, L. (2004). *V.I.K. (Very Important Kids): Development of a school-based intervention to prevent weight-related disorders.* Paper presented at the Academy for Eating Disorders International Conference on Eating Disorders, Orlando, FL.

Jackson, T., Grilo, C. M., & Masheb, R. M. (2000). Teasing history, onset of obesity, current eating disorder psychopathology, body dissatisfaction, and psychological functioning in binge eating disorder. *Obesity Research, 8*(6), 451–458.

Lieberman, M., Gauvin, L., Bukowski, W. M., & White, D. R. (2001). Interpersonal influence and disordered eating behaviors in adolescent girls: The role of peer modeling, social reinforcement, and body-related teasing. *Eating Behaviors, 2*(3), 215–236.

Lunner, K., Werthem, E. H., Thompson, J. K., Paxton, S. J., McDonald, F., & Halvaarson, K. S. (2000). A cross-cultural examination of weight-related teasing, body image, and eating disturbance in Swedish and Australian samples. *International Journal of Eating Disorders, 28*(4), 430–435.

Neumark-Sztainer, D., Falkner, N., Story, M., Perry, C., Hannan, P. J., & Mulert, S. (2002). Weight-teasing among adolescents: Correlations with weight status and disordered eating behaviors. *International Journal of Obesity and Related Metabolic Disorders, 26*(1), 123–131.

Neumark-Sztainer, D., Story, M., & Faibisch, L. (1998). Perceived stigmatization among overweight African American and Caucasian adolescent girls. *Journal of Adolescent Health, 23*(5), 264–270.

Neumark-Sztainer, D., Story, M., Faibisch, L., Ohlson, J., & Adamiak, M. (1999). Issues of self-image among overweight African American and Caucasian adolescent girls: A qualitative study. *Journal of Nutrition Education, 31*(6), 311–320.

Neumark-Sztainer, D., Story, M., & Harris, T. (1999). Beliefs and attitudes about obesity among teachers and school health care providers working with adolescents. *Journal of Nutrition Education, 31*, 3–9.

Price, J., Desmond, S., & Ruppert, E. (1990). Elementary physical education teachers' perceptions of childhood obesity. *Health Education, 21*(6), 26–32, 63.

Shroff, H., & Thompson, J. K. (2004). Body image and eating disturbance in India: Media and interpersonal influences. *International Journal of Eating Disorders, 35*(2), 198–203.

Sobal, J., Nicolopoulos, V., & Lee, J. (1995). Attitudes about overweight and dating among secondary students. *International Journal of Obesity, 19*, 376–381.

Stice, E., Cameron, R. P., Killen, J. D., Hayward, C., & Taylor, C. B. (1999). Naturalistic weight-reduction efforts prospectively predict growth in relative weight and onset of obesity among female adolescents. *Journal of Consulting and Clinical Psychology, 67*(6), 967–974.

Stice, E., & Whitenton, K. (2002). Risk factors for body dissatisfaction in adolescent girls: A longitudinal investigation. *Developmental Psychology, 38*(5), 669–678.

Teachman, B. A., Gapinski, K. D., Brownell, K. D., Rawlins, M., & Jeyaram, S. (2003). Demonstrations of implicit anti-fat bias: The impact of providing causal information and evoking empathy. *Health Psychology, 22*(1), 68–78.

Thompson, J. K., Coovert, M. D., Richards, K. J., Johnson, S., & Cattarin, J. (1995). Development of body image, eating disturbance, and general psychological functioning in female adolescents: Covariance structure modeling and longitudinal investigations. *International Journal of Eating Disorders, 18*(3), 221–236.

van den Berg, P., Wertheim, E. H., Thompson, J. K., & Paxton, S. J. (2002). Development of body image, eating disturbance, and general psychological functioning in adolescent females: A replication using covariance structure modeling in an Australian sample. *International Journal of Eating Disorders, 32*(1), 46–51.

PART II

■ ■ ■ ■

Origins, Explanations, and Measurement

CHAPTER 6

■ ■ ■

Attributions and Weight-Based Prejudice

CHRISTIAN S. CRANDALL
APRIL HORSTMAN RESER

One of the best-established relations in the study of attitudes toward fat people is that attributions of controllability—seeing fat people as responsible for their weight—is an excellent predictor of prejudice. The more people believe that weight is a function of willpower, exercise, diet, or self-indulgence, the more negative an attitude they express (Cahnman, 1968; Crandall, 1994; DeJong, 1980; Weiner, Perry, & Magnusson, 1988). In this chapter, we review the close relationship between attributions and prejudice toward fat people, and consider the history of theory and research in this area. The evidence is quite reliable and speaks in nearly one voice, and the journey takes us through surprising terrain, including cultural differences, political ideology, and self-justification, to examine the relationship between explanations and affect.

First, it is important to define prejudice, as "a negative evaluation of a social group, or a negative evaluation of an individual that is significantly based on the individual's group membership" (Crandall & Eshleman, 2003, p. 414). Prejudice is defined by the presence of *negative affect*, and whether or not one's stereotypes are accurate, or one's explanations of weight's cause scientifically supported, is not, in itself, prejudice. We seek to understand the negative affect toward fat people, and do not seek to sort out what is considered acceptable or unacceptable prejudice.

PREJUDICE, DISCRIMINATION, AND OBESITY

There is ample evidence of prejudice against fat people, and in the context of this volume, we need not review this at great length (see Chapters 1–5). But it is the prevalence and power of this prejudice, and its concomitant discrimination that makes research in anti-fat attitudes so important. In their social lives, fat people, as compared to thin people, are rated as less likable (Goodman, Richardson, Dornbusch, & Hastorf, 1963), have fewer romantic contacts (Halpern, Udry, Campbell, & Suchindran, 1999), are perceived as less sexual (Regan, 1996), and report more sexual problems (Jagstaidt, Golay, & Pasini, 1997). In their work life, they are less likely to be hired (Puhl & Brownell, 2001), receive lower wages (Frieze, Olson, & Good, 1990), and advance more slowly in their careers (Rothblum, Brand, Miller, & Oetjen, 1990). They are less likely to attend top colleges (Canning & Mayer, 1966), and receive less support from their parents to pay for higher education when they do (Crandall, 1991, 1995).

ATTRIBUTION AND PREJUDICE

What Are Attributions?

Attributions are causal explanations about the social world (Heider, 1958). We may infer that a person behaves aggressively because she is mean, because she has been made angry, because she has a brain tumor, because she is drunk, because she misunderstands the situation, or because she is acting in a play. Each of these explanations lead to different evaluations of the woman, and in each case the attribution is based on the kinds of information that are available about the causes of her aggression. Attribution theorists have suggested that people act like naive psychologists, trying to ascertain why people act the way they do and what outcomes they receive. Attributions are judgments about the causes of outcomes, and they have substantial consequences for emotions and motivation.

Attribution's Link to Prejudice

Prejudice and negative attitudes toward targets have been linked to attributions of controllability across a wide range of domains. The more people are held responsible for their negative outcomes, the more negative affect is expressed toward them, including welfare recipients, the poor, homosexuals, those with HIV/AIDS, individuals suffering from depression, individuals with alcohol dependence, spousal-abuse victims, targets of rape and sexual harassment, people with physical and mental illnesses, blacks, Asians, Jews, women, and innumerable other groups (see Crandall & Moriarty, 1995; Ryan, 1976; Weiner, 1995, among many others).

The way one accounts for successes and failures (such as being thin or fat) influences how people are evaluated, and the explanation one generates determines the reaction one has. To the extent that fat is seen as a bad thing, attributing individual responsibility to fatness—be it a lack of willpower, gluttony, or laziness—leads to a negative evaluation and forms the basis for prejudice against fat people (Crandall et al., 2001).

It is the attribution of controllability, or the judgment of responsibility, that leads to a moral evaluation of the person (Weiner, 1995); this notion of responsibility introduces a component of moral judgment. Cahnman (1968) was among the first to recognize the close relationship between attributions and moral judgment:

> Contrary to those that are blind, one-legged, paraplegic, or dark-pigmented, the obese are presumed to hold their fate in their own hands; if they were only a little less greedy or lazy or yielding to impulse or obliviousness of advice, they would restrict excessive food intake, resort to strenuous exercise, and as a consequence of such deliberate action, they would reduce. . . . While blindness is considered a misfortune, obesity is branded as a defect. (p. 294)

The importance of this distinction is the difference between sin (which is controllable) and sickness (which is uncontrollable). Sinners are certainly more punishable than the sick (Weiner, 1993). Research in our lab and others over the last decade has shown that belief in the controllability of fatness is a primary and proximal cause of prejudice.

Some research carried out with a different hypothesis in mind supports the importance of attributions in prejudice. Research suggests that taking the perspective of a stigmatized target reduces the prejudice toward that target (e.g., Batson et al., 1997; Batson and colleagues were studying empathy). However, there is reason to believe that perspective taking changes the kinds of attributions that are made—shifting from person attributions to situational attributions (Regan & Totten, 1975), and this shift in attributions may be more powerful than the effect of empathy (Vescio, Sechrist, & Paolucci, 2003).

ATTRIBUTIONS AND ANTI-FAT PREJUDICE

Crandall (1994) developed the Anti-Fat Attitudes (AFA) questionnaire about attitudes toward fatness, with a wide range of items that developed into three subscales. One measured prejudice toward fat people

(*Dislike*), one measured concern about one's own weight (*Fear of Fat*), and one measured the judgment of responsibility or the attribution of controllability (*Willpower*). Across about a dozen samples, *Willpower* has proved a very reliable predictor of *Dislike* (average r = .48).

Several experiments have shown the same relation. DeJong (1980) had participants evaluate either a photograph of a normal weight or overweight woman. The overweight woman was rated as more self-indulgent and lacking self-discipline when she gave no reason for her weight, as compared to when her weight was ascribed to a "glandular disorder." The woman with the glandular disorder was rated more likable than the woman with no favorable attribution. Weiner et al. (1988) manipulated the perceived controllability of obesity. They briefly described an obese target, who either had a "glandular dysfunction" or engaged in "excessive eating without exercise." In the excessive eating condition, people made attributions of responsibility and the targets were less liked; they incited more anger and received less help than when a biological cause was indicated.

The correlations between judgments of responsibility and anti-fat attitudes and the experiments in which changing attributions led to more positive attitudes provide powerful converging evidence that attributions play an important role in determining attitudes. The experiments make a strong case that attributions cause attitudes. In this experimental research, attributions were changed for a particular target of interest (e.g., toward a person in a photo, toward a target described by a vignette), but the attributions of nonresponsibility probably did not generalize to all fat people.

THERAPEUTIC EXPERIMENTS: CHANGING ATTRIBUTIONS ABOUT FATNESS

Attributions toward particular individuals can be changed; it is harder to change the attributions for a group as a whole. Several researchers have tried to change attributions toward fat people as a group, with some success.

Wiese, Wilson, Jones, and Neises (1992) created an educational intervention on the causes of obesity for first-year medical students. Compared to a control group, students who had received the intervention were more likely to attribute the cause of obesity to genetic (i.e., uncontrollable) causes. Although the stigmatization of obesity was not reduced by their intervention, endorsement of negative stereotypical beliefs about obese people was reduced.

Robinson, Bacon, and O'Reilly (1993) examined women with negative body image who participated in a program designed to enhance self-esteem and body image. Therapeutic sessions included changing attributions about controllability of weight, along with discussion about beauty standards, experiential exercises, minimizing the disability of fatness, and encouraging political activism and consumer pressure techniques. They found that negative evaluation of fat people reduced over the course of therapy, including both attributions (e.g., blameworthy, willpower) and evaluation (e.g., irritable, cold).

Crandall (1994) directly addressed the issue of changing attributions. Under the guise of a study of reading and oral comprehension, participants read either a brief article about the important role of genetics and physiology in weight, or an article about the physiology of stress. They received a summary of this information orally, and then filled out a "memory test" that included the AFA. Participants in the Weight condition scored lower in both *Willpower* and *Dislike* than the Stress condition. Although not in the original report, Crandall's (1994) participants came back 1 week later and filled out the same questionnaire again; the reduction in attribution and prejudice both persisted over the week. (These significance of these effects slipped from $p < .05$ down to $p < .09$ due to participant attrition from Time 1 to Time 2; the effect size was the same for both weeks.)

Teachman, Gapinski, Brownell, Rawlins, and Jeyaram (2003) manipulated attributions about obesity's cause by having participants read a newspaper article about research describing the cause of obesity. In one version, obesity was ascribed to genetics, while another version attributed obesity to overeating/lack of exercise; in a control condition no article was read. Participants in the "overeating" condition reported more implicit bias in a computer task than in the "genetic" condition; they equated "good" with "thin" and "bad" with "fat" more readily than in the control or genetic conditions. The genetic condition did not, however, reduce bias when compared to the control conditions, suggesting that it may be easier to increase the expression of anti-fat prejudice than reduce it.

WHERE EXPLANATIONS COME FROM: ATTRIBUTION AND IDEOLOGY

If prejudice toward fat people comes from attributions, where do the attributions come from? Attitudes toward fat people are not particularly special, unusual, or idiosyncratically different from all other social attitudes, with a unique structure and completely independent source. Crandall and colleagues (Crandall, 1994; Crandall & Martinez, 1996; Crandall & Schiffhauer, 1998) have argued that attributions for fatness come from a connected set of convictions, attitudes, and values that form a reasonably coherent belief system—attributions come from ideology. An ideology is set of doctrines or beliefs that form the psychological basis of a political, economic, or social system; this ideology supplies the background beliefs that inform attributions about weight.

Many different values and beliefs are correlated with anti-fat prejudice, including belief in a just world, right-wing authoritarianism, the Modern Racism Scale, support for capital punishment, the Protestant work ethic, the belief that poverty is under people's control, support for traditional sex roles in marriage, and conservative political ideology (e.g., Crandall, 1994; Crandall & Biernat, 1990; Crandall & Martinez, 1996). These beliefs and values are consistent with the notion that people are responsible for what happens to them, that they deserve what they get, and that they are in control of what happens to them in life. People have characteristic ways of viewing the world, and this viewpoint includes characteristic ways of making attributions, which can lead to prejudices (Duckitt, Wagner, du-Plessis, & Birum, 2002). The more one's worldview promotes beliefs in individual responsibility, the more one reports anti-fat attitudes.

Conservative political ideology is perhaps the most interesting component of the ideological network, which reliably correlates with anti-fat attitudes (e.g., Biernat, Vescio, & Theno, 1996; Crandall & Biernat, 1990). Members of Republican college groups report more attributions of responsibility and more anti-fat attitudes than members of Democratic student groups (Crandall, 1994). One of the most important components of conservative political ideology is the notion of individual responsibility and freedom. Individuals are thought to be free to make their own choices in virtually any arena of life, but they also must bear responsibility for those choices. Conservatives are more likely to believe that most outcomes in life reflect the kinds of choices people have made, to endorse a belief in the just world, and to hold people responsible for their less-than-ideal fates (Lane, 2001). Political conservatism is associated with high levels of attribution of responsibility not only for poverty but also for being on welfare, levels of income, business success, and physical sickness, leading to more negative evaluations of the less fortunate (Skitka, Mullen, Griffin, Hutchinson, & Chamberlin, 2002; Williams, 1984; Zucker & Weiner, 1993). To the extent that political beliefs contain a strong component of attributions, then political ideology will play a strong role in determining attributions of causality for a wide variety of phenomena, which will in turn influence levels of prejudice and tolerance. Anti-fat attitudes are merely one manifestation of these relations.

CULTURE, ATTRIBUTIONS, AND ANTI-FAT ATTITUDES

Attributions of responsibility are clearly important to anti-fat attitudes, but individual responsibility is a meme, a culturally embedded way of seeing things. The emphasis on personal responsibility is key to Western individualism, but it is not a necessary component of all cultures. The more collectivist the country, the less that individualism matters (Triandis, 1993) and the less that attributions of responsibility for weight should matter in evaluations of people's weight.

To test this idea, Crandall & Martinez (1996) compared anti-fat attitudes in the United States (Florida and Kansas) to attitudes in Mexico City. Mexicans were less likely than Americans to report that overweight people were at fault for their weight, and that fatness was a failure of willpower. They also reported more positive views about fat people, and were less concerned about their own weight.

Crandall et al. (2001) looked at an expanded model of attributions and prejudice across cultures. They hypothesized that any given prejudice might result from two factors: (1) a judgment that the group or characteristic has a negative cultural value (e.g., fat is "a bad thing"), and (2) attributions of responsibility that are made. This attribution–value model suggests that being personally responsible for a negative characteristic leads to prejudice. The authors compared attributions for fatness and cultural values of fatness in six countries, three from individualistic cultures (United States, Australia, Poland) and three from collectivist cultures (Venezuela, India, Turkey). Findings supported the attribution–value model: Attributions and values predicted prejudice, but attributions were clearly more important in the individualistic countries.

Culture matters to anti-fat attitudes, but not all cultural differences are about attributions. Hebl and Heatherton (1998) found that black women and white women both reported that thin women depicted in photographs were more attractive than fat women. However, black women did not downgrade fat women's intelligence, job success, or happiness. Cultural/ethnic differences within local subcultures affect stereotyping and prejudice processes, with little implication of attributional processes.

ATTRIBUTIONS ABOUT WEIGHT AND THE SELF

Attribution theory is remarkable for its ability to cross the self/other perception line; the rules that govern perception of other people apply to perception of the self. There is research on attributions about weight, and its consequence for well-being and self-esteem, which supports this contention.

Crandall and Biernat (1990) found that politically conservative fat women, who were more likely to make attributions of responsibility, endorsed more negative attitudes toward fat people. They also reported lower self-esteem than politically conservative women who were not fat, and lower self-esteem than politically liberal women of all weight categories.

Pierce and Wardle (1997) found that overweight children who attributed their weight to controllable causes (eat too much, do not exercise enough) had lower self-esteem than children who attributed their weight to external causes (genetics, medical status).

Crocker, Cornwell, and Major (1993) found that when overweight and normal-weight women were given negative feedback from a "dating partner," overweight women attributed the feedback to their weight, but did not blame the dating partner evaluator for his reaction. This attribution was associated with more negative mood for overweight women than those in the other conditions.

Ideological variables associated with attributions of responsibility also play a role in determining self-esteem. Crocker and Major (1989) have argued that when one attributes negative feedback from the world to one's stigma (e.g., being fat), then the self can be protected from incorporating negative appraisals. But such attributions can be a double-edged sword—to the extent that mistreatment is justified, attributions of bad treatment to the stigma of weight may decrease self-esteem (Crocker & Major, 1994).

Quinn and Crocker (1999) found that Protestant Ethic (PE), an ideological variable closely related to belief in individual responsibility for life's outcomes (such as fatness), was associated with lower levels of well-being among women, but this relationship existed only among fat women. High levels of PE were associated with *increased* well-being among thinner women participants. They argued that belief in a "personal responsibility ideology" like PE leads to self-blame for weight among fat women, which reduces self-esteem. In a follow-up experiment, Quinn and Crocker primed fat and average-weight women with either PE ideology (having participants read excerpts from a political speech advocating the importance of personal responsibility for both positive and negative outcomes), or a more accepting, inclusive ideology (reading excerpts from a political speech advocating that "Americans need to combine our differences into unity"). When overweight women were primed with the harsh standards of a PE ideology, their self-esteem decreased and anxiety increased compared to women who read about the tolerant ideology (who slightly improved in well-being). The primes had little effect on normal-weight women.

In general, attributions about controllability and responsibility for the self mimic these attributions for others. When concluding that another individual is personally responsible for being fat, negative affect toward the target results, in the form of negative evaluations and prejudice. When concluding that oneself is personally responsible for being fat, negative affect toward the self results, in the form of anxiety, depression, and low self-esteem.

ATTRIBUTIONS AS CAUSES OR CONSEQUENCES OF EMOTION

Attributions lead to affective consequences.The dominant model in attribution theory comes from Weiner's (1993, 1995) work and is well supported by research showing that information leads to a particular attribution, which leads reliably to a specific emotional state, which in turn determines what kinds of action (e.g., helping, aggression, attraction) will follow.

Although many experiments have established that attributions *can* lead to emotions, they do not establish that this is the only causal pathway. Indeed, the father of attribution theory, Fritz Heider (1958) argued that there is a pressure to bring perceptual elements into harmony, to have a consistency between a person and his or her behaviors. When a person for whom we feel affection acts rudely, we are likely to infer that the slight was unintentional (avoiding a person attribution) and thus we do not form a unit relation between the negative behavior and our friend (see also Malle & Knobe, 1997). When making moral judgments, good behaviors lead to perceptions of targets as good people, but we also believe that good people's behavior is driven by good intentions. If we like and trust a friend, we will explain ambiguous behavior in a way that preserves our positive evaluation of him or her; not only does perception lead to evaluation, but evaluation can lead to perception (Heider, 1954/1958, p. 31).The judgment of people as good or bad will affect how we make attributions for their behavior, and will affect our feelings about anything that we perceive to be in relationship to them. Attribution and affect are bidirectional and motivated by a desire for consistency.

Whenever causes are ambiguous, the attributions we choose will be partly determined by our preexisting feelings toward people or groups. To the extent that we are biased against a group, our attributions for their behavior and outcomes will be unfavorable. Among those who do not like fat people, attributions of controllability will be adopted.

ATTRIBUTIONS AS JUSTIFICATION OF PREJUDICE

The presence of a correlation between attributions and attitudes in anti-fat prejudice research should not be assumed as evidence that attributions lead to prejudice. To the contrary, there is much research and theory on how attributions, stereotypes, and ideological beliefs serve as justifications for prejudice—the beliefs legitimize the prejudice (see Jost & Major, 2001, for many relevant reviews).

Crandall and Eshleman (2003) have developed a justification-suppression model (JSM) of the expression of prejudice, which focuses on the relative processes of causing, suppressing, and releasing suppressed prejudice. The JSM suggests that many social, cultural, and cognitive factors create a variety of prejudices—racial, ethnic, religious, sexual, or anti-fat—which the JSM calls "genuine" prejudice. This is genuine prejudice in the sense that is an authentically negative reaction that is not managed, suppressed, or manipulated, but is primary and powerful. Genuine prejudice is usually suppressed, due to social norms, personal standards, or inconsistent beliefs and values. Suppression processes reduce the appearance of prejudice, but prejudice that is suppressed can be still expressed, if it is *justified.* Justification processes release the expression of prejudice. Beliefs, ideologies, and attributions can liberate prejudice, leading to public expression of prejudice. Justification makes prejudices legitimate, and allows the expression of prejudice without guilt or shame.

In this context, one may consider the attribution–attitude link as evidence of both cause and justification of prejudice. Attributions of controllability lead to prejudice against fat people—several experiments have shown that the relationship can work in this way (e.g., Crandall, 1994; DeJong, 1980; Weiner et al., 1988). However, these experiments do not rule out the role of attributions as justifications, and to the extent that prejudices toward fat people can be derived in other ways (e.g., social consensus, peer influence, normative factors, cultural socialization, evaluative conditioning, rejection of deviance, and narrow aesthetic training), attributions are likely to serve as justifications for prejudice.

Even though attribution theory promotes attribution as causes, or independent variables, we should caution that theorists tend to promote their favorite variables as privileged and powerful. It is something of a demotion for attributions to be treated merely as a symptom of other psychological processes. Attributions are both causes and consequences of prejudice, and much work still remains to distinguish these patterns.

There is more to learn about the role of attributions as justifications, and how to compare the public face of expression with the private representation of affect. In Western societies, attributions of responsibility have a powerful legitimization function. But we do not know whether people are aware of this process, or can distinguish between attributions that *legitimize* and attributions that *cause* prejudice.

CONCLUSIONS

Attributions of controllability lead to prejudice, and attributions of controllability about weight lead to prejudice toward fat people. If attributions are an important cause of prejudice, what causes attributions? The background and context of attributions are an individual's entire network of beliefs and values. Attributions do not spring up separately and disconnected from each other, but they have an internal consistency, relate to each other in predictable ways, and make coherent sense. Attributions are ideological.

As discussed in this chapter, attributions also come from prejudice. People will make attributions for the controllability of poverty or unemployment of fat people, or their negative health outcomes, to the extent that they dislike them. Alternatively, a sympathetic observer will emphasize genetics and physiology as causes of fatness and correlated health variables.

Attributions clearly matter, but they are certainly not the only factor in anti-fat prejudice. Prejudices increase and decrease over time, based on a wide variety of historical, economic, cultural, and social issues; fat prejudice is no exception to this. In some cases, the mere proximity, unrelated to choice or control, of a fat person to another person is enough to create discrimination (Hebl & Mannix, 2003). Deviation of the physical body from "normal" may be enough to generate a "disease avoidance" mechanism that affects anxiety, attitudes, and prejudice (Kurzban & Leary, 2001; Park, Faulkner, & Schaller, 2003).

Nevertheless, attributional approaches give an excellent proximal account of anti-fat attitudes and are an essential part of understanding this prejudice. In some cases, attributions are likely to serve as justifications for more ultimate causes, such as culture or evolutionary processes. In other cases, the attributions themselves are likely to form the foundation of prejudice. Attributional approaches integrate well theoretically with other approaches, and are certain to play a key role in any comprehensive account of prejudice against fat people.

REFERENCES

Batson, C. D., Polycarpou, M. P., Harmon-Jones, E., Imhoff, H. J, Michener, E. C., Bednar, L. L., et al. (1997). Empathy and attitudes: Can feeling for a member of a stigmatized group improve feelings toward the group? *Journal of Personality and Social Psychology, 72,* 105–118.

Biernat, M., Vescio, T. K., & Theno, S. A. (1996). Violating American values: A "value congruence" approach to understanding outgroup attitudes. *Journal of Experimental Social Psychology, 32*, 387–410.

Cahnman, W. J. (1968). The stigma of obesity. *The Sociological Quarterly, 9*, 283–299.

Canning, H., & Mayer, J. (1966). Obesity: Its possible effect on college acceptance. *New England Journal of Medicine, 275,* 1172–1174.

Crandall, C. S. (1991). Do heavyweight students have more difficulty paying for college? *Personality and Social Psychology Bulletin, 17,* 606–611.

Crandall, C. S. (1994). Prejudice against fat people: Ideology and self-interest. *Journal of Personality and Social Psychology, 66,* 882–894.

Crandall, C. S. (1995). Do parents discriminate against their own heavyweight daughters? *Personality and Social Psychology Bulletin, 21,* 724–735.

Crandall, C. S., & Biernat, M. R. (1990). The ideology of anti-fat attitudes. *Journal of Applied Social Psychology, 20*, 227–243.

Crandall, C. S., D'Anello, S., Sakalli, N., Lazarus, E., Nejtardt, G. W., & Feather, N. T. (2001). An attribution-value model of prejudice: Anti-fat attitudes in six nations. *Personality and Social Psychology Bulletin, 27,* 30–37.

Crandall, C. S., & Eshleman, A. (2003). A justification-suppression model of the expression and experience of prejudice. *Psychological Bulletin, 129,* 414–446.

Crandall, C. S., & Martinez, R. (1996). Culture, ideology, and anti-fat attitudes. *Personality and Social Psychology Bulletin, 22*, 1165–1176.

Crandall, C. S., & Moriarty, D. (1995). Physical illness stigma and social rejection. *British Journal of Social Psychology, 34,* 67–83.

Crandall, C. S., & Schiffhauer, K. L. (1998). Anti-fat prejudice: Beliefs, values and American culture. *Obesity Research, 6,* 458–461.

Crocker, J., Cornwell, B., & Major, B. (1993). The stigma of overweight: Affective consequences of attributional ambiguity. *Journal of Personality and Social Psychology, 64*, 60–70.

Crocker, J., & Major, B. (1989). Social stigma and self-esteem: The self-protective properties of stigma. *Psychological Review, 96*, 608–630.

Crocker, J., & Major, B. (1994). Reactions to stigma: The moderating role of justifications. In M. P. Zanna & J. M. Olson (Eds.), *The psychology of prejudice: The Ontario symposium* (Vol. 7, pp. 289–314). Hillsdale, NJ: Erlbaum.

DeJong, W. (1980). The stigma of obesity: The consequences of naive assumptions concerning the causes of physical deviance. *Journal of Health and Social Behavior, 21*, 75–87.

Duckitt, J., Wagner, C., du-Plessis, I., & Birum, I. (2002). The psychological bases of ideology and prejudice: Testing a dual process model. *Journal of Personality and Social Psychology, 83,* 75–93.

Frieze, I. H., Olson, J. E., & Good, D. C. (1990). Perceived and actual discrimination in the salaries of male and female managers. *Journal of Applied Social Psychology, 20*, 46–67.

Goodman, N., Richardson, S. A., Dornbusch, S. M., & Hastorf, A. H. (1963). Variant reactions to physical disabilities. *American Sociological Review, 28*, 429–435.

Halpern, C. T., Udry, J. R., Campbell, B., & Suchindran, C. (1999). Effects of body fat on weight concerns, dating, and sexual activity: A longitudinal analysis of black and white adolescent girls. *Developmental Psychology, 35*, 721–736.

Hebl, M. R., & Heatherton, T. F. (1998). The stigma of obesity in women: The difference is black and white. *Personality and Social Psychology Bulletin, 24*, 417–426.

Hebl, M. R., & Mannix, L. M. (2003). The weight of obesity in evaluating others: A mere proximity effect. *Personality and Social Psychology Bulletin, 29*, 28–38.

Heider, F. (1958). Consciousness, the perceptual world and communication with others. In R. Tagiuri & L. Petrullo (Eds.), *Person perception and interpersonal behavior* (pp. 27–32). Stanford, CA: Stanford University Press. (Original work published 1954)

Heider, F. (1958). *The psychology of interpersonal relations*. New York: Wiley.

Jagstaidt, V., Golay, A., & Pasini, W. (1997). Relationships between sexuality and obesity in male patients. *New Trends in Experimental and Clinical Psychiatry, 13*, 105–110.

Jost, J., & Major, B. (Eds.). (2001). *The psychology of legitimacy: Emerging perspectives on ideology, justice, and intergroup relations*. New York: Cambridge University Press.

Kurzban, R., & Leary, M. R. (2001). Evolutionary origins of stigmatization: The functions of social exclusion. *Psychological Bulletin, 127*, 187–208.

Lane, R. E. (2001). Self-reliance and empathy: The enemies of poverty—and of the poor. *Political Psychology, 22*, 473–492.

Malle, B. F., & Knobe, J. (1997). The folk concept of intentionality. *Journal of Experimental Social Psychology, 33*, 101–121.

Park, J. H., Faulkner, J., & Schaller, M. (2003). Evolved disease-avoidance processes and contemporary anti-social behavior: Prejudicial attitudes and avoidance of people with physical disabilities. *Journal of Nonverbal Behavior, 27*, 65–87.

Pierce, J. W., & Wardle, J. (1997). Cause and effect beliefs and self-esteem of overweight children. *Journal of Child Psychology and Psychiatry and Allied Disciplines, 38*, 645–650.

Puhl, R., & Brownell, K. D. (2001). Bias, discrimination, and obesity. *Obesity Research, 9*, 788–805.

Quinn, D. M., & Crocker, J. (1999). When ideology hurts: Effects of belief in the Protestant ethic and feeling overweight on the psychological well-being of women. *Journal of Personality and Social Psychology, 77*, 402–414.

Regan, D. T., & Totten, J. (1975). Empathy and attribution: Turning observers into actors. *Journal of Personality and Social Psychology, 32*, 850–856.

Regan, P. C. (1996). Sexual outcasts: The perceived impact of body weight and gender on sexuality. *Journal of Applied Social Psychology, 26*, 1803–1815.

Robinson, B. E., Bacon, J. G., & O'Reilly, J. (1993). Fat phobia: Measuring, understanding, and changing anti-fat attitudes. *International Journal of Eating Disorders, 14*, 467–480.

Rothblum, E. D., Brand, P. A., Miller, C. T., & Oetjen, H. A. (1990). The relationship between obesity, employment discrimination, and employment-related victimization. *Journal of Vocational Behavior, 37*, 251–266.

Ryan, W. J. (1976). *Blaming the victim.* New York: Vintage.

Skitka, L. J., Mullen, E., Griffin, T., Hutchinson, S., & Chamberlin, B. (2002). Dispositions, scripts, or motivated correction?: Understanding ideological differences in explanations for social problems. *Journal of Personality and Social Psychology, 83*, 470–487.

Teachman, B. A., Gapinski, K. D., Brownell, K. D., Rawlins, M., & Jeyaram, S. (2003). Demonstrations of implicit anti-fat bias: The impact of providing causal information and evoking empathy. *Health Psychology, 22*, 68–78.

Triandis, H. C. (1993). *Culture and social behavior.* New York: McGraw-Hill.

Vescio, T. K., Sechrist, G. B., & Paolucci, M. P. (2003). Perspective taking and prejudice reduction: The mediational role of empathy arousal and situational attributions. *European Journal of Social Psychology, 33*, 455–472.

Weiner, B. (1993). On sin versus sickness: A theory of perceived responsibility and social motivation. *American Psychologist, 48*, 957–965.

Weiner, B. (1995). *Judgments of responsibility: A foundation for a theory of social conduct.* New York: Guilford Press.

Weiner, B., Perry, R. P., & Magnusson, J. (1988). An attributional analysis of reactions to stigmas. *Journal of Personality and Social Psychology, 55*, 738–748.

Wiese, H. J. C., Wilson, J. S., Jones, R. A., & Neises, M. (1992). Obesity stigma reduction in medical students. *International Journal of Obesity, 16*, 859–868.

Williams, S. (1984). Left-right ideological differences in blaming victims. *Political Psychology, 5*, 573–581.

Zucker, G. S., & Weiner, B. (1993). Conservatism and perceptions of poverty: An attributional analysis. *Journal of Applied Social Psychology, 23*, 925–943.

CHAPTER 7

■ ■ ■

Social Consensus and the Origins of Stigma

GRETCHEN B. SECHRIST
CHARLES STANGOR

There is no more powerful social psychological principle than the fact that our attitudes, beliefs, and behaviors are profoundly influenced by our perceptions of the attitudes, beliefs, and behaviors of others we care about (Allport, 1935; Asch, 1952; Festinger, 1957; Hardin & Higgins, 1996; Sherif, 1936; Turner, 1991). Other people influence our attitudes toward trivial matters such as the perceived physical attractiveness of someone in a photo (Baron et al., 1996), judgments about the length of a line (Asch, 1956), and how much a pinpoint of light moves in a dark room (Sherif, 1936), as well as more important attitudes and behaviors, including one's political orientation (Newcomb, 1943; 1963), drug use (Chassin, Presson, Montello, Sherman, & McGrew, 1986), sexual behavior (Berndt & Savin-Williams, 1993), school achievement and college aspirations (Epstein, 1983), tendency to engage in binge eating (Crandall, 1988), and willingness to give another person severe electrical shocks (Milgram, 1974). The goal of this chapter is to review relevant research and theories demonstrating how perceptions of other people's beliefs—*social consensus information*—influence one aspect of social life: the development, maintenance, and change of stereotypes and prejudice.

The idea that consensus is an important component of stereotyping is not unique—many definitions of stereotypes include social agreement on the content of the belief as a defining feature (e.g., Devine, 1989; Gardner, 1994; Katz & Braly, 1933; Stangor & Lange, 1994; Stangor & Schaller, 1996). Because social stereotypes have important implications for social interaction, and because they tend to be socially shared by members of the same social groups, it seems reasonable to expect that stereotypes, like other attitudes, will develop and change in part through perceptions of the beliefs of other relevant individuals. Hence, examining perceptions of other people's beliefs seems essential to fully understanding the origins of as well as to developing ways to change stereotypes and prejudice.

SHERIF AND SHERIF'S GROUP-NORM THEORY

The notion that prejudice and stereotypes are developed and maintained as a result of social consensus information is the basis of Sherif and Sherif's (1953) group-norm theory. According to this theory, prejudice develops as a result of the group socialization process, which involves group formation, identification, and continuous interaction. During and after group formation, group members learn appropriate group attitudes and behaviors from each other. Group members pressure each other to conform to group norms and standards and ignore, punish, or reject those individuals who deviate from group values (Schachter, 1951). This theory predicts that changing group attitudes is more effective than changing individual attitudes because individual beliefs are based on group norms (see also Allport, 1954). In support of their theory, Sherif, Sherif, and colleagues (Sherif, Harvey, White, Hood, & Sherif, 1961; Sherif & Sherif, 1953) conducted a series of experiments with boys at summer camp to demonstrate how quickly group norms can develop and create prejudice. After the boys at the camp were divided into two groups, and as competition between the groups increased, prejudiced norms quickly followed. The boys increasingly favored their own group, as expressed in both attitude and behavior, even though the outgroup consisted of children who had been close friends of the boys prior to the start of the study. Thus, as a result of the norms created by the highly identified and cohesive groups, stereotypes and prejudice were developed.

Other classic experiments concur. Pettigrew (1958) found that participants who were especially responsive to the norms of the white society in South Africa were more likely to endorse anti-African attitudes, regardless of their individual personality characteristics. In addition, the expression of prejudice may differ depending on the salient norms present in the immediate environment. For instance, Watson (1950) found that individuals who had recently moved to New York City and had interacted with anti-Semitic people became more anti-Semitic in their attitudes. Pettigrew (1958) found that white Southern men became less prejudiced against blacks after entering the Army, where the social norms were less discriminatory than their home environments. Research with West Virginia coal miners showed that individuals' racial attitudes were more favorable at work, where white and black coal miners were integrated, than when they were home or in their communities, where whites and blacks were segregated (Minard, 1952).

Recent research is consistent with classic studies. Wittenbrink and Henly (1996, Experiment 3) demonstrated that high-prejudice participants expressed more favorable attitudes toward African Americans when provided with positive, as opposed to negative, feedback about the beliefs of others; low-prejudice individuals did not change as a result of the opinion feedback. In addition, Haslam, Oakes, McGarty, Turner, Reynolds, and Eggins (1996) found that people changed their stereotypes of national groups to be more similar to the beliefs allegedly held by members of a desirable ingroup (other nonprejudiced students at one's college), and they changed their stereotypes away from those allegedly held by an undesirable outgroup (prejudiced people). Crandall, Eshleman, and O'Brien (2002) demonstrated that participants followed social norms not only in their expression of prejudice, but in their evaluations of discrimination scenarios and reactions to hostile jokes. Prejudiced-based jokes were tolerated only when consistent with social norms (Study 3). If norms to suppress expression of prejudice were salient, such jokes were considered offensive.

RESEARCH FROM OUR LAB

We (Sechrist & Stangor, 2001; Stangor, Sechrist, & Jost, 2001a, 2001b) conducted a number of studies designed to test the influence of social consensus information on intergroup beliefs. In three experiments, Stangor, Sechrist, and Jost (2001a) examined how perceptions about the beliefs of relevant ingroup members influence racial stereotypes and attitudes. In one experiment, European American students first indicated their beliefs about positive and negative stereotypes of African Americans, and then estimated the beliefs of fellow students at their university. One week later, participants received (false) information indicating that, according to our prior research, other students were either more or less favorable in their evaluation of African Americans than the participants had originally estimated. Ostensibly as a result of a computer error, participants were then asked to estimate their racial beliefs again. We found that the participants expressed significantly more positive attitudes toward African Americans when they had learned that other people held more favorable stereotypes than they had originally estimated and more negative attitudes when told others held less favorable stereotypes. These changes were strong and remained persistent when assessed 2 weeks later (Stangor et al., 2001b). In a second experiment we found that consensus effects were stronger for people exposed to information about the opinions of ingroup rather than outgroup members, and that this change occurred even when assessed in private on a different measure, and at an unrelated experimental session.

In addition to creating new intergroup beliefs, we also assessed the hypothesis that perceived consensus information increases the extent to which intergroup beliefs are resistant to change (Stangor et al., 2001a, Experiment 3). One week after estimating their own attitudes toward African Americans, participants were provided with information that their beliefs were either shared or not shared by other students at their university. Then, in an attempt to change beliefs, they were given allegedly "objective" information about the actual traits possessed by African Americans, supposedly as determined by actual research. Perceptions of agreement with others strengthened racial stereotypes, such that participants given information that others shared their beliefs (high perceived consensus) showed less opinion change, on both positive and negative stereotypes, in comparison with participants given information that others did not agree with their beliefs (low perceived consensus).

Research from our lab also demonstrates that social consensus information influences implicit attitude and behavioral measures. In Experiment 1 (Sechrist & Stangor, 2001), we found that high-prejudice participants who were provided with information that other students at their university shared their (negative) beliefs subsequently sat farther away from an African American individual than participants who were informed that their beliefs were not shared. Low-prejudice participants provided with information that their (favorable) beliefs were shared by others sat closer than did participants who were informed that their beliefs were not shared. The correlation between expressed attitudes (on the Pro-black scale; Katz & Hass, 1988) and behavior (seating distance) was greater for participants in conditions where their beliefs were supported by their ingroup. Thus, perceived group beliefs appear to increase attitude–behavior consistency in the domain of racial relations, and this occurred even on a nonreactive behavior (the participants did not know that their seating distance was being observed).

In a second experiment (Sechrist & Stangor, 2001), we examined whether learning that one's racial attitudes are consistent with group beliefs would alter the mental representation of those beliefs (become more closely associated with the category label in memory), and thus be more quickly activated upon exposure to the relevant category label. This prediction was based on stereotype models which suggest that stereotypes are mentally associated with category labels in memory (Dovidio, Evans, & Tyler, 1986; Stangor & Lange, 1994; Wittenbrink, Judd, & Park, 1997), and thus come to mind when the category is activated. We found that participants who learned that their stereotypes of African Americans were shared with others (consistent with the ingroup norm) were faster at identifying those same stereotypes as words after being primed with a word associating them with African Americans (black) than after neutral primes, but this difference did not occur for participants who had just learned that their stereotypes were inconsistent with their ingroup's beliefs. As expected, stereotypes that are perceived as shared by the group are highly cognitively accessible, in the sense that they come to mind quickly on exposure to the category label, and thus facilitate their identification as words.

SUBTLE SOCIAL CONSENSUS

These studies support the norm theories by demonstrating that the beliefs of others, especially other ingroup members, influence intergroup attitudes and behaviors. Social consensus is typically provided about the beliefs of other groups of people (i.e., other students at one's university, other members of one's national group). Several studies suggest that merely overhearing information about the beliefs of one other ingroup member may substantially change racial beliefs. For example, Henderson-King and Nisbett (1996) found that simply overhearing that an African American had committed an assault (a stereotype-consistent act) increased the extent to which whites perceived blacks as antagonistic and hostile (see also Greenberg & Pyszczynski, 1985; Kirkland, Greenberg, & Pyszczynski, 1987).

Blanchard, Crandall, Brigham, and Vaughn (1994) had white participants hear another student from their college either condone or condemn racism before completing five questions regarding how their college should respond to acts of racism. Hearing another student condemn racism increased anti-racist opinions and hearing someone condone racism reduced anti-racist expressions, in comparison to a control condition in which no information about others' opinions was provided. This occurred whether responses were spoken publicly in the presence of the person making the comment and the experimenter, or were written privately on a questionnaire and sealed in an envelope, suggesting that social consensus information influences people's privately expressed or internal attitudes toward racism (see also Blanchard, Lilly, & Vaughn, 1991; Monteith, Deenan, & Tooman, 1996). Taken together, these studies suggest that simply overhearing a negative belief expressed by a single ingroup member is sufficient to create a social norm of racial antipathy.

COMMUNICATING SOCIAL NORMS

Recently researchers have focused on the importance of communication in stereotype change and development. Prejudice is communicated in everyday interaction, including interactions with parents, peers, ingroup members, and the mass media. Prejudice appears in both blatant and subtle forms, including direct expression of attitudes toward members of other groups, jokes, and facial expressions (Ruscher, 2001). For example, stereotypes and prejudices of parents and children are correlated (Epstein & Komorita, 1966; Fagot, Leinbach, & O' Boyle, 1992). Derogatory nicknames or labels used to refer to members of different social groups also provide social consensus information regarding prejudice (Palmore, 1962; Stangor & Schaller, 1996; Valentine, 2004). Mass media provides information about the stereotypes of different social groups in television shows (e.g., Hartmann & Husband, 1974; Wilson & Gutierrez, 1985), advertising (e.g., Bell, 1992; Pasadeos, 1987), and children's school texts (Stinton, 1980; Zimet, 1976). Such information may contribute to the development of stereotypes and prejudice by creating a misperception regarding societal norms or pluralistic ignorance (Prentice & Miller, 1993). Prejudiced communication, whether it be a derogatory nickname, a prejudice-based joke, or an explicit expression of attitudes, is important because it reflects categorization of ingroups and outgroups and is a method for ingroup members to indicate that they too hold such beliefs (Ruscher, 2001).

According to Schaller and Conway (1999), the content of interpersonal communications has an important influence on stereotypes. Ruscher and colleagues found that when given a consensus motivation or goal, such as being asked to achieve a consensus and to think as a team, dyads focused their conversation around stereotype-consistent information (Ruscher, 2001; Ruscher & Hammer, 1994; Ruscher, Hammer, & Hammer, 1996). When a negative stereotype is revealed about a target person, dyads talk about the stereotype and focus on information to support the stereotype in forming impressions of that person. The assumption is that members of the dyads wish to agree and be liked by each other, and use negative stereotypes as a means of achieving consensus. The consensus of the stereotype is validating, increasing favorable impressions made by the individual on other ingroup members and making stereotypes harder to change.

WHY CONFORM TO SOCIAL NORMS?

In fact, the validating nature of social consensus is just one of the many benefits of following group norms. According to Festinger's (1954) theory of social comparison, people have a need to evaluate and compare their opinions in order to establish a sense of validity or correctness. The knowledge that other people hold similar beliefs provides social validation (Hardin & Higgins, 1996); hence, social consensus information offers individuals the opportunity to evaluate and validate their beliefs.

There are additional benefits of social consensus that encourage individuals to internalize and conform to social norms. It gives individuals the possibility for social acceptance and approval, such that individuals like and are more attracted to people who hold similar attitudes (Asch, 1956; Byrne & Clore, 1970; Schachter, 1951). The sharing of beliefs is one means of perceiving oneself as similar to others and may strengthen one's perceptions of similarity, which in turn maintains effective group functioning (Bar-Tal, 2000; Cartwright & Zander, 1968). This helps to explain why individuals are especially influenced by ingroup members or individuals with whom they identify, value, or are similar to (Haslam et al., 1996; Martin, 1988; van Knippenberg & Wilke, 1988). Consistent with social identity and self-categorization theories, research has shown that individuals, in becoming prototypical ingroup members or in adopting their group membership as an integral part of their self-concepts, tend to become more extreme in their attitudes or change their attitudes to be consistent with a valued or salient ingroup (Haslam et al., 1996; Mackie, 1986; Newcomb, 1943; Turner, 1991).

CONCLUSION

Like most attitudes and beliefs, stereotypes and prejudice are based to large extent upon perceived social consensus. Prejudice is a social norm—we become prejudiced if we think other people are too. Theories and research provide strong evidence for the importance of social consensus in stereotype and prejudice development, maintenance, and change. Numerous studies suggest that social consensus, from the mass media to the beliefs of other people, and especially other ingroup members, to the beliefs of a single individual, may have an important influence on our attitudes toward others.

Considering the role of stereotyping in conformity also helps explain why what is acceptable in one time or place may be unacceptable elsewhere. When norms change, so does prejudice. Although social norms can create prejudice, they can also reduce it. Conformity does not always imply prejudice—many group norms, and indeed the American credo itself, are based on tolerance, egalitarianism, and the humanity of all people, regardless of race, religion, ethnicity, belief, social station, or class (and perhaps at some point, weight).

Most research on social consensus has focused on development and change of prejudice directed at African Americans (e.g., Sechrist & Stangor, 2001; Stangor, Sechrist, & Jost, 2001a; Wittenbrink & Henly, 1996). Some research has examined prejudice directed at different nationalities (Haslam et al., 1996) and gay men (Monteith et al., 1996). Recently, this perspective has been extended to account for stereotypes of and prejudice against obese individuals (Puhl, Schwartz, & Brownell, in press; see Puhl, Chapter 20, this volume). That the results of such studies will demonstrate the influence of social consensus is expected, as findings from this theoretical perspective should extend to other social groups as well, including religious groups, racial groups, and class.

The social consensus perspective is valuable because it helps explain the development and change of stereotypes and prejudice, but also because it addresses why and how individuals develop strong negative attitudes about groups with which they interact frequently or not at all (Katz & Braly, 1933; Maio, Esses, & Bell, 1994). Interventions designed to promote positive intergroup attitudes may be particularly effective by providing individuals with information about the favorable intergroup attitudes of other people, especially people with whom they identify. Focusing on social norms avoids the practical difficulties of approaches assuming that stereotypes are formed and changed primarily through intergroup contact. According to the intergroup contact literature, attitudes change through exposure to outgroup members only in limited conditions, and contact rarely leads to change in attitudes toward the whole group (Hewstone & Brown, 1986; Rothbart & John, 1985; Stephan, 1985). In focusing interventions on whole groups and the norms of these groups, perhaps new norms can be created that promote equality, benevolence, and acceptance.

REFERENCES

Allport, G. W. (1935). Attitudes. In C. Murchison (Ed.), *A handbook of social psychology* (pp. 798–844). Worcester, MA: Clark University Press.

Allport, G. W. (1954). *The nature of prejudice.* Cambridge, MA: Addison-Wesley.

Asch, S. E. (1952). *Social psychology.* New York: Prentice-Hall.

Asch, S. E. (1956). Studies of independence and conformity: A minority of one against a unanimous majority. *Psychological Monographs, 70*(9, Whole No. 416).

Baron, R. S., Hoppe, S. I., Kao, C. F., Brunsman, B., Linneweh, B., & Rogers, D. (1996). Social corroboration and opinion extremity. *Journal of Experimental Social Psychology, 32*, 537–560.

Bar-Tal, D. (2000). *Shared beliefs in a society.* Thousand Oaks, CA: Sage.

Bell, J. (1992). In search of a discourse on aging: The elderly on television. *Gerontologist, 32*, 305–311.

Berndt, T. J., & Savin-Williams, R. C. (1993). Peer relations and friendships. In P. H. Tolan & B. J. Cohler (Eds.), *Handbook of clinical research and practice with adolescents* (pp. 203–219). New York: Wiley.

Blanchard, F. A., Crandall, C. S., Brigham, J. C., & Vaughn, L. A. (1994). Condemning and condoning racism: A social context approach to interracial settings. *Journal of Applied Psychology, 79*, 993–997.

Blanchard, F. A., Lilly, T., & Vaughn, L. A. (1991). Reducing the expression of racial prejudice. *Psychological Science, 2*, 101–105.

Byrne, D., & Clore, G. L. (1970). A reinforcement model of evaluative processes. *Personality: An International Journal, 1*, 103–128.

Cartwright, D., & Zander, A. (1968). *Group dynamics: Research and theory.* New York: Harper & Row.

Chassin, L., Presson, C. C., Montello, D., Sherman, S. J., & McGrew, J. (1986). Changes in peer and parent influence during adolescence: Longitudinal versus cross-sectional perspectives on smoking initiation. *Developmental Psychology, 22*, 327–334.

Crandall, C. S. (1988). Social contagion of binge eating. *Journal of Personality and Social Psychology, 550*, 588–598.

Crandall, C. S., Eshleman, A., & O'Brien, L. (2002). Social norms and the expression and suppression of prejudice: The struggle for internalization. *Journal of Personality and Social Psychology, 82*, 359–378.

Devine, P. G. (1989). Stereotypes and prejudice: Their automatic and controlled components. *Journal of Personality and Social Psychology, 56*, 5–18.

Dovidio, J., Evans, N., & Tyler, R. (1986). Racial stereotypes: The contents of their cognitive representations. *Journal of Experimental Social Psychology, 22*, 22–37.

Epstein, J. L. (1983). The influence of friends on achievement and affective outcomes. In J. L. Epstein & N. Karweit (Eds.), *Friends in school: Patterns of selection and influence in secondary schools* (pp. 177–200). New York: Academic Press.

Epstein, R., & Komorita, S. S. (1966). Prejudice among Negro children as related to parental ethnocentrism. *Journal of Personality and Social Psychology, 4,* 643–647.

Fagot, B. I., Leinbach, M. D., & O'Boyle, C. (1992). Gender labeling, gender, stereotyping, and parenting behaviors. *Developmental Psychology, 28*, 225–230.

Festinger, L. (1954). A theory of social comparison processes. *Human Relations, 7,* 117–140.

Festinger, L. (1957). *A theory of cognitive dissonance.* Evanston, IL: Row-Peterson.

Gardner, R. C. (1994). Stereotypes as consensual beliefs. In M. P. Zanna & J. M. Olson (Ed.), *The psychology of prejudice: The Ontario symposium* (Vol. 7, pp. 1–31). Hillsdale, NJ: Erlbaum.

Greenberg, J., & Pyszczynski, T. (1985). The effects of an overheard ethnic slur on evaluations of the target: How to spread a social disease. *Journal of Experimental Social Psychology, 21*, 61–72.

Hardin, C., & Higgins, T. (1996). Shared reality: How social verification makes the subjective objective. In R. M. Sorrentino & E. T. Higgins (Eds.), *Handbook of motivation and cognition: Foundations of social behavior* (pp. 28–84). New York: Guilford Press.

Hartmann, P., & Husband, C. (1974). *Racism and the mass media.* London: Davis-Poynter.

Haslam, S. A., Oakes, P. J., McGarty, C., Turner, J. C., Reynolds, K. J., & Eggins, R. A. (1996). Stereotyping and social influence: The mediation of stereotype applicability and sharedness by the views of in-group and out-group members. *British Journal of Social Psychology, 35*, 369–397.

Henderson-King, E. I., & Nisbett, R. E. (1996). Anti-black prejudice as a function of exposure to the negative behavior of a single black person. *Journal of Personality and Social Psychology, 71*, 654–664.

Hewstone, M., & Brown, R. J. (1986). Contact is not enough: An intergroup perspective on the "contact hypothesis." In M. Hewstone & R. J. Brown (Eds.), *Contact and conflict in intergroup encounters* (pp. 1–44). Oxford, UK: Blackwell.

Katz, D., & Braly, K. W. (1933). Racial stereotypes of one hundred college students. *Journal of Abnormal and Social Psychology, 28*, 280–290.

Katz, I., & Hass, R. G. (1988). Racial ambivalence and American value conflict: Correlational and priming studies of dual cognitive structures. *Journal of Personality and Social Psychology, 55*, 893–905.

Kirkland, S. L., Greenberg, J., & Pyszczynski, T. (1987). Further evidence of the deleterious effects of overheard ethnic slurs: Derogating beyond the target. *Personality and Social Psychology Bulletin, 13*, 216–227.

Mackie, D. M. (1986). Social identification effects in group polarization. *Journal of Personality and Social Psychology, 50*, 720–728.

Maio, G. R., Esses, V. M., & Bell, D. W. (1994). The formation of attitudes toward new immigrant groups. *Journal of Applied Social Psychology, 24*, 1762–1776.

Martin, R. (1988). Ingroup and outgroup minorities: Differential impact upon public and private responses. *European Journal of Social Psychology, 18*, 39–52.

Milgram, S. (1974). *Obedience to authority: An experimental view.* New York: Harper & Row.
Minard, R. D. (1952). Race relationships in the Pocohontas coal field. *Journal of Social Issues, 8*, 29–44.
Monteith, M. J., Deneen, N. E., & Tooman, G. D. (1996). The effect of social norm activation of the expression of opinions concerning gay men and blacks. *Basic and Applied Social Psychology, 18*, 267–288.
Newcomb, T. M. (1943). *Personality and social change: Attitude formation in a student community.* Oxford, UK: Dryden.
Newcomb, T. M. (1963). Persistence and regression of changed attitudes: Long range studies. *Journal of Social Issues, 19*, 3–14.
Palmore, E. B. (1962). Ethnophaulisms and ethnocentrism. *American Journal of Sociology, 67*, 442–445.
Pasadeos, Y. (1987). Changes in television newscast advertising, 1974–1985. *Communication Research Reports, 4*, 43–46.
Pettigrew, T. F. (1958). Personality and sociocultural factors and intergroup attitudes: A cross-national comparison. *Journal of Conflict Resolution, 2*, 29–42.
Prentice, D. A., & Miller, D. T. (1993). Pluralistic ignorance and alcohol use on campus: Some consequences of misperceiving the social norm. *Journal of Personality and Social Psychology, 64*, 243–256.
Puhl, R. M., Schwartz, M. B., & Brownell, K. D. (in press). Impact of perceived consensus on stereotypes about obese people: A new approach for reducing bias. *Health Psychology.*
Rothbart, M., & John, O. P. (1985). Social categorization and behavioral episodes: A cognitive analysis of the effects of intergroup contact. *Journal of Social Issues, 41*, 81–104.
Ruscher, J. B. (2001). *Prejudiced communication: A social psychological perspective.* New York: Guilford Press.
Ruscher, J. B., & Hammer, E. D. (1994). Revising disrupted impressions through conversation. *Journal of Personality and Social Psychology, 66*, 530–541.
Ruscher, J. B., Hammer, E. Y., & Hammer, E. D. (1996). Forming shared impressions through conversation: An adaptation of the continuum model. *Personality and Social Psychology Bulletin, 7*, 705–720.
Schachter, S. (1951). Deviation, rejection, and communication. *Journal of Abnormal and Social Psychology, 46*, 190–207.
Schaller, M., & Conway, L. G. (1999). Influence of impression-management goals on the emerging contents of group stereotypes: Support for a social-evolutionary process. *Personality and Social Psychology Bulletin, 25*, 819–833.
Sechrist, G. B., & Stangor, C. (2001). Perceived consensus influences intergroup behavior and stereotype accessibility. *Journal of Personality and Social Psychology, 80*, 645–654.
Sherif, M. (1936). *The psychology of social norms.* New York: Harper.
Sherif, M., Harvey, O. J., White, J., Hood, W., & Sherif, C. (1961). *Intergroup conflict and cooperation: The robber's cave experiment.* Norman: University of Oklahoma Institute of Intergroup Relations.

Sherif, M., & Sherif, C. W. (1953). *Groups in harmony and tension: An integration of studies on intergroup relations*. New York: Octagon Books.

Stangor, C., & Lange, J. (1994). Mental representations of social groups: Advances in conceptualizing stereotypes and stereotyping. *Advances in Experimental Social Psychology, 26*, 367–416.

Stangor, C., & Schaller, M. (1996). Stereotypes as individual and collective representations. In C. N. Macrae, C. Stangor, & M. Hewstone (Eds.), *Stereotypes and stereotyping* (pp. 3–40). New York: Guilford Press.

Stangor, C., Sechrist, G. B., & Jost, J. T. (2001a). Changing racial beliefs by providing consensus information. *Personality and Social Psychological Bulletin, 27*, 484–494.

Stangor, C., Sechrist, G. B., & Jost, J. T. (2001b). Social influence and intergroup attitudes: The role of perceived social consensus. In J. Forgas & K. Williams (Eds.), *Social influence* (pp. 235–252). Philadelphia: Psychology Press.

Stephan, W. G. (1985). Intergroup relations. In G. Lindzey & E. Aronson (Eds.), *The handbook of social psychology* (3rd ed., Vol. 2, pp. 599–658). New York: Random House.

Stinton, J. (1980). *Racism and sexism in children's books*. London: Writers & Readers.

Turner, J. C. (1991). *Social influence*. Milton Keynes, UK: Open University Press.

Valentine, T. M. (2004). *Language and prejudice*. New York: Pearson Longman.

van Knippenberg, A., & Wilke, H. (1988). Social categorization and attitude change. *European Journal of Social Psychology, 18*, 395–406.

Watson, J. (1950). Some social and psychological situations related to change in attitude. *Human Relations, 3*, 15–56.

Wilson, C. C., & Gutierrez, F. (1985). *Minorities and the media*. Beverly Hills, CA: Sage.

Wittenbrink, B., & Henly, J. R. (1996). Creating social reality: Informational social influence and content of stereotypic beliefs. *Personality and Social Psychology Bulletin, 22*, 598–610.

Wittenbrink, B., Judd, C. M., & Park, B. (1997). Evidence for racial prejudice at the implicit level and its relationship with questionnaire measures. *Journal of Personality and Social Psychology, 72*, 262–274.

Zimet, S. (1976). *Print and prejudice*. London: Hodder & Stoughton.

CHAPTER 8

■ ■ ■

Theories of Stigma

Limitations and Needed Directions

EDEN B. KING
MICHELLE R. HEBL
TODD F. HEATHERTON

The meaning of the term "stigma" dates back to ancient Greece, where a mark was branded or cut into the body to depict one as a slave or criminal. Following these early influences, Goffman (1963) defined stigma as an attribute that is discrediting and prevents an individual from full social acceptance. In Goffman's typology, stigmas can be separated into "discredited" stigmas, or stigmas that are known to others (e.g., skin color), and "discreditable" stigmas, or stigmas that can be concealed (e.g., homosexuality). More recently, Crocker, Major, and Steele (1998) defined stigma as an attribute that conveys a devalued social identity across most social contexts. They identified the prototypical features of devaluation as being the target of negative stereotypes, being rejected socially, being discriminated against, and being economically disadvantaged.

In the 21st-century United States, obesity clearly fits both definitions of stigma. Using Goffman's terminology, obesity is a discredited stigma that is overtly visible to others and prevents obese individuals from social acceptance. Consonant with more recent definitions (e.g., Crocker et al., 1998), obese individuals are devalued across almost every social context, from the workplace (Roehling, 1999) to social settings (DeJong & Kleck, 1981). Despite its increasing prevalence (see Wadden,

Brownell, & Foster, 2002), obesity has been unaffected by changes toward "political correctness" and remains as one of the most negative stigmas in contemporary society (Crandall & Martinez, 1996). Particularly telling is the fact that, whereas members of many stigmatized groups reject the opinions of others and maintain their sense of self-worth, obese individuals hold negative attitudes toward themselves (Crandall & Biernat, 1990; Crocker, Cornwell, & Major, 1993).

While there is congruence in beliefs about the obesity stigma, there is a general lack of theories to organize our understanding of this stigma. General theories of stigmatization might enable researchers to more clearly understand why obesity stigma is particularly pernicious, to predict contexts in which individuals are especially vulnerable to the stigma, and ultimately to avoid or remediate its negative effects. In this chapter, we discuss modern theories of stigma and their potential applications to the stigma of obesity. We also consider the limitations of each theory in the context of obesity stigma. Finally, we offer directions in which researchers can begin to respond to unanswered questions regarding the stigma of obesity.

CURRENT THEORIES

A great deal of social psychological research has considered specific aspects of stigmatization. For example, researchers have identified individual differences associated with prejudice (e.g., Pratto, Sidanius, Stallworth, & Malle, 1994), a movement from overt to subtle forms of discrimination (e.g., Hebl, Foster, Mannix, & Dovidio, 2002), negative consequences of discrimination (e.g., King, Hebl, George, & Matusik, 2005) and the social costs of making claims of discrimination (Kaiser & Miller, 2001). These studies have built a body of knowledge about particular cognitive, affective, and behavioral components of prejudice (i.e., stereotypes, prejudice, discrimination). However, there have been relatively few attempts to develop overarching, comprehensive theories to understand, explain, and predict stigmatization (cf. Hebl, King, & Knight, 2005). In this chapter, we briefly discuss five contemporary theories of stigmatization that address elements of stigmatization: the stereotype content model, intergroup emotions theory, a sociofunctional approach, system justification explanation, and the justification-suppression model. We do not claim that this is an exhaustive list of such theories, but that each has made an important contribution to an understanding of stigma and represent perspectives that may be informative to the study of the obesity stigma.

Stereotype Content Model

The primary cognitive factor affecting the process of stigmatization is stereotyping. Recently, a group of researchers (Fiske, Cuddy, Glick, & Xu, 2002) began to investigate the content of stereotypes. They argued that the content of all stereotypes varies along two dimensions of more and less socially desirable traits: warmth and competence. For example, the stereotype of Asian American individuals is high on the competence dimension but low on the warmth dimension. The authors also proposed that the content of stereotypes is derived from social structures such that social status is correlated with the positivity of stereotypes. Fiske and her colleagues further suggested that the unique point at which a particular stereotype falls on the dimensions of warmth and competence is associated with specific affective reactions (i.e., prejudices). The associated emotional reaction to the Asian American stereotype would be expected to be envious prejudice. As proposed, a study of nine participant samples showed that the content of stereotypes for feminists, housecleaners, gay men and lesbians, and other stigmatized groups fell into four clusters along the dimensions of warmth and competence.

Although their investigation did not include stereotypes of obese individuals, the model proposed by Fiske and her colleagues can be applied to the stigma of obesity. Following this model, predictions can be made about the content of stereotypes about obese individuals as well as the reactions that are most likely to emerge as a function of obesity stigma. Discussions of the stigma of obesity typically rely on the dimensions of visibility and controllability (see Crocker et al., 1998). There is evidence that obesity may be a particularly negative stigma because it is both visible and perceived to be controllable (Weiner, Perry, & Magnusson, 1988). Previous research shows that being overweight is associated with perceptions of being lazy, undisciplined, and gluttonous (DeJong & Kleck, 1981; Harris, Harris, & Bochner, 1982; Hebl & Kleck, 2002), implying that stereotypes about obese individuals are likely to be low in both warmth and competence dimensions. Consistent with expectations about the negativity of the stigma of obesity, the stereotype content model suggests that stereotypes low on both warmth and competence may be associated with the most negative stigmas. Furthermore, if stereotypes of obese individuals conform to these expectations, the model suggests that affective reactions to obese individuals will consist of disgust and contempt. Although the theory's creators did not consider the stigma of obesity in their initial investigation, the stereotype content model can be utilized in expanding knowledge about the content of and emotional reactions to stereotypes of obese individuals.

Intergroup Emotions Theory

The intergroup emotions theory approach considers emotions as sources of behavior in the process of stigmatization by combining appraisal and self-categorization theories (see Mackie, Devos, & Smith, 2000; Smith & Henry, 1996). Appraisal theories of emotion suggest that emotions are triggered by an individual's interpretation of whether or not a particular event favors or harms the self (Frijda, 1986). The concept of the self, according to self-categorization theory (Turner, 1985), includes the group with which the individual identifies. In other words, individuals perceive that their group membership is part of their self. Smith and Henry (1996) suggested that emotions become tied to events that individuals perceive to favor or harm their group. From this perspective, prejudice is driven by specific emotional reactions to an outgroup that are generated by appraisals of the outgroup. Generally, when individuals or groups have power relative to others, anger emerges, as opposed to fear or contempt (Frijda, 1986). Anger, in turn, leads to offensive action tendencies such as attacking or confronting the outgroup member (Mackie et al., 2000). In other words, when individuals feel that their ingroup is more powerful than an outgroup, their emotional response (i.e., anger) may lead to action tendencies that are manifested in discrimination toward members of that outgroup.

This contemporary theoretical approach to intergroup relations may be useful in building a framework for understanding the stigma of obesity. Relative to obesity, thinness is valued as a societal ideal (Hebl & King, 2005). Identification with the high-status group (i.e., thin individuals) may trigger specific emotions (i.e., anger) toward the low-status group (i.e., obese individuals). According to the intergroup emotions approach, anger toward obese individuals may be manifested in negative, offensive action tendencies such as confrontation and overt degradation. The theory of intergroup emotions suggests that discrimination toward obese individuals may derive from unfavorable appraisals of interactions with obese individuals and resultant angry emotional responses.

It is critical to note that the predictions regarding the stigma of obesity that follow from an intergroup emotions approach are potentially contradictory to those made by the stereotype content model. Although both theories predict negative emotional reactions to obese individuals, the intergroup emotions theory suggests that anger emerges, whereas the stereotype content model suggests that disgust should surface. The qualitative difference between these emotions may be subtle, but the implications for remediation of the stigma of obesity could be great. Strategies targeted to diminish anger might differ significantly from strategies designed to lessen disgust. Mackie et al.'s (2000) research shows that particular types of intergroup emotions elicit particular kinds of behaviors (i.e., offensive or nonoffensive). It follows that behavioral manifestations of stigma may differ as a function of the emotion evoked. Given the importance of emotional responses, and the inconsistent predictions made by each of these theories, future research should consider which emotions are most salient in response to obese individuals.

Sociofunctional Approach

Whereas the stereotype content model specifies the components of stigma and the accompanying emotional responses, the intergroup emotions approach goes deeper in an attempt to understand why specific emotions emerge as a function of intergroup relations. The sociofunctional, or biocultural, approach focuses even more intensely on addressing the question of why stigmatization occurs. This approach is grounded in the assumption that stigmatizing others can serve meaningful purposes to the stigmatizer (Neuberg, Smith, & Asher, 2000). Following an evolutionary line of reasoning, Neuberg and his colleagues argue that stigmatization is rooted in an inherent biological need to live in effective groups in order to promote the survival of their genetic makeup. Individuals or groups who are perceived to threaten the survival of one's ingroup will be stigmatized. Neuberg further posits that individuals will attempt to minimize perceived threat from stigmatized outgroups with specific emotional (i.e., prejudice) and behavioral (i.e., discrimination) responses. Thus, the process of stigmatization may arise in order to ensure the "survival of the fittest."

Applying a biocultural approach to stigmatization is inherently controversial. Although Neuberg and his colleagues (2000) reject biological determinism and the implicit valuation of adaptive behaviors, the fact that in this framework those who stigmatize may be those most likely to survive can be seen as problematic. Application of this theory to the stigma of obesity may be even more troublesome, as it could be interpreted to support the avoidance (at best) or destruction (at worst) of obese individuals. However, the renewed interest in evolutionary explanations for psychological phenomena encourages exploration of the biological functionality of the stigmatization of obese individuals. On the one hand, proponents of this approach might argue that obesity is often genetically based and has been linked with severely negative health outcomes (see Wadden et al., 2002). It therefore may be functionally adaptive to avoid obese individuals in the process of mate selection. Consistent with this approach, obese individuals could arguably consume more resources than other individuals, making it more difficult to support the interests of the group as a whole. This might violate the norms of reciprocity and increase the likelihood of stigmatization (Neuberg et al., 2000). On the other hand, Kurzban and Leary (2001) admit that a biocultural approach cannot explain the stigma against obesity. Obesity is relatively new condition in evolutionary terms in that it is only within the last several hundred years that leisure has been coupled with excess food. Thus, evolutionary theories may have little value in understanding the stigma of obesity. Given these potentially popular and controversial evolutionary arguments, and the inherent challenge for prevention or remediation of stigma, future research should consider the stigma of obesity from a sociofunctional perspective.

System Justification Approach

A broad theoretical approach that has been applied to intergroup relations is predicated on the assumption that people justify and perpetuate the status quo (Jost & Banaji, 1994). According to the system justification approach, individuals of both high- and low-status groups reinforce existing social arrangements. Jost and his colleagues (Jost & Banaji, 1994; Jost, Pelham, & Carvallo, 2002) offered cognitive reasons (e.g., need for cognitive closure, uncertainty reduction) and motivational ones (e.g., belief in a just world, illusion of control) for participating in system justification. Extended to social stigma, this rationale suggests that both perpetrators and targets of stigmatization are likely to express preference for nonstigmatized (i.e., high-status) group members. This preference may, in turn, lead to the perpetuation of the existing status differences. Applied to the stigma of obesity, the system justification approach may explain why obese individuals perceive their stigma negatively. Whereas members of some stigmatized groups (e.g., African American individuals) maintain high self-esteem despite their stigma (Crocker & Major, 1989), obese individuals tend to view themselves negatively and have low self-esteem (Crandall & Biernat, 1990; Crocker et al., 1993). From a system justification perspective, obese individuals may share the thoughts and feelings of their stigmatizers and may engage in behaviors that reinforce the existing social structure and stigma of obesity. Following this approach, a first step toward remediation of the obesity stigma may be to change the reinforcing thoughts, feelings, and behaviors of obese individuals themselves. The perpetuation of the obesity stigma, and the potential for its prevention, explained by a system justification theory make this an important area for research.

Justification-Suppression Model

In a departure from theories that consider the "what" (i.e., content) and the "why" (e.g., threat, survival) of stigmatization, Crandall and Eshleman (2003) proposed a model that examines the "when" of prejudice. In their justification-suppression model (JSM) of prejudice, Crandall and Eshleman describe a psychological process in which three sources of variation (i.e., genuine prejudice, suppression, justification) account for conditions under which prejudice may or may not be expressed regardless of the content or reason for stigmatization. They begin with the assumption that individuals face the conflicting demands of wanting to express their true emotions and wanting to maintain egalitarian values. The core emotional component of prejudice, termed "genuine prejudice" in Crandall and Eshleman's model, consists of "pure, unadulterated, original, unmanaged, and unambivalently negative feelings toward members of a devalued group" (p. 422). The egalitarian component of prejudice consists of a "motivated attempt to reduce the expression or awareness of prejudice" (p. 423). This component of the JSM, termed "suppression," can lessen the likelihood that an individual will express his or her genuine prejudice. However, "justifications" for prejudice can increase the likelihood of prejudice expression by undoing suppression and releasing prejudice. According to the JSM, the expression of prejudice is a function of the variation in genuine prejudice, suppression of prejudice, and justification for prejudice.

This integrative model of the expression of prejudice points to specific methods for investigation and remediation of the stigma of obesity. In particular, the JSM specifies that the expression of prejudice is lessened to the extent that suppression is maximized and justification is minimized. Crandall and Eshleman outline specific methods by which to achieve these ideal states. They suggest that prejudice suppression can be enhanced by extensive practice, egalitarian goal commitment, and improved cognitive resources. Furthermore, the negative effects of justification may be eliminated by avoiding the cognitions and values that serve to justify prejudice. Following the JSM, researchers of the stigma of obesity might investigate methods by which to bolster suppression in critical contexts. In the case of workplace discrimination (e.g., Roehling, 1999) it may be important that employers get trained to minimize their reliance on stereotypes of obese individuals when making job decisions. Some targets of stigmatization may limit the effects of justification by acknowledging their stigma (Hebl & Kleck, 2002), but obese individuals may need to develop other strategies to reduce justification (see Miller &

Myers, 1998). The JSM provides an overarching framework through which to investigate the occurrence and prevention of the expression of prejudice toward obese individuals.

LIMITATIONS AND FUTURE DIRECTIONS

Taken together, the stereotype content model, intergroup emotions theory, sociofunctional theory, the system justification approach, and the justification-suppression model contribute to an understanding of obesity as a stigma. However, there are critical limitations to these theories and to the current state of research regarding the stigma obesity.

Theory Limitations

The theoretical frameworks presented in this chapter consist of contemporary explanations for components of the process of stigmatization. Each theory has strengths, but also is limited in its utility to the study of the obesity stigma by two important factors. First, across theories, there is not enough focused consideration of the remediation of stigma. For example, the stereotype-content model is a descriptive account of a wide range of stereotypes but does not specify intervening processes. Similarly, the intergroup emotions, system justification, and sociofunctional theories provide compelling rationales for the existence of stigmatization, but do not address remediation. The JSM does illustrate general methods by which to reduce the expression of prejudice, but may be too broad to offer specific solutions. Researchers are beginning to build an understanding of the stigma of obesity, but there is simply not enough known about the prevention and remediation of its negative consequences.

Second, there is no specific consideration of the stigma of obesity in any of these models. More generally, there is no specific theory of the stigma of obesity. In and of itself, this is both a positive and negative feature. On the one hand, knowledge can be drawn from overarching, parsimonious theories and applied to the stigma of obesity. On the other hand, findings that hold for most stigmatized groups may not translate for obese individuals. For example, the consequences of stigma acknowledgment are different for disabled individuals and obese individuals (Hebl & Kleck, 2002). This suggests that the generalizability of theories of stigma to obesity must be thoroughly tested, and that theories specific to the stigma of obesity must be developed.

Research Limitations

In addition to the theoretical limitations, current research on the stigma of obesity is restricted in several important ways. First, and perhaps most importantly, there is a general lack of research on obesity as a stigma. At this point, we know that obese individuals are stigmatized, that there are consequences of this stigmatization, and that there are processes by which obese individuals can cope with stigmatization. However, given the increasing prevalence and stigmatization of obesity, the specificities and intricacies of these conclusions and answers to other research questions must be investigated. Second, there is no clear definition of what constitutes obesity in the context of stigmatization. Research generally relies upon self-report weight-to-height ratios (i.e., body mass index, BMI) that can be considered a categorical index that distinguishes between underweight, average, overweight, and obese individuals, or it can be used as a continuous, linear variable. We are unaware of any research that investigates whether the stigma of obesity operates in a categorical or continuous fashion. It may be that as BMI increases, so does the negativity of the stigma. It may also be that there is a distinct threshold beyond which the obesity stigma becomes salient, or that overweight individuals are stigmatized to the same extent as are obese individuals. Overweight and obese individuals may also carry their weight in different areas (e.g., legs, bust) which may be differentially stigmatizing. Being overweight may also serve as a general attractiveness cue. Clear operationalization of obesity is necessary for building an understanding of its stigma.

Third, there has been a lack of attention paid to the potential effects of context or situation on the stigma of obesity. Preliminary research findings suggest that perceptions of the stigma of obesity may be worse in some situations (e.g., wearing a bathing suit) than others (e.g., wearing a sweater) (Hebl, King, & Lin, 2004). It is likely that the situation surrounding an obese individual will affect perceptions of that individual. For example, because obesity is perceived to be controllable, an obese individual may be regarded more positively when they are working out in a gym than when they are eating dinner with friends. Future research should identify and investigate important dimensions of situations that influence the stigma of obesity.

Fourth, subcultural differences in the stigma of obesity may hold the key to remediation and coping with the stigma of obesity but have only begun to be considered. As an example, initial evidence suggests that African American individuals are generally resilient to the stigma of obesity, but that contextual factors may penetrate their protective exteriors (e.g., Hebl & Heatherton, 1998; Hebl & King, 2005). Examination of the factors that lead members of some subcultures to stigmatize obesity and others to develop resilience may inform an understanding of the origin and development of the stigma.

A fifth and final limitation of the current body of research on the stigma of obesity is its reliance on lab studies and questionnaire data. Although this data helps build a foundation for understanding obesity, it is often limited in either its generalizability or lack of control, respectively. Through experimental field research, obesity stigma has been found to play a meaningful role in multiple interpersonal contexts, including job decisions (Hebl & Mannix, 2003), customer service (King, Shapiro, Hebl, Singletary, & Turner, in press), and health care (Hebl & Xu, 2001). Research should continue in this tradition and explore the antecedents, manifestations, and consequences of the stigma of obesity across contexts with multiple methods.

CONCLUSIONS

In this chapter, we presented five contemporary theoretical approaches to stigmatization and discussed their applicability to the stigma of obesity. We outlined several consequential limitations of these theories and of current research in this area and provided directions for future research. In so doing, we have attempted to help direct the attention of researchers to an important practical problem. Obesity and negative attitudes and behaviors toward obese individuals are increasing concurrently. Thus, it is vital that theory and research continue to strive toward building a comprehensive understanding of the stigma of obesity.

REFERENCES

Crandall, C. S., & Biernat, M. (1990). The ideology of anti-fat attitudes. *Journal of Applied Social Psychology, 20*, 227–243.

Crandall, C. S., & Eshleman, A. (2003). A justification-suppression model of the expression and experience of prejudice. *Psychological Bulletin, 129*, 414–446.

Crandall, C. S., & Martinez, R. (1996). Culture, ideology, and antifat attitudes. *Personality and Social Psychology Bulletin, 22*, 1165–1176.

Crocker, J., Cornwell, B., & Major, B. (1993). The stigma of overweight: Affective consequences of attributional ambiguity. *Journal of Personality and Social Psychology, 60*, 218–228.

Crocker, J., & Major, B. (1989). Social stigma and self-esteem: The self-protective properties of stigma. *Psychological Review, 96*, 608–630.

Crocker, J., Major, B., & Steele, C. (1998). Social stigma. In D. T. Gilbert, & S. T. Fiske (Eds.), *The handbook of social psychology* (Vol. 2, 4th ed., pp. 504–553). New York: McGraw-Hill.

DeJong, W., & Kleck, R. E. (1981). The social psychological effects of overweight. In C. P. Herman, M. P. Zanna, & E. T. Higgins (Eds.), *Physical appearance, stigma, and social behavior* (pp. 65–87). Hillsdale, NJ: Erlbaum.

Fiske, S. T., Cuddy, A. J. C., Glick, P., & Xu, J. (2002). A model of (often mixed) stereotype content: Competence and warmth respectively follow from perceived status and competition. *Journal of Personality and Social Psychology, 82*, 878–902.

Frijda, N. H. (1986). *The emotions*. Cambridge, UK: Cambridge University Press.

Goffman, E. (1963). *Stigma: Notes on the management of spoiled identity.* New York: Simon & Schuster.

Harris, M. B., Harris, R. J., & Bochner, S. (1982). Fat, four-eyed, and female: Stereotypes of obesity, glasses, and gender. *Journal of Applied Social Psychology, 12,* 503–516.

Hebl, M., Foster, J. M., Mannix, L. M., & Dovidio, J. F. (2002). Formal and interpersonal discrimination: A field study examination of applicant bias. *Personality and Social Psychological Bulletin, 28*, 815–225.

Hebl, M. R., & Heatherton, T. F. (1998). The stigma of obesity in women: The difference is black and white. *Personality and Social Psychology Bulletin, 24*, 417–426.

Hebl, M. R., & King, E. B. (2005). *When is thin "in" for black women?: Ego-defensive and status value explanations.* Unpublished manuscript, Rice University.

Hebl, M. R., King, E. B., & Knight, J. L. (2005). *Stigma at work: A multilevel, dual perspective theory. Unpublished manuscript*, Rice University.

Hebl, M. R., King, E. B., & Lin, J. (2004). The swimsuit becomes us all: Gender, ethnicity, and vulnerability to self-objectification. *Personality and Social Psychology Bulletin, 30*, 1322–1331.

Hebl, M. R., & Kleck, R. E. (2002). Acknowledging one's stigma in the interview setting: Effective strategy or liability? *Journal of Applied Social Psychology, 32*, 223–249.

Hebl, M., & Mannix, L. (2003). The weight of obesity in evaluating others: A mere proximity effect. *Personality and Social Psychological Bulletin, 29*, 28–38.

Hebl, M. R., & Xu, J. (2001). Weighing the care: Physicians' reactions to the size of a patient. *International Journal of Obesity and Related Metabolic Disorders, 25*, 1246–1252.

Jost, J. T., & Banaji, M. R. (1994). The role of stereotyping in system justification and the production of false consciousness. *British Journal of Social Psychology, 33*, 1–27.

Jost, J. T., Pelham, B. W., & Carvallo, M. R. (2002). Non-conscious forms of system justification: Implicit and behavioral preferences for higher status groups. *Journal of Experimental Social Psychology, 83*, 586–602.

Kaiser, C. R., & Miller, C. T. (2001). Stop complaining! The social costs of making attributions to discrimination. *Personality and Social Psychology Bulletin, 27*, 254–263.

King, E. B., Hebl, M. R., George, J. M., & Matusik, S. F. (2005). *Negative consequences of perceived gender discrimination*. Unpublished manuscript, Rice University.

King, E. B., Shapiro, J. R., Hebl, M. R., Singletary, S., & Turner, S. (in press). The stigma of obesity in customer service: A mechanism of remediation and bottom-line consequences. *Journal of Applied Psychology.*

Kurzban, R., & Leary, M. R. (2001). Evolutionary origins of stigmatization: The functions of social exclusion. *Psychological Bulletin, 127*, 187–208.

Mackie, D. M., Devos, T., & Smith, E. R. (2000). Intergroup emotions: Explaining offensive action tendencies in an intergroup context. *Journal of Personality and Social Psychology, 79*, 602–616.

Miller, C. T., & Myers, A. M. (1998). Compensating for prejudice: How heavyweight people (and others) control outcomes despite prejudice. In J. K. Swim & C. Stangor (Eds.), *Prejudice: The target's perspective* (p. 191–217). San Diego, CA: Academic Press.

Neuberg, S. L., Smith, D. M., & Asher, T. (2000). Why people stigmatize: Toward a biocultural framework. In T. F. Heatherton, R. E. Kleck, M. R. Hebl, & J. G. Hull (Eds.), *The social psychology of stigma* (p. 31–61). New York: Guilford Press.

Pratto, F., Sidanius, J., Stallworth, L. M., & Malle, B. F. (1994). Social dominance orientation: A personality variable predicting social and political attitudes. *Journal of Personality and Social Psychology, 67*, 741–763.

Roehling, M. V. (1999). Weight-based discrimination in employment: Psychological and legal aspects. *Personnel Psychology, 5*, 969–1016.

Smith, E. R., & Henry, S. (1996). An in-group becomes part of the self: Response time evidence. *Personality and Social Psychology Bulletin, 22*, 635–642.

Turner, J. C. (1985). Social categorization and the self-concept: A social-cognitive theory of group behavior. In E. J. Lawler (Ed.), *Advances in group process: Theory and research* (Vol. 2, pp. 77–122). Greenwich, CT: JAI Press.

Wadden, T. A., Brownell, K. D., & Foster, G. D. (2002). Obesity: Responding to the global epidemic. *Journal of Consulting and Clinical Psychology, 70*, 510–525.

Weiner, B., Perry, R. P., & Magnusson, J. (1988). An attributional analysis of reactions to stigmas. *Journal of Personality and Social Psychology, 55*, 738–748.

CHAPTER 9

■ ■ ■

Measurement of Bias

BETHANY A. TEACHMAN
ROBYN K. MALLETT

Understanding the assessment of obesity stigma requires familiarity with the measurement of bias against marginalized groups more broadly. In this chapter, we outline the terminology used to describe bias, offer a historical perspective on the measurement of bias with particular emphasis on the role of indirect and automatic measures (reflections of bias that are involuntary or outside conscious awareness), and then describe the primary approaches that have been used to measure stigma of obesity.

Measurement of stigma derives in part from its defining features. Goffman (1963) defined social stigma as any aspect of an individual that is deeply discrediting and thereby allows others to discount that individual as "tainted" (p. 3). Jones and colleagues elaborated by specifying six dimensions on which an individual could be discredited (Jones et al., 1984): (1) concealability—whether one can hide a stigma from others; (2) course—the way that a stigma changes over time; (3) disruptiveness—how much the stigma interferes with social interactions; (4) aesthetic qualities—the extent to which the stigma makes an individual repellent or upsetting to others; (5) origin—who is responsible for the stigma or how it was acquired; and (6) peril—the type and degree of danger that the stigma poses for others. Measurement of weight stigma has been influenced by each of these features: (1) Obesity is not concealable; (2) weight often fluctuates over time, so obese people may view their status as temporary (Quinn & Crocker, 1998); (3) weight frequently plays a role in social interactions (e.g., Harris, 1990); (4) fat is often deemed aesthetically unpleasing or even repellent (see W. I. Miller, 1997); (5) despite strong evidence for the role of biological and environmental factors, people are often held personally responsible for being overweight (e.g., Quinn & Crocker, 1999); and (6) peoplc are judged negatively for even socializing with obese persons (e.g., Hebl & Mannix, 2003), suggesting some degree of associated peril.

Because stigma has the potential to render the possessor as less than "a whole and usual person" (Goffman, 1963, p. 3), a great deal of research has focused on bias, or the way that thoughts, feelings, and behaviors may be altered because of a stigmatizing mark. Research on biased *cognitions* focuses on *stereotypes*; research on bias in *affect* or emotional reactions focuses on *prejudice*; and research on bias in *behavior* focuses on *discrimination* (Fiske, 1998).

HISTORICAL PERSPECTIVE ON BIAS MEASUREMENT

As the nature of prejudice changed, so did its measurement. In the early 1900s, prejudice was blatant and measurement was direct. Katz and Braly (1933) investigated the content of stereotypes by simply presenting individuals with dozens of adjectives and asking them to indicate the extent to which each adjective was descriptive of members of various races. Adorno (Adorno, Frenkel-Brunswik, Levinson, & Sanford, 1950) was one of the first to investigate the nature of prejudiced individuals. Drawing from psychoanalytic theory, he proposed that the authoritarian personality (characterized by excessive conformity and submission to authority) was at the heart of prejudice, and he specified several correlates of prejudice, including religiosity and cognitive rigidity. Bogardus (1933) created one of the first measures of discrimination in the form of the social distance scale, which required individuals to select the forms of contact that he or she would be comfortable having with members of various races, occupations, and religions (e.g., ranging from "I'd exclude them from my country" to I would consort with them "as close kin by marriage").

Early bias research typically focused on race-related bias. The Civil Rights movement and subsequent social change in the 1960s modified social norms and curtailed the expression of blatant prejudice. Although bias and hostility toward individuals from different social groups diminished in overt forms, it remained in subtle, more covert forms. For example, although many whites claimed they were not biased against blacks, they resisted school integration. This made clear the need for investigation of the discrepancy between overt and covert or subtler forms of bias. This was accomplished initially by changing the content of the questions to disguise the true meaning of the items. Specifically, subtle scales measure three components: (1) denial of continued discrimination, (2) antagonism toward the target group's demands, and (3) lack of support for policies designed to help the target group (Swim, Aikin, Hall, & Hunter, 1995). For example, rather than asking whites how much they liked blacks—a fairly overt measure of bias—the questions asked about values or policy preferences (McConahay, 1983).

Recognizing that some individuals would attempt to disguise their true attitudes in response to changing social norms, researchers developed alternatives to the traditional self-report questionnaires. Assuming that some individuals might not realize they act in discriminatory ways, some researchers looked to aspects of interpersonal communication, including tone of voice, speech content, facial expression, and body language to assess bias (Babad, Bernieri, & Rosenthal, 1989), while others assessed the likelihood of helping an individual from a different social group (e.g., Gaertner & Dovidio, 1977). One ingenious measure that distinguished overt and covert attitudes was the bogus pipeline (Jones & Sigall, 1971), which misled participants to believe that their untrue responses could be detected via physiological responses to stimuli.

INDIRECT MEASURES OF BIAS

In the 1990s, Devine and colleagues further clarified the difference between overt and covert forms of bias with the dissociation model, which posits that although people may harbor prejudice at an automatic (involuntary and immediate) level, they can consciously control the *expression* of prejudice (Devine, 1989). The model suggests that stereotypes are automatically activated when an individual sees a member of a stereotyped group, but that individuals can respond without prejudice by controlling the automatically activated stereotype. Devine's (1989) dissociation model advanced bias measurement by challenging researchers to create measures that assessed automatic cognitions using advances in technology (i.e., computers).

One method of assessing automatic attitudes is to present individuals with faces or words that belong to their own or a different social group very rapidly (called priming), and then measure the speed of response to a subsequent word or nonword (e.g., Fazio, Jackson, Dunton, & Williams,1995; Wittenbrink, Judd, & Park, 1997). For instance, when presented with words or faces related to blacks, whites respond more quickly to negative than positive stereotypical attributes (Dovidio, Evans, & Tyler, 1986). Other research has used a lexical decision task to assess automatic bias. The lexical decision task requires participants to indicate as quickly and as accurately as possible whether an item is a real word or a nonword. The response latency or reaction time to make this judgment is interpreted as an indication of the cognitive resources required to attend to and evaluate the item. For example, after being presented with a black face, individuals who were biased against blacks should take longer to identify a positive word as being a real word but should take less time to identify a negative word as a real word (e.g., Gaertner & McLaughlin, 1983).

A more recent development is the Implicit Association Test (IAT; Greenwald, McGhee, & Schwartz, 1998). The IAT is a measure widely used to reflect automatic memory-based associations. It requires participants to classify words or pictures into superordinate categories (e.g., "fat people" vs. "thin people"). Simultaneously, the task requires categorization of stimuli into descriptor category pairs, such as good versus bad (an attitude measure) or motivated versus lazy (a stereotype measure). There are both computerized and paper-and-pencil versions of the IAT; both assume that classification is facilitated when categories are paired so that they match a person's automatic associations in memory. The instrument has adequate psychometric properties (see Greenwald & Nosek, 2001).

Bias researchers have also begun to consider how targets of stereotypes, prejudice, and discrimination perceive the bias against them (Swim & Stangor, 1998). A variety of methods have been developed to assess a person's experience, including in-depth interviews, focus groups, and reactions to contrived situations in a laboratory setting. Daily diaries are another unique method in that the observers are not researchers but are members of the target group of interest (C. T. Miller & Myers, 1998).

OBESITY BIAS MEASUREMENT

As evident from even this brief review, there is a rich and dynamic history to the measurement of stereotypes, prejudice, and discrimination. Relative to this history, assessment of stigma of obesity is relatively new. Nevertheless, researchers have used a variety of explicit (self-reported or endorsed), automatic (outside of conscious control or awareness), and behavioral indicators to capture the pervasive negativity toward overweight persons.

Applications of these measures need to be understood in the context of the unique features of weight stigma, relative to measurement of stigmatization of other marginalized groups. In particular, it is still comparatively acceptable to report anti-fat views (Kilbourne, 1994). In addition, the rising rates of obesity (Berkow, 1997) mean that not only is obesity a highly visible stigma, but is increasingly normative. Further, unlike many marginalized groups, there is less direct legal protection for obese individuals who have been discriminated against (McDermott, 1995) because the Americans with Disabilities Act does not identify weight as a protected characteristic (see Johnson & Wilson, 1995; Roehling, 1999), though the legal status of weight discrimination may be changing (Adamitis, 2000; Solovay, 2000). This lack of social and legal protection may help explain why the majority of explicit measures of weight stigma find that both obese and average-weight people report similar levels of anti-fat views, suggesting that no protective ingroup bias exists (Crandall, 1994; Wang, Brownell, & Wadden, 2004). Finally, unlike race, gender, and other marginalized designations, weight is seen as an attribute over which people have control (Quinn & Crocker, 1999; Weiner, Perry, & Magnusson, 1988).

Explicit/Questionnaire Measures

One of the more popular questionnaire measures of weight bias is Crandall's (1994) Anti-fat Attitudes Test, which was originally designed to evaluate parallels between anti-fat views and symbolic (covert) racism. The 13-item scale includes three subscales: dislike of fat people (e.g., "Fat people make me feel somewhat uncomfortable"), fear of fat (e.g., "I feel disgusted with myself when I gain weight"), and beliefs about the controllability of weight or about willpower (e.g., "People who weigh too much could lose at least some part of their weight through a little exercise"). The measure has adequate psychometric properties, though to increase internal consistency, Quinn and Crocker (1999) added items to the Dislike and Controllability subscales.

A number of other attitude questionnaires have been used to assess stigmatization of obesity, but unfortunately, most of the measures have only been used in a small number of studies, and there is limited psychometric information (e.g., on reliability and validity) available for many of the scales. Allison, Basile, and Yuker (1991) developed companion scales, the 8-item Beliefs About Obese Persons Scale and 20-item Attitudes Toward Obese Persons Scale. One advantage of these scales is that normative data is available for college students and for members of the National Association to Advance Fat Acceptance. Bagley, Conklin, Isherwood, Pechiulis, and Watson (1989) developed the Attitudes Toward Obese Adult Patients with a particular focus on assessing nurse's attitudes toward their overweight patients, and Price and colleagues developed a series of measures for health professionals and school officials (e.g., Price, Desmond, Ruppert, & Stelzer, 1989). Bray (1972) developed the 47-item Bray Obesity Attitude Scale, which was later revised by Sims (1979) to test attitudes across different ethnic and racial groups. Other obesity attitude measures include sentence completion measures (Canning & Mayer, 1966), ratings of line drawings, and rankings of sketches of various physiques (e.g., Richardson, Goodman, Hastorf, & Dornbusch, 1961).

Some researchers have focused on adjective ratings to reflect stereotypes about "fat people" (e.g., Staffieri, 1967). Often, vignettes or some kind of personal descriptions are presented, and then participants are asked to rate the presented character on various attributes (see Counts, Jones, Frame, Jarvie, & Strauss, 1986; Harris, Harris, & Bochner, 1982). The focus in this case is on an individual overweight person. To evaluate stereotypes about overweight people as a group, researchers have sometimes used semantic-differential scales, frequently evaluating attitudes toward fat people relative to thin people. For instance, Teachman, Gapinski, Brownell, Rawlins, and Jeyaram (2003) asked participants to rate their feelings about "fat people" and about "thin people" on negative and positive attributes, and then calculated a difference score between the items. In contrast, the Fat Phobia Scale (Robinson, Bacon, & O'Reilly, 1993), one of the more rigorously developed instruments, has been used to assess group-level weight bias in a nonrelative way. This 50-item, semantic-differential scale asks participants to rate their feelings about what "fat people are like" on a series of different opposing dimensions (e.g., smart vs. stupid). This and other nonrelative measures (e.g., Harris, Walters, & Waschull, 1991) simplify interpretation, but leave open the question of what constitutes the baseline evaluation.

Few studies have measured stigma of obesity by directly asking overweight persons about their experiences of discrimination, although it appears that participants can readily recall instances of perceived prejudice and discrimination. For instance, 96% of overweight adolescents reported experiences of stigma in qualitative clinical interviews (Neumark-Sztainer, Story, & Faibisch, 1998).

Implicit Measures

Most research on anti-fat biases has used explicit measures of attitudes and stereotypes, but new evidence suggests that anti-fat bias can be activated without conscious intention (and perhaps outside of awareness), and can even differ in important ways from explicit views. This incongruence may arise because automatic responses to marginalized groups can occur outside of conscious control or awareness, or because individuals are motivated to deny these responses, perhaps to appear or to actually be fair-minded.

Bessenoff and Sherman (2000) used a lexical decision task to demonstrate that implicit anti-fat evaluations predict how far participants choose to sit from an overweight woman, whereas explicit attitudes do not. In their study, participants were presented with pictures of fat and thin women, and then evaluated fat-stereotypical, thin-stereotypical, and stereotype-irrelevant words. Not surprisingly, the authors found greater implicit activation of negative evaluations to fat compared to thin women. Researchers have also recently applied the IAT to measure implicit anti-fat biases, based on the idea that classification of words and pictures is faster when categories are paired so that associations with obesity reflect the person's automatic evaluations. Teachman and Brownell (2001) found strong implicit bias even among health professionals who specialize in obesity treatment and who did not explicitly report negative attitudes. In addition, Grover, Keel, and Mitchell (2003) found that implicit anti-fat attitudes were ubiquitous across both average-weight and overweight women and men. Similarly, Teachman et al. (2003) found strong evidence of implicit anti-fat/pro-thin stereotypes of overweight people as lazy, stupid, and worthless among both the general population and college students. Finally, Geier, Schwartz, and Brownell (2003) demonstrated implicit anti-fat biases following presentation of "beforc and after" diet advertisements.

Behavioral/Rejection Measures

Rather than relying on direct evaluation of obese persons, many studies have used more indirect (but arguably more externally valid) behavioral indicators of rejection across domains from health care to housing, employment, school, and relationships. The measures range from microlevel indicators, such as proximity of a chair to an overweight confederate (Bessenoff & Sherman, 2000) or time before salespersons respond to overweight customers (Pauley, 1989), to macrolevel surveys with nationally representative samples illustrating the negative relationship between weight and wages (e.g., Pagan & Davila, 1997; Register & Williams, 1990).

There have been a number of studies demonstrating discrimination against overweight persons in the workplace (see review by Roehling, 1999), including field studies like the surveys cited earlier and experimental studies that involve judgments about hypothetical job applicants or employees whose weight status is manipulated (e.g., Brink, 1988; Klassen, Jasper, & Harris, 1993; Pingitore, Dugoni, Tindale, & Spring, 1994). Participants are typically given a résumé or videotape presentation of a candidate, and weight is either embedded in the résumé or is manipulated verbally or through a photo or videotape of the applicant (e.g., using theatrical prostheses; Pingitore et al., 1994). Job applicants are then rated on a variety of features, including desirability for hiring, personal attributes, fitness for the job, professional qualifications, perceived skills, and professional ethics. These measures indicate that obese persons routinely experience discrimination in the workplace at all stages of the employment process: They are less likely to be hired (Klesges et al., 1990; Roe & Eickwort, 1976); their wages are lower and they experience discrimination on the job (Rothblum, Brand, Miller, & Oetjen, 1990); and promotions occur less frequently (Larkin & Pines, 1979). In an intriguing variation on the job applicant paradigm, Hebl and Mannix (2003) found that average-weight applicants perceived to be in a social relationship with an obese person were stigmatized themselves.

Analogous approaches have been used to measure weight stigma across other life domains. To demonstrate housing discrimination, Karris (1977) had obese and average-weight college students inquire in person about apartments for rent, and showed that landlords were less willing to rent the apartment to obese potential tenants. In relationships, overweight persons are less likely to be trusted or be chosen as friends or romantic partners (DeJong & Kleck, 1986; Harris, 1990). Similar rejecting views have been assessed in the health care field, including negative attitudes by nurses (Maroney & Golub, 1992), medical students (Wiese, Wilson, Jones, & Neises, 1992), doctors (Klein, Najman, Kohrman, & Munro, 1982; Teachman & Brownell, 2001), and psychotherapists (Davis-Coelho, Waltz, & Davis-Coelho, 2000). In school settings, weight bias has been measured through sociometric nominations by classmates indicating which children are liked and disliked (Cohen, Klesges, Summerville, & Meyers, 1989), which children are desirable playmates (Jarvie, Lahey, Graziano, & Framer, 1983; Strauss, Smith, Frame, & Forehand, 1985), and which children are "mean" or "nice" (Cramer & Steinwert, 1998). These studies show that weight bias can be demonstrated in children as young as 3 years old, and that school-based discrimination continues across developmental stages (e.g., parents are less willing to finance their overweight daughters' college education; Crandall, 1995).

RECOMMENDATIONS FOR FUTURE RESEARCH

Although measurement of weight bias is still a relatively young field, much has been learned about the numerous ways that overweight persons routinely experience stereotypes, prejudice, and discrimination. We conclude this chapter with suggestions for future studies on the measurement of weight bias, based on both current gaps in the obesity literature and exciting advances in stigma research:

1. Evaluating the psychometric properties of the many anti-fat questionnaires will help to establish "gold-standard" measures that have strong reliability and validity.
2. Further research on measures of the experience of obese persons is needed. This includes assessing awareness and sensitivity to stigma and their consequences for behavior, thoughts, and feelings, as well as methods used by overweight persons to cope with or respond to perceived bias (e.g., C. T. Miller & Myers, 1998).
3. It will be important to assess how attitudes versus beliefs, and implicit versus explicit bias measures, predict discriminatory behaviors against overweight persons.
4. As the field becomes more adept at reducing the stigma of obesity, developing instruments that are sensitive to change will be critical. For example, establishing measures of interactions between obese and average-weight individuals can foster recognition of covert forms of bias.
5. It will be helpful to more consistently use standard criteria for "overweight" and "obese" to facilitate comparison across studies.

We look forward to seeing how the measurement of weight bias will evolve, given the remarkable advances in the fields of stigma, assessment, and obesity research in recent years.

REFERENCES

Adamitis, E. M. (2000). Appearance matters: A proposal to prohibit appearance discrimination in employment. *Washington Law Review, 75*, 195–223.

Adorno, T. W., Frenkel-Brunswik, E., Levinson, D. J., & Sanford, R. N. (1950). *The authoritarian personality*, New York: Harper.

Allison, D. B., Basile, V. C., & Yuker, H. E. (1991). The measurement of attitudes toward and beliefs about obese persons. *International Journal of Eating Disorders, 5*, 599–607.

Babad, E., Bernieri, F., & Rosenthal, R. (1989). Students as judges of teachers' verbal and nonverbal behavior. *American Educational Research Journal, 28*, 211–234.

Bagley, C. R., Conklin, D. N., Isherwood, R. T., Pechiulis, D. R., & Watson, L. A. (1989). Attitudes of nurses toward obesity and obese patients. *Perceptual and Motor Skills, 68*, 954.

Berkow, R. (Ed.). (1997). *Merck manual of medical information.* Whitehouse Station, NJ: Merck Research Laboratories.

Bessenoff, G. R., & Sherman, J. W. (2000). Automatic and controlled components of prejudice toward fat people: Evaluation versus stereotype activation. *Social Cognition, 18*, 329–353.

Bogardus, E. S. (1933). A social distance scale. *Sociology and Social Research, 17*, 265–271.

Bray, C. R. (1972). *The development of an instrument to measure attitudes toward obesity*. Unpublished doctoral dissertation, University of Mississippi.

Brink, T. L. (1988). Obesity and job discrimination: Mediation via personality stereotypes. *Perceptual and Motor Skills, 66*, 494.

Canning, H., & Mayer, J. (1966). Obesity: Its possible effect on college acceptance. *New England Journal of Medicine, 275*, 1172–1174.

Cohen, R., Klesges, R. C., Summerville, M., & Meyers, A. W. (1989). A developmental analysis of the influence of body weight on the sociometry of children. *Addictive Behaviors, 14*, 473–476.

Counts, C. R., Jones, C., Frame, C. L., Jarvie, G. J., & Strauss, C. C. (1986). The perception of obesity by normal-weight versus obese school-age children. *Child Psychiatry and Human Development, 17*, 113–120.

Cramer, P., & Steinwert, T. (1998). Thin is good, fat is bad: How early does it begin? *Journal of Applied Developmental Psychology, 19*, 429–451.

Crandall, C. S. (1994). Prejudice against fat people: Ideology and self-interest. *Journal of Personality and Social Psychology, 66*, 882–894.

Crandall, C. S. (1995). Do parents discriminate against their heavyweight daughters? *Personality and Social Psychology Bulletin, 21*, 724–735.

Davis-Coelho, K., Waltz, J., & Davis-Coelho, B. (2000). Awareness and prevention of bias against fat clients in psychotherapy. *Professional Psychology: Research and Practice, 31*, 682–684.

DeJong, W., & Kleck, R. E. (1986). The social psychological effects of overweight. In C. P. Herman, M. P. Zanna, & E. T. Higgins (Eds.), *The Ontario Symposium: Vol. 3. Physical appearance, stigma, and social behavior* (pp. 65–87). Hillsdale, NJ: Erlbaum.

Devine, P. G. (1989). Stereotypes and prejudice: Their automatic and controlled components. *Journal of Personality and Social Psychology, 56*, 5–18.

Dovidio, J. F., Evans, N., & Tyler, R. B. (1986). Racial stereotypes: The contents of their cognitive representations. *Journal of Experimental Social Psychology, 22*, 22–37.

Fazio, R. H., Jackson, J. R., Dunton, B. C., & Williams, C. J. (1995). Variability in automatic activation as an unobtrusive measure of racial attitudes: A bona fide pipeline? *Journal of Personality and Social Psychology, 69*, 1013–1027.

Fiske, S. T. (1998). Stereotyping, prejudice, and discrimination. In D. T. Gilbert, S. T. Fiske, & G. Lindzey (Eds.), *The handbook of social psychology, Vol. 2* (4th ed., pp. 357–411). New York: McGraw-Hill.

Gaertner, S. L., & Dovidio, J. (1977). The subtlety of white racism, arousal, and helping behavior. *Journal of Personality and Social Psychology, 117*, 69–77.

Gaertner, S. L., & McLaughlin, J. P. (1983). Racial stereotypes: Associations and ascriptions of positive and negative characteristics. *Social Psychology Quarterly, 46*, 23–30.

Geier, A. B., Schwartz, M. B., & Brownell, K. D. (2003). "Before and after" diet advertisements escalate weight stigma. *Eating and Weight Disorders, 8*, 282–288.

Goffman, E. (1963). *Stigma: Notes on the management of spoiled identity.* Englewood Cliffs, NJ: Prentice-Hall.

Greenwald, A. G., McGhee, D. E., & Schwartz, J. L. K. (1998). Measuring individual differences in implicit cognition: The implicit association test. *Journal of Personality and Social Psychology, 74,* 1464–1480.

Greenwald, A. G., & Nosek, B. A. (2001). Die Gesundheit des Implicit Association Test im Alter von dre: Jahren [Health of the Implicit Association Test at age 3]. *Zeitschrift Fuer Experimentelle Psychologie, 48*, 85–93.

Grover, V. P., Keel, P. K., & Mitchell, J. P. (2003). Gender differences in implicit weight identity. *International Journal of Eating Disorders, 34,* 125–135.

Harris, M. B. (1990). Is love seen as different for the obese? *Journal of Applied Social Psychology, 20,* 1209–1224.

Harris, M. B., Harris, R. J., & Bochner, S. (1982). Fat, four-eyed and female: Stereotypes of obesity, glasses and gender. *Journal of Applied Social Psychology, 6*, 503–516.

Harris, M. B., Walters, L. C., & Waschull, S. (1991). Altering attitudes and knowledge about obesity. *Journal of Social Psychology, 131,* 881–884.

Hebl, M. R., & Mannix, L. M. (2003). The weight of obesity in evaluating others: A mere proximity effect. *Personality and Social Psychology Bulletin, 29*, 28–38.

Jarvie, G. J., Lahey, B., Graziano, W., & Framer, E. (1983). Childhood obesity: What we know and what we don't know. *Developmental Review, 2,* 237–273.

Johnson, T., & Wilson, M. C. (1995). An analysis of weight-based discrimination: Obesity as a disability. *Labor Law Journal*, *46*, 238–244.

Jones, E. E., Farina, A., Hastorf, A. H., Markus, H., Miller, D. T., & Scott, R. A. (1984). *Social stigma: The psychology of marked relationships.* New York: Freeman.

Jones, E. E., & Sigall, H. (1971). The bogus pipeline: A new paradigm for measuring affect and attitude. *Psychological Bulletin, 76,* 349–364.

Karris, J. (1977). Prejudice against obese renters. *Journal of Social Psychology, 101*, 159–160.

Katz, D., & Braly, K. (1933). Racial stereotypes in one hundred college students. *Journal of Abnormal and Social Psychology, 28,* 280–290.

Kilbourne, J. (1994). Still killing us softly: Advertising and the obsession with thinness. In P. Fallon, M. A. Katzman, & S. C. Wooley (Eds.), *Feminist perspectives on eating disorders* (pp. 395–418). New York: Guilford Press.

Klassen, M. L., Jasper, C. R., & Harris, R. J. (1993). The role of physical appearance in managerial decisions. *Journal of Business and Psychology, 8*, 181–198.

Klein, D., Najman, J., Kohrman, A. F., & Munro, C. (1982). Patient characteristics that elicit negative responses from family physicians. *Journal of Family Practice, 14*, 881–888.

Klesges, R. C., Klein, M., Hanson, C. L., Eck, L. H., Ernst, J., O'Laughlin, D., et al. (1990). The effects of applicant's health status and qualifications on simulated hiring decisions. *Journal of Obesity, 14, 527–535.*

Larkin, J. C., & Pines, H. A. (1979). No fat persons need apply: Experimental studies of the overweight stereotype and hiring preference. *Sociology of Work and Occupations, 6,* 312–327.

Maroney, D., & Golub, S. (1992). Nurses' attitudes toward obese persons and certain ethnic groups. *Perceptual and Motor Skills, 75*, 387–391.

McConahay, J. B. (1983). Modern racism and modern discrimination: The effects of race, racial attitudes, and context on simulated hiring decisions. *Personality and Social Psychology Bulletin, 9,* 551–558.

McDermott, C. M. (1995). Should employers be allowed to weigh obesity in their employment decisions? *Cook v. Rhode Island, Department of Mental Health, Retardation and Hospitals. The University of Kansas Law Review, 44*, 199–216.

Miller, C. T., & Myers, A. M. (1998). Compensating for prejudice: How heavyweight people (and others) control outcomes despite prejudice. In J. K. Swim & C. Stangor (Eds.), *Prejudice: The target's perspective* (pp. 191–218). San Diego, CA: Academic Press.

Miller, W. I. (1997). *The anatomy of disgust.* Cambridge, MA: Harvard University Press.

Neumark-Sztainer, D., Story, M., & Faibisch, L. (1998). Perceived stigmatization among overweight African-American and Caucasian adolescent girls. *Journal of Adolescent Health, 23*, 264–270.

Pagan, J. A., & Davila, A. (1997). Obesity, occupational attainment, and earnings. *Social Science Quarterly, 78,* 756–770.

Pauley, L. (1989). Customer weight as a variable in salespersons' response time. *Journal of Social Psychology, 129*, 713–714.

Pingitore, R., Dugoni, B. L., Tindale, R. S., & Spring, B. (1994). Bias against overweight job applicants in a simulated employment interview. *Journal of Applied Psychology, 79*, 909–917.

Price, J. H., Desmond, S. M., Ruppert, E. S., & Stelzer, C. M. (1989). Pediatricians' perceptions and practices regarding childhood obesity. *American Journal of Preventative Medicine, 5,* 95–103.

Quinn, D. M., & Crocker, J. (1998). Vulnerability to the affective consequences of the stigma of overweight. In J. K. Swim & C. Stangor (Eds.), *Prejudice: The target's perspective* (pp. 125–143). San Diego, CA: Academic Press.

Quinn, D. M., & Crocker, J. (1999). When ideology hurts: Effects of belief in the Protestant ethic and feeling overweight on the psychological well-being of women. *Journal of Personality and Social Psychology, 77*, 402–414.

Register, C. A., & Williams, D. R. (1990). Wage effects of obesity among young workers. *Social Science Quarterly, 71,* 130–141.

Richardson, S. A., Goodman, N., Hastorf, A. H., & Dornbusch, S. M. (1961). Cultural uniformity in reaction to physical disabilities. *American Sociological Review,* 241–247.

Robinson, B. E., Bacon, J. G., & O'Reilly, J. (1993). Fat phobia: Measuring, understanding and changing anti-fat attitudes. *International Journal of Eating Disorders, 14*, 467–480.

Roe, D. A., & Eickwort, K. R. (1976). Relationships between obesity and associated health factors with unemployment among low income women. *Journal of American Medical Women's Association, 31*, 193–204.

Roehling, M. V. (1999). Weight-based discrimination in employment: Psychological and legal aspects. *Personnel Psychology, 52,* 969–1017.

Rothblum, E. D., Brand, P. A., Miller, C. T., & Oetjen, H. A. (1990). The relationship between obesity, employment discrimination, and employment-related victimization. *Journal of Vocational Behavior, 37,* 251–266.

Sims, H. J. (1979). *A study to identify and evaluate the attitudes toward obesity among three ethnic groups of women in Oklahoma: Black, white, and Indian.* Unpublished doctoral dissertation, University of Oklahoma.

Solovay, S. (2000). *Tipping the scales of justice: Fighting weight-based discrimination.* Amherst, NY: Prometheus Books.

Staffieri, J. (1967). A study of social stereotype of body image in children. *Journal of Personality and Social Psychology, 7,* 101–104.

Strauss, C. C., Smith, K., Frame, C., & Forehand, R. (1985) Personal and interpersonal characteristics associated with childhood obesity. *Journal of Pediatric Psychology, 10,* 337–343.

Swim, J. K., Aikin, K. J., Hall, W. S., & Hunter, B. A. (1995). Sexism and racism: Old-fashioned and modern prejudices. *Journal of Personality and Social Psychology, 68,* 199–214.

Swim, J. K., & Stangor, C. (1998). *Prejudice: The target's perspective.* San Diego, CA: Academic Press.

Teachman, B., & Brownell, K. (2001). Implicit associations toward obese people among treatment specialists: Is anyone immune? *International Journal of Obesity, 25,* 1–7.

Teachman, B. A., Gapinski, K., Brownell, K., Rawlins, M., & Jeyaram, S. (2003). Demonstrations of implicit anti-fat bias: The impact of providing causal information and evoking empathy. *Health Psychology, 22,* 68–78.

Wang, S. S., Brownell, K. D., & Wadden, T. A. (2004). The influence of the stigma of obesity on overweight individuals. *International Journal of Obesity and Related Metabolic Disorders, 28,* 1333–1337.

Weiner, B., Perry, R. P., & Magnusson, J. (1988). An attributional analysis of reactions to stigmas. *Journal of Personality and Social Psychology, 55,* 738–748.

Wiese, H. J. C., Wilson, J. F., Jones, R. A., & Neises, M. (1992). Obesity stigma reduction in medical students. *International Journal of Obesity, 16,* 859–868.

Wittenbrink, B., Judd, C. M., & Park, B. (1997). Evidence for racial prejudice at the implicit level and its relationship with questionnaire measures. *Journal of Personality and Social Psychology, 72,* 262–274.

PART III

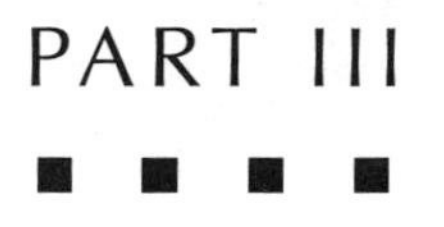

Consequences of Weight Bias

CHAPTER 10

■ ■ ■

Effects of Weight-Related Teasing in Adults

J. KEVIN THOMPSON
SYLVIA HERBOZO
SUSAN HIMES
YUKO YAMAMIYA

Given the high value society places on physical attractiveness, it is not surprising that one's physical appearance influences the reactions of others and elicits different types of feedback (Thompson, Heinberg, Altabe, & Tantleff-Dunn, 1999). According to Lerner's developmental view, social interactions and feedback about one's body during socialization are interpersonal experiences that shape one's body image (Lerner & Jovanovic, 1990). There is evidence suggesting that parents and peers may directly and/or indirectly promote societal standards of physical attractiveness through negative verbal commentary or teasing (Keery, van den Berg, & Thompson, 2004). Such interpersonal influences may make individuals more sensitive to sociocultural pressures for thinness and attractiveness (Thompson et al., 1999), and these experiences may particularly affect overweight or obese individuals, an observation noted almost 40 years ago by Stunkard and Mendelson (1967).

In this chapter, we examine the role of a specific form of societal pressure that is a form of stigmatization—appearance-based teasing—and how being the recipient of such feedback may contribute to elevated body dissatisfaction. We cover not only the occurrence of teasing for individuals who are overweight or obese, but also examine its prevalence in other samples, measurement issues, and experimental studies. We close with recommendations for future work in the area.

TEASING: DEFINITION, EARLY FINDINGS, AND MEASUREMENT

Although almost all of the work in the area of commentary on physical appearance has involved the assessment and evaluation of "teasing," it should be noted that verbal feedback may be quite pointed and cruel; therefore, we have often used the more general term of "negative verbal commentary" to characterize this construct. Additionally, as noted later in this chapter, feedback may also be nonverbal, and a relatively unexplored area of commentary involves "positive" commentary. However, the bulk of work in this area has examined the issue of verbal "teasing" about appearance, so we begin with an overview of this work.

In an early nationwide survey conducted in *Psychology Today*, Cash, Winstead, and Janda (1986) found that women with a childhood history of appearance-related teasing were more likely to be dissatisfied with their appearance as adults. A more recent nationwide survey conducted in *Psychology Today* (Garner, 1997) provides additional evidence that teasing strongly influences one's body satisfaction. Of the 4,000 respondents, 44% of the women and 35% of the men reported that "being teased by others" shaped their body image during childhood and adolescence. Several of the respondents' comments also illustrate the extent to which their body image was affected by previous appearance-related teasing. For example, a 37-year-old woman wrote, "No matter how thin I become, I always feel like the fat kid everyone made fun of" (p. 42). A 59-year-old man reported, "Being teased when I was a child made me feel bad about my body for years and years" (p. 42).

The potential negative consequences of being teased early in life on adult body image have also been demonstrated in correlational studies and in research examining eating-disturbed versus asymptomatic samples. In a sample of college women, Thompson and Psaltis (1988) found that both teasing frequency and the "effect" of teasing (i.e., how distressed participants were by the feedback) were strongly associated with general physical appearance satisfaction and eating disturbance. Thompson (1991) found that college females with eating disturbance experienced more teasing and a greater effect of teasing compared to asymptomatic college females. The college females with eating disturbance also reported less general appearance satisfaction.

These early surveys and research studies utilized single-item indices of teasing, but were the impetus for the development of more sophisticated questionnaire measures for the assessment of the construct. We now briefly review the measures developed for the measurement of teasing and related aspects of negative verbal commentary, followed by a presentation of recent work with these psychometrically evaluated measures. Table 10.1 contains a brief description of these scales. The Physical Appearance Related Teasing Scale (PARTS) measures Weight/Size Teasing and General Appearance Teasing (Thompson, Fabian, Moulton, Dunn, & Altabe, 1991). The Perception of Teasing Scale (POTS), was a revision and extension of the PARTS that consists of Weight-Related Teasing and Competency Teasing subscales (Thompson, Cattarin, Fowler, & Fisher, 1995). This scale included separate ratings for an item's frequency and effect (which reflected the severity of the respondent's reaction to the teasing comment). Advantages of the POTS over the PARTS include the measurement of teasing specifically related to an overweight or obese status and the ability to partial out competency teasing from appearance-based teasing.

The Appearance Teasing Inventory (ATI) was developed by Cash (1995) to obtain both descriptive and quantitative information about the history of appearance-related teasing and the effects of such teasing. A modified version of the ATI enables respondents to differentiate between recurrent appearance-related teasing and criticism. In the ATI, respondents identify the targets of teasing or criticism (i.e., specific physical attributes), duration, frequency, and emotional effect at the time. Researchers have also examined more subtle aspects of negative appearance-related feedback than teasing. Tantleff-Dunn, Thompson, and Dunn (1995) developed the Feedback on Physical Appearance Scale (FOPAS) to measure the frequency of verbal as well as nonverbal feedback (i.e., facial expressions and gestures) regarding one's physical appearance.

CONTEMPORARY RESEARCH ON TEASING

In the first study to use the PARTS, Thompson and Heinberg (1993) found that weight and size teasing uniquely predicted body dissatisfaction for college females. In a study focusing on ethnic differences among college women using the PARTS, Akan and Grilo (1995) found that weight and size teasing was related to body dissatisfaction in African American and Caucasian females. No such associations were found with Asian American females; however, this ethnic group also reported significantly less teasing

Cash (1995) used the ATI to examine the influence of appearance-related teasing and criticism on women's body image development. The

TABLE 10.1. Measures of Teasing and Appearance-Related Feedback

Name of Instrument	Author(s)	Description	Scale type	Psychometric properties	α and n	Author address
Appearance Teasing Inventory (ATI)	Cash (1995)	Measures descriptively and quantitatively one's past experiences of teasing and appearance-related criticism, including targets of teasing/criticism (i.e., specific body parts), duration, frequency, and their emotional effects	▪ 6 items ▪ Combination of 5-point Likert-type, open-ended, and checklist	▪ Good internal consistency for a sample of college female students ▪ Good convergent validities with measures of body image, appearance schematicity, and the PARTS	$\alpha = .83$ $n = 152$	Thomas F. Cash, PhD Department of Psychology Old Dominion University Norfolk, VA 23529
Feedback on Physical Appearance Scale (FOPAS)	Tantleff-Dunn, Thompson, and Dunn (1995)	Measures the frequency of verbal and nonverbal feedback (i.e., facial expressions and gestures) one has received regarding physical appearance and the specific sources of the feedback (e.g., romantic partner, parents)	▪ 8 items ▪ 5-point Likert-type	▪ Good internal consistency and test–retest reliability for a sample of female and male college students ▪ Good convergent validities with measures of body image, eating disturbance, self-esteem, and depression	$\alpha = .84$ $n = 74$ (M) and 89 (F)	Stacey Dunn, PhD Department of Psychology University of Central Florida 4000 Central Florida Blvd. Orlando, FL 32816-1360

Perception of Teasing Scale (POTS)	Thompson, Cattarin, Fowler, and Fisher (1995)	Measures one's past experiences of weight-related and competency-based teasing in terms of frequency, effect, and the specific sources of teasing (e.g., peers, parents)	■ 11 items ■ 5-point Likert-type	■ Good internal consistency for a sample of college female students ■ Good convergent validities with measures of body dissatisfaction, physical appearance-related anxiety, eating disturbance, and self-esteem	α = .84–.88 n = 223	J. Kevin Thompson, PhD Department of Psychology University of South Florida 4202 Fowler Ave. Tampa, FL 33620-8200
Physical Appearance Related Teasing Scale (PARTS)	Thompson, Fabian, Moulton, Dunn, and Altabe (1991)	Measures the frequency of one's past teasing experiences regarding weight, size, and general appearance	■ 18 items ■ 5-point Likert-type	■ Good internal consistency and 2-week test–retest reliability for a sample of college females ■ Good convergent validity with measures of body image, eating disturbance, social comparison, depression, and self-esteem	α = .71–.91 n = 153	J. Kevin Thompson, PhD Department of Psychology University of South Florida 4202 Fowler Ave. Tampa, FL 33620-8200

results indicated that 72% of the women had been teased or criticized about their appearance for an average duration of 5.8 years. In terms of frequency, 46% of the women teased or criticized said it had occurred moderately often (26%), often (14%), or very often (6%). The most reported focus of teasing or criticism was facial attributes (41%), followed by weight (39%). Peers in general (60%) were most commonly identified as the perpetrators of teasing or criticism. Also, peers in general, specific peer(s), and friends were collectively (62%) found to be the "worst" perpetrators. The negative effects of being teased or criticized are apparent in the following findings: 71% of the women reported that these experiences were moderately upsetting or more upsetting; 71% said that these experiences had influenced their current body image to some extent; and 70% noted that they think about these past experiences. Interestingly, the occurrence of appearance-related teasing or criticism was not related to current body image. Instead, the prevalence (i.e., duration in years × frequency rating) and the emotional impact (i.e., distressfulness of appearance-related teasing) and criticism were significantly associated with body image, specifically appearance evaluation and situational body-image dysphoria. This latter finding highlights the importance of assessing the emotional impact of previous appearance-related teasing or criticism experiences.

In a similar study, Rieves and Cash (1996) investigated the influence of several social developmental factors, including appearance-related teasing and criticism, on women's body image. The PARTS was used as the primary measure of appearance-related teasing and the ATI was used to obtain qualitative information. Rieves and Cash (1996) found that 72% of women were teased (39%) or criticized (12%) about their appearance, or both (21%), during their childhood or adolescence. Of those teased or criticized, 55% reported that these experiences occurred "sometimes" to "moderately often" and for an average length of 6.6 years. Seventy-one percent of these women also reported that such experiences were "moderately" to "extremely" upsetting and 38% felt they had a negative impact on their body-image development. As in the study by Cash (1995), features of the face and head (45%) and weight (36%) were the most frequently teased or criticized physical attributes. In addition, "peers in general" were the most common (62%) as well as the worst perpetrators (28%) of teasing or criticism about appearance. Friends (47%) and family members (22–41%) were also frequent perpetrators. However, of the respondents with one or more brothers, an overwhelming majority (79%) mentioned brothers as teasers, and approximately one-third said they were the worst perpetrators. Furthermore, appearance-related teasing as assessed by the PARTS was related to appearance evaluation, maladaptive appearance assumptions, body-image dysphoria, and overweight preoccupation.

Cross-cultural studies also document the role of teasing in body-image disturbance. Mautner, Owen, and Furnham (2000) examined college females from the United States, Italy, and England. As in the study by Stormer and Thompson (1996), history of weight-related teasing, as measured by the POTS, predicted body-image disturbance across all three Western cultures. No cultural differences in the relationship between teasing history and body-image disturbance were found. Shroff and Thompson (2004) conducted a cross-cultural study in which they evaluated the relationships among body mass index (BMI), history of weight-related teasing, media internalization, and body-image and eating disturbance in an Indian sample. Weight-related teasing was assessed using the POTS and was found to mediate the relationship between BMI and body dissatisfaction, suggesting that it is not weight per se (BMI) that leads to body dissatisfaction, but whether weight-based teasing has occurred.

An evaluation of obese individuals suggests that teasing may be particularly problematic. Using the PARTS, Grilo and colleagues (Grilo, Wilfley, Brownell, & Rodin, 1994) found that greater frequency of weight and size teasing was associated with more negative appearance evaluation and body dissatisfaction. Wardle, Waller, and Fox (2002) studied the relationship between age of onset of obesity, body dissatisfaction, history of weight- and size-related teasing, and self-esteem among obese females. Women who reported being overweight by age 16 were identified as the early-onset group. Wardle et al. (2002) used the Weight and Size-Related Teasing frequency scale of the POTS and found that the early-onset group was exposed to more teasing during childhood.

In a sample of obese males and females, Womble et al. (2001) examined a psychosocial model of binge eating and used the POTS to evaluate teasing history as one of the variables in the model. Other psychosocial variables included were depression, body dissatisfaction, neuroticism, dietary restraint, self-esteem, and weight cycling. The psychosocial model proposed by Womble and colleagues was the best fitting model, explaining over 60% of the variance for binge eating in both obese male and female samples.

Researchers have also examined the effects of appearance-related teasing for populations with eating disorder. Jackson, Grilo, and Masheb (2002) studied the relationship between appearance-related teasing history and eating dysfunction in females with bulimia nervosa compared to females with binge-eating disorder. The PARTS was used to differentiate the effects of teasing regarding weight and size versus general appearance. The findings indicated that females with bulimia nervosa experienced more weight- and size-related teasing but similar amounts of general appearance-related teasing in comparison to females with binge-eating disorder.

In contrast to the literature on appearance-related feedback among female adults, very little is known about the potential negative effects of such interpersonal experiences for males. Using the POTS and PARTS, Gleason, Alexander, and Somers (2000) investigated the effect of three types of childhood teasing (competency, weight, and appearance) on self-esteem and body image in a sample of college females and males. More frequent teasing during childhood significantly predicted lower self-esteem and poorer body image for both females and males. An interesting finding was that certain types of teasing influenced the females and males in different ways. For instance, teasing about competence was predictive of self-esteem in males whereas teasing about both appearance and competence was predictive of self-esteem in females. Teasing about weight was the only predictor of body-image disturbance for both females and males.

Little research has focused on the examination of teasing in an experimental setting, perhaps due to the difficulty in constructing a context that would not be distressing to participants. Tantleff-Dunn and Thompson (1998) examined the effects of body-image anxiety and appearance-related feedback on recall, judgment, and subsequent affective responses using two videotaped vignettes with college females. Each vignette consisted of a social interaction between a male and female acquaintance, with the male providing subtle appearance-related feedback (verbal or nonverbal) or non-appearance-related feedback to the female. After watching the videos, free recall of the social interaction and perceived reaction (ranging from negative to positive) of the women in the video were assessed. Mood reaction to the vignettes was also examined. Free recall of the appearance-related feedback was not significantly different for females with high or low levels of body-image anxiety. However, females with high body-image anxiety found incidents of appearance-related feedback to be more negative for the female recipient than the non-appearance-related feedback. This difference was not found for the females with low body-image anxiety. Also, compared to females with low body-image anxiety, those with high body-image anxiety experienced higher levels of anger after viewing the appearance-related feedback video. Tantlefff-Dunn and Thompson (1998) concluded that the reactions of the females with high body-image anxiety may have been influenced by a cognitive bias, leading them to perceive certain social interactions in a more negative manner.

Furman and Thompson (2002) studied the influence of teasing history on one's mood and body satisfaction after reading vignettes in which another female is the target of the teasing. The female in the vignette either received a teasing comment regarding her physical appearance or abilities during a social interaction. Unexpectedly, the results indicated that history of teasing, as assessed by the PARTS, was not a significant predictor for mood responses in the negative appearance or abilities scenarios. Only eating disturbance uniquely predicted mood reactions for both scenarios. Given the limited research involving manipulation of appearance-related feedback, it is evident that more experimental studies are needed.

THEORETICAL MODELS OF NEGATIVE VERBAL COMMENTARY

The role of the media as a potential factor leading individuals to tease others has received perhaps the most research attention. Fat stigmatization is often presented in the form of humor through entertainment media. Television programs and movies often portray teasers and their targets of fat disparagement as engaged in various fat joke dialogues. Although fat stereotyping in media has not been extensively studied, a small number of studies and content analyses document the presence of fat disparagement material.

Fouts and colleagues have extensively examined positive and negative verbal commentary received by characters in prime-time television situation comedies. In an initial study, they found that overweight characters, primarily female overweight characters, are underrepresented on television (Fouts & Burggraf, 1999). In a second study, Fouts and Burggraf (2000) found that overweight female characters received more negative comments from male characters, and those negative comments were reinforced by audience laughter. Negative references to overweight men were not associated with audience laughter (Fouts & Vaughn, 2002). Finally, Fouts and Burggraf (1999, 2000) found that the thinner the female, the more positive comments she received from the male characters; conversely, the higher the weight of the female character, the more negative comments she received from male characters. Males with heavier bodies did not receive significantly more negative comments than other males; audience laughter was only associated with men making disparaging comments about themselves (Fouts & Vaughn, 2002). Thus, Fouts argues that popular prime-time programs reinforce discriminatory behavior against women based on weight and size, while heavy males receive little punishment or rejection; therefore, the analyses support the existence of a double standard in popular media programs.

According to Fairclough's (1989) theory of critical discourse analysis, the media expresses and reproduces the power of the dominant societal class; they constrain language content by excluding some views and reproduce societal norms of power by promoting or discussing others. When media portrays powerful thin individuals teasing less powerful overweight targets in the form of humor, the media promotes the idea that such behavior is normative and acceptable; in effect, they reproduce social hierarchies of power. To date, however, there is no evidence from controlled evaluations that exposure to media representations of fat stigmatization or ridicule in the form of teasing drives individuals to engage in similar behaviors.

Generally, little theoretical work has been developed to further our understanding of why people tease and why this experience affects people in a negative manner. Thompson et al. (1999) briefly discuss the possible role that social dominance and conformity may play as motivators driving the instigator (teaser) to engage in such behavior. Perhaps the most extensive model of teasing was provided by Keltner, Capps, Kring, Young, and Heery (2001), yet this is a general model of teasing with no particular components related to appearance-based commentary. In sum, much more theoretical work needs to be articulated to guide empirical work in this area.

RECENT TRENDS AND DIRECTIONS FOR FUTURE RESEARCH

Teasing measures have recently been created to assess constructs other than teasing directed at weight or other appearance attributes. For instance, Herbozo and Thompson (2004) developed the Verbal Commentary on Physical Appearance Scale, which has a subscale that assesses positive body-related comments. Lundgren, Anderson, Thompson, Shapiro, and Paulosky (2004) modified the POTS to allow for the assessment of teasing focused on thinness or an underweight status. Iyer and Haslam (2003) modified the POTS to evaluate the role of racial teasing on body image and eating disturbance among South-Asian American college females. The modified 8-item scale assessed perceived frequency and effect of teasing regarding one's race or ethnicity. Items focused on name calling, behavior-related teasing, appearance-related teasing, and social exclusion. Sarwer and colleagues (2003) have also recently found that women who seek breast augmentation surgery had a greater history of appearance-based teasing than a control group of nonseekers.

There is still much work to be done in the area to expand our understanding of the putative negative effects of teasing. For instance, as noted by Neumark-Sztainer and Eisenberg (Chapter 5, this volume), there are few prospective studies on teasing with adolescents, and we could find no prospective studies with adult samples. Second, although Thompson et al. (1999) suggested several avenues for treatment approaches, such as reframing, role playing, and assertiveness training, we could find no controlled treatment studies of teasing. Third, much more needs to be done to explore potential moderators that would help indicate factors that potentiate or mitigate the negative effects of teasing. For instance, Thompson et al. suggested that attributional style might moderate effects, such that someone with a tendency to internalize negative events might suffer more from teasing experiences. A second personality variable that might explain unique variance in predicting the effects of teasing is fear of negative appearance evaluation (Lundgren, Anderson, & Thompson, 2004). Finally, controlled experimental studies and theoretical models are needed to further explore the contextual and individual factors that not only help explain who responds negatively to teasing and under what specific circumstances, but also point the way toward potential treatment interventions.

REFERENCES

Akan, G., & Grilo, C. (1995). Sociocultural influences on eating attitudes and behaviors, body image, and psychological functioning: A comparison of African-American, Asian-American and Caucasian college women. *International Journal of Eating Disorders, 18*, 181–187.

Cash, T. F. (1995). Developmental teasing about physical appearance: Retrospective descriptions and relationships with body image. *Social Behavior and Personality, 23*, 123–130.

Cash, T. F., Winstead, B. A., & Janda, L. H. (1986). Body Image Survey report: The great American shape-up. *Psychology Today, 24*, 30–37.

Fairclough, N. (1989). *Language and power.* New York: Longman Group UK.

Fouts, G., & Burggraf, K. (1999). Television situation comedies: Female body images and verbal reinforcements. *Sex Roles, 40*, 473–481.

Fouts, G., & Burggraf, K. (2000). Television situation comedies: Female weight, male negative comments, and audience reactions. *Sex Roles, 42*, 925–932.

Fouts, G., & Vaughan, K. (2002). Television situation comedies: Male weight, negative references, and audience reactions. *Sex Roles, 46*, 439–442.

Furman, K., & Thompson, J. K. (2002). Body image, teasing, and mood alterations: An experimental study of exposure to negative verbal commentary. *International Journal of Eating Disorders, 32*, 449–457.

Garner, D. M. (1997, January/February). The Body Image Survey. *Psychology Today*, 32–84.

Gleason, J.H., Alexander, A. M., & Somers, C. L. (2000). Later adolescents' reactions to three types of childhood teasing: Relations with self-esteem and body image. *Social Behavior and Personality, 28*, 471–480.

Grilo, C. M., Wilfley, D. E., Brownell, K. D., & Rodin, J. (1994). Teasing, body image, and self-esteem in a clinical sample of obese women. *Addictive Behaviors, 19*, 443–450.

Herbozo, S., & Thompson, J. K. (2004). *The Verbal Commentary on Physical Appearance Scale*. Unpublished manuscript, University of South Florida.

Iyer, D. S., & Haslam, N. (2003). Body image and eating disturbance among South Asian-American women: The role of racial teasing. *International Journal of Eating Disorders, 34*, 142–147.

Jackson, T. D., Grilo, C. M., & Masheb, R. M. (2002). Teasing history and eating disorder features: An age- and body mass index-matched comparison of bulimia nervosa and binge-eating disorder. *Comprehensive Psychiatry, 43*, 108–113.

Keery, H., van den Berg, P., & Thompson, J. K. (2004). An evaluation of the Tripartite Influence Model of body image and eating disturbance with adolescent females. *Body Image: An International Journal of Research, 1*, 237–251.

Keltner, D., Capps, L., Kring, A. M., Young, R. C., & Heery, E. A. (2001). Just teasing: A conceptual analysis and empirical review. *Psychological Bulletin, 127*, 229–248.

Lerner, R. M., & Jovanovic, J. (1990). The role of body image in psychosocial development across the life span: A developmental contextual perspective. In T. F. Cash & T. Pruzinsky (Eds.), *Body images: Development, deviance, and change* (pp. 110–127). New York: Guilford Press.

Lundgren, J. D., Anderson, D. A., & Thompson, J. K. (2004). Fear of negative appearance evaluation: Development and evaluation of a new construct for risk factor work in the field of eating disorders. *Eating Behaviors, 5*, 75–84.

Lundgren, J. D., Anderson, D. A., Thompson, J. K., Shapiro, J. R., & Paulosky, C. A. (2004). A modification of the Perception of Teasing Scale. *Eating and Weight Disorders: Studies on Anorexia, Bulimia, and Obesity, 9*, 139–146.

Mautner, R. D., Owen, S. V., & Furnham, A. (2000). Cross-cultural explanations of body-image disturbance in Western cultural samples. *International Journal of Eating Disorders, 28*, 165–172.

Rieves, L., & Cash, T. F. (1996). Social developmental factors and women's body-image attitudes. *Journal of Social Behavior and Personality, 11*, 63–78.

Sarwer, D., B., LaRossa, D., Bartlett, S. P., Low, D. W., Bucky, L. P., & Whitaker, L. A. (2003). Body image concerns of breast augmentation patients. *Plastic and Reconstructive Surgery, 112*, 83–90.

Shroff, H., & Thompson, J. K. (2004). Body image and eating disturbance in India: Media and interpersonal influences. *International Journal of Eating Disorders, 35*, 198–203.

Stormer, S. M., & Thompson, J. K. (1996). Explanations of body image disturbance: A test of maturational status, negative verbal commentary, social comparison, and sociocultural hypotheses. *International Journal of Eating Disorders, 19,* 193–202.

Stunkard, A. J., & Mendelson, M. (1967). Obesity and body image: I. Characteristics of disturbances in the body image of some obese persons. *American Journal of Psychiatry, 123,* 1296–1300.

Tantleff-Dunn, S., & Thompson, J. K. (1998). Body image and appearance-related feedback: Recall, judgment, and affective response. *Journal of Social and Clinical Psychology, 17*, 319–340.

Tantleff-Dunn, S., Thompson, J. K., & Dunn, M. F. (1995). Development and validation of the Feedback on Physical Appearance Scale (FOPAS). *Eating Disorders: The Journal of Treatment and Prevention, 3,* 341–350.

Thompson, J. K. (1991). Body shape preferences: Effects of instructional protocol and level of eating disturbance. *International Journal of Eating Disorders, 10*, 193–198.

Thompson, J. K., Cattarin, J., Fowler, B., & Fisher, E. (1995). The Perception of Teasing Scale (POTS): A revision and extension of the Physical Appearance Related Teasing Scale (PARTS). *Journal of Personality Assessment, 65*, 146–157.

Thompson, J. K., Fabian, L. J., Moulton, D. O., Dunn, M. E., & Altabe, M. N. (1991). Development and validation of the Physical Appearance Related Teasing Scale. *Journal of Personality Assessment, 56*, 513–521.

Thompson, J. K., & Heinberg, L. J, (1993). Preliminary test of two hypotheses of body-image disturbance. *International Journal of Eating Disorders, 14*, 59–63.

Thompson, J. K., Heinberg, L. J, Altabe, M. N., & Tantleff-Dunn, S. (1999). *Exacting beauty: Theory, assessment, and treatment of body image disturbance.* Washington, DC: American Psychological Association.

Thompson, J. K., & Psaltis, K. (1988). Multiple aspects and correlates of body figure ratings: A replication and extension of Fallon and Rozin (1985). *International Journal of Eating Disorders, 7,* 813–818.

Wardle, J., Waller, J., & Fox, E. (2002). Age of onset and body dissatisfaction in obesity. *Addictive Behaviors, 27, 561–573.*

Womble, L. G., Williamson, D. A., Martin, C. K., Zucker, N. L., Thaw, J. M. Netemeyer, R., et al. (2001). Psychosocial variables associated with binge eating in obese males and females. *International Journal of Eating Disorders, 30*, 217–221.

CHAPTER 11

■ ■ ■

Social Consequences of Weight Bias by Partners, Friends, and Strangers

JEFFERY SOBAL

Body size is a highly salient social characteristic, and individuals and groups with deviant bodies experience bias, stigma, and discrimination. There are many dimensions and components of deviant body size, including weight (being seen as too fat or too thin) and height (being seen as too short and too tall). While thin, short, and tall people experience bias and discrimination (e.g., Harmatz, Gronendyke, & Thomas, 1985; Roberts & Herman, 1986; Way, 1995), the focus of this review is on social consequences of weight bias for overweight individuals.

Overweight biases have many consequences, including creating problems in navigating and negotiating formal arenas of public life such as schooling, employment, and health care. For example, considerable analysis describes stigmatization of obese workers by employers (e.g., DeJong & Kleck, 1986), but little work carefully examines weight bias by coworkers. Similarly, educational discrimination against obese applicants by institutional admissions committees is well documented (e.g., Sobal, 2004), but less investigation of weight bias between schoolmates and school staff has been conducted. Finally, an extensive body of evidence shows that health care providers discriminate against obese patients (e.g., Puhl & Brownell, 2001, 2003), but much less attention is given to weight bias among medical practitioners (but see Parham, 1999).

The social consequences of weight bias in informal, private arenas of life are less explicitly and empirically considered, such as dating and marital relationships, friendships and social networks, and interactions and encounters with strangers. These areas represent a more diffuse and sometimes less dramatic aspect of the social marginality of obese individuals that is no less important to quality of life than the more easily quantifiable and legally accountable arenas of education, work, and medical treatment. The consequences of weight bias in these three informal social areas will be reviewed here, examining partners, friends, and strangers.

PARTNERS: DATING, MARRIAGE, AND FAMILY RELATIONSHIPS

Entry into romantic relationships and marriage is substantially more difficult for obese individuals, particularly for women (Regan, 1996). Body weight is an important aspect of attractiveness to potential romantic partners (e.g., Hayes & Ross, 1987; Lewis, Cash, Jacobi, & Bubb-Lewis, 1997). For example, heavier adolescent boys (but not girls) reported feeling that they had less personal romantic appeal (French, Perry, Leon, & Fulkerson, 1996). Obese individuals are widely seen as less desirable dating/courtship partners (Sobal & Bursztyn, 1998; Sobal, Nicolopoulos, & Lee, 1995; Venes, Krupka, & Gerard, 1982) and heavier girls (and sometimes boys) begin dating later, date less often, and date less attractive partners (Bullen, Monello, Cohen, & Mayer, 1963; Cawley, 2001; Cawley, Joyner, & Sobal, 2006; Halpern, Udry, Campbell, & Suchindran, 1999; Kallen & Doughty, 1984; Pearce, Boegers, & Prinstein, 2002). Furthermore, personal advertisements for romantic partners also reveal bias against obese individuals (e.g., Sitton & Blanchard, 1995; Stack, 1996). Obese women marry later and marry less desirable partners (Fu & Goldman, 1996; Garn, Sullivan, & Hawthorne, 1989a, 1989b; Gortmaker, Must, Perrin, Sobol, & Dietz, 1993), even though obese young women do not have lower marital aspirations than thinner women (Ball, Crawford, & Kenardy, 2004). Married people, especially men, tend to have higher relative body weights than those who are not married (Sobal, 1984; Sobal, Rauschenbach, & Frongillo, 1992), and people tend to gain weight after they marry (Sobal, Rauschenbach, & Frongillo, 2003). Overall, bias against obese girls and women (and to a lesser extent obese boys and men) leads to difficulty in entering romantic and marital relationships, and marriage itself may lead to weight gain.

Once obese individuals do marry, however, they tend to report that their relationships with their spouses are of comparable quality with those of their thinner counterparts. Cross-sectional community and population studies of marital quality and weight find few significant differences between a person's weight and their marital satisfaction, conflict, and problems (S. Cohen, Schwartz, Bromet, & Parkinson, 1991; Gallo, Troxel, Matthews, & Kuller, 2003; Klesges, Klem, & Klesges, 1992; Sobal, Rauschenbach, & Frongillo, 1995). However, weight changes (including both weight gains and weight losses) may be associated with marital problems (Margolin & White, 1987), and some individuals in clinical studies who make considerable weight changes may experience marital difficulties and even marital termination (e.g., Herpertz et al., 2003). Falkner et al. (1999) reported that over 10% of men and women reported weight mistreatment by a spouse; the percentage of heavier individuals reporting mistreatment is even higher. Myers and Rosen (1999) found that obese individuals reported that an average of once a year they experienced name calling from their partners because of their weight. Overall, this suggests that while obese individuals may have a restricted market of available marital partners and take a longer time to marry, most tend to report they are satisfied with their marital relationship; however, some experience a range of effects from the weight biases of their partners.

Family relationships of obese people often include stigmatization by other family members (Falkner et al., 1999), particularly where only one person in the family unit is obese (Sobal, Rauschenbach, & Frongillo, 1995). This is especially an issue for obese children and obese women, who may elect to eat separately from other family members (Zdrodwski, 1996) or become scapegoats for problems rooted in the family system (e.g., Beck & Terry, 1985; Ganley, 1986; Kinston, Loader, & Miller, 1987; Kinston, Loader, Miller, & Rein, 1988). In contrast, other studies found that families with an obese member revealed few problematic family dynamics or impaired functioning (e.g., Valtolina & Marta, 1998). However, for other obese individuals the family may be a refuge from bias in the larger community (Sobal, Rauschenbach, & Frongillo, 1995). Overall, the extent that families may serve as a source of or buffer from obesity bias, the types of family bias, and the types of individuals most subject to family bias are not clear at this time.

In summary, courtship, marital, and family relationships are difficult for obese individuals to initiate and establish. However, once marital and family relationships are established and a functioning family system develops, spousal and family relationships may operate smoothly (unless changes or disruptions of the system occur). Thus, social consequences of weight bias occur in relationships with romantic and marital partners, although they may be conditional on age and gender and be more likely to emerge in times of change than in stable situations.

FRIENDS: FRIENDSHIPS, SOCIAL NETWORKS, AND SOCIAL SUPPORT

Friendship formation is sometimes more difficult for obese individuals, especially women and children, although existing data on this topic includes mixed results. Stereotypes about obese individuals begin in children at an early age and include the perception that obese people have few friends, have difficulty making friends, are less popular, are less liked, receive more peer rejection, have fewer social skills, and are more lonely (e.g., Brylinsky & Moore, 1994; Davison & Birch, 2004; Davis-Pyles, Conger, & Conger, 1990; Harris, Harris, & Bochner, 1982; Harris & Smith, 1983; Hill & Silver, 1995; C. C. Strauss, Smith, Frame, & Forehand, 1985; Wardle, Volz, & Golding, 1995). However, some studies find that obese individuals are reported as being no less friendly (Davis-Pyles et al., 1990; DeJong, 1980; Sallade, 1973) or even friendlier than those who are not obese (e.g., Tiggemann & Rothblum, 1988). Some research reports that obese people have fewer friends, fewer close friendships, spend less time with friends, and are less likely to be "best friends" (Falkner et al., 2001; French et al., 1996; Harris & Smith, 1983; Matthews & Westie, 1966; Staffieri, 1967), while other investigations report that obese youth do have friends (Hoerr, Kallen, & Kwantes, 1995) and that few differences by weight occur in the number of friendships (Dietz, 1990; Jarvie, Lahey, Graziano, & Framer, 1983; Miller, Rothblum, Brand, & Felicio, 1995). Overall, the stigma of obesity may make it more difficult for children and adults to develop and participate in friendships, although that is not a consistent finding in existing research.

Gender and age conditionalities appear to exist in weight–friendship patterns, with obese women more frequently reporting an absence of close friends (Harmatz et al., 1985; Sarlio-Lahteenkorva & Lahelma, 1999). Falkner et al. (1999) reported that 5% of women and 7.5% of men reported weight-related mistreatment by friends; this treatment was more common among heavier than thinner individuals. However, some studies question the presence and persistence of overweight influences on friendships beyond elementary school. For example, Cohen and colleagues (R. Cohen, Klesges, Summerville, & Meyers, 1989) found less liking (but not disliking) for overweight first- and third-grade boys (but not girls), but no differences in liking according to the weight of fifth-grade boys or girls (R. Cohen et al., 1989). Similarly, while heavier preadolescent girls were judged by peers as less attractive, they were not less likely to be chosen as friends (Phillips & Hill, 1998). Being a target for teasing and bullying is a negative friendship interaction, with overweight adolescents more likely to be victims of withdrawing friendship, rumors, teasing, and physical aggression (Janssen, Craig, Boyce, & Pickett, 2004). Over half of overweight adolescent boys and girls reporting being teased (Neumark-Sztainer et al., 2002). Overall, gender and life course patterns appear to occur with friendship among obese individuals, but further specific longitudinal analyses are needed to better clarify these patterns and their temporal trajectories.

Social networks are systems of formal and informal ties that individuals have with others, and have a variety of characteristics such as being larger or smaller, homogeneous or heterogeneous, and others (Wellman & Berkowitz, 1988). Some sociometric studies of adolescents report that obese individuals tend to be socially isolated and marginalized, have smaller social networks, and also are more peripheral and less central in social network relationships (R. S. Strauss & Pollack, 2003). Similarly, analysis of a large sample of Swedish adults found that obese individuals more often lived alone, and had lower contact with friends, coworkers, and neighbors (Kuskowska-Wolk & Rossner, 1990). Some research finds that obese adolescents participated in fewer organizations and are less involved in organizations than their thinner counterparts (Bullen et al., 1963; R. S. Strauss & Pollack, 2003). However, other comparisons among adults report that social network size did not differ between obese and nonobese women (Ball et al., 2004; Miller et al., 1995). Some studies have reported that obese people report greater loneliness (Horchner, Tuinebreijer, Kelder, & Urk, 2002; Schumaker, Krejci, Small, & Sargent, 1985). One study of obese adults reported that positive attitudes and beliefs toward obese persons were associated with having more obese friends (Allison, Basile, & Yuker, 1990). Overall, it is not yet clear how much obesity is associated with social exclusion and how different characteristics of social networks are associated with body weight for various ages, genders, and other types of individuals.

Social networks provide social support, and more restricted and less diverse social networks offer less and lower quality social support of various types (tangible resources, information, emotional help, and appraisal) (S. Cohen, Underwood, & Gottleib, 2000). Some studies report no differences between obese and nonobese adults in social support (Miller et al., 1995). However, widespread social stigmatization appears to lead obese individuals to experience exclusion from valued "ingroups" into devalued "outgroups" (Puhl & Brownell, 2003) and results in less social support for obese people. Social withdrawal is a common coping method used by obese individuals to avoid exposure to stigmatization from a variety of sources by self-isolation and self-segregation (e.g., Millman, 1980; Sobal, 2004), which contributes to fewer friendships, smaller social networks, and less social support. The presence of social support from a close confidant may buffer effects of obesity on physical functioning capacity (Surtees, Wainwright, & Khaw, 2004). Social support from sources such as partners, family, and groups may play a role in facilitating weight management (Black, Gleser, & Kooyers, 1990; Kelsey, Earp, & Kirkley, 1997; McLean, Griffin, Toney, & Hardeman, 2003; Parham, 1993). Overall, it is not currently clear how social support operates to exacerbate or buffer the effects of bias in obese individuals.

In summary, friendships, social networks, and social support offer important forms of social capital for children and adults to draw upon to cope with routine hassles as well as major stressful life events. These relational realms appear to be difficult arenas for many obese individuals to participate in, and may or may not provide social reinforcement or social refuges from the effects of bias in other aspects of society.

STRANGERS: INTERPERSONAL INTERACTIONS AND PUBLIC ENCOUNTERS

Stigmatization of obese individuals is a routine experience in their everyday life as they participate in "mixed interactions" with those who are not obese (Goffman, 1963). Such contacts are often awkward and tense for both obese people and those they are dealing with, with considerable anxiety and discomfort about weight issues continually present in these social interactions (Hebl, Tickle, & Heatherton, 2000). Two major categories of this type of social relationships include formal interactions and informal encounters.

Formal interpersonal interactions in everyday life are often problematic for obese individuals (Allon, 1981; Sobal, 2004). For example, relationships between various service providers and customers are difficult for obese people in both roles. Obese customers experience slower reaction times from salesclerks (Pauley, 1989), and obese salespeople provide negative images for the stores in which they work (Klassen, Clayson, & Jasper, 1996). Similarly, obese renters suffer discrimination from potential landlords (Karris, 1977). Additionally, obese individuals are often denied access to public accommodations in transportation, eating, and entertainment settings because of their size (e.g., O'Hara, 1996). Overall, these formal interactions are sometimes difficult for obese individuals to navigate, although the frequency, intensity, and specific types of such interactional biases have yet to be well documented or explained.

Public encounters with strangers may be difficult experiences for obese individuals, who are under continual scrutiny in the public gaze and always under threat of various forms of stigmatizing acts (e.g., Crossrow, Jeffery, & McGuire, 2001; Joanisse & Synnott, 1999; Sobal, 1991). Mistreatment by a stranger is often particularly upsetting (Falkner et al., 1999). Stigmatizing acts may be active and overt or passive and covert, and include actions that are verbal (such as teasing, joking, or ridicule) or nonverbal (such as staring, hostility, gestures, shunning, or avoidance) (Sobal, 1991, 2004). A study of a small sample of obese people found that they reported experiencing negative comments from children and adults, staring and laughing, and unsolicited advice from strangers an average of once a year (Myers & Rosen, 1999). Rand and MacGregor (1990) reported that 84% of obesity surgery patients did not like to be seen in public. Mistreatment of women, but not men, due to weight is most commonly perpetrated by strangers (Falkner et al., 1999), with 12.5% of women and 4% of men reporting such harassment; the percentage of heavier individuals reporting harassment is even higher. For example, strangers often verbally reprimand the food choices of obese women eating in public places such as at work, in fast food and other restaurants, at social events, or on the street (Zdrodowski, 1996). Obese individuals experience public distress because of their weight that diminishes their quality of life (Kolotkin, Crosby, Kosloski, & Williams, 2001). Overall, obese people may encounter many weight-biased individuals during their daily routines, and the visibility of their body weights may subject them to acts of verbal degradation, physical challenges, and other forms of bias.

In summary, interactions and encounters in public and private are situations where many obese individuals are at continual risk of stigmatization and discrimination. Eating is a particularly problematic act for obese people (English, 1991) and is often subject to criticism, castigation, and condemnation. The frequency, extent, types, and conditions for such biases is not clear, and further research in this area is needed.

CONCLUSION

People create social distance between themselves and others with stigmatized conditions such as obesity (Albrecht, Walker, & Levy, 1982; Goffman, 1963). A substantial and fairly consistent body of evidence has accumulated to suggest that obese individuals face bias, stigmatization, and discrimination in education, employment, and health care (Puhl & Brownell, 2001; Sobal, 2004). However, fewer analyses have examined the social consequences of weight bias in relationships with partners, friends, and strangers in public and private interactions that occur in arenas where stigmatization is often more insidious, subtle, and implicit, and therefore difficult to study. The overall patterns of interactions of obese individuals with romantic partners, spouses, friends, and strangers leads to some negative social consequences of weight, although there are mixed findings and conditional results in each of these areas among the relatively small number of available studies on these topics.

Clear gaps exist in research on these phenomena. The body of studies is gendered, with a focus on studying girls and women rather than boys and men. Also, most studies of friendship and dating were conducted with adolescents, rather than adults and the elderly, and most studies of interactions with strangers were only done with adult samples. The bulk of existing literature about weight bias is culture- and subculture-bound, and ethnic subgroups and other societies may have substantially different patterns of stigmatization in various settings and situations that may provide important insights about the dynamics of weight stigmatization (e.g., Hebl & Heatherton, 1998). Although empirical studies of the social consequences of obesity in dating/marriage, friendship/networks, and interactions/encounters have been done for more than half a century (e.g., Hanley, 1951), it is not clear whether there are historical or temporal trends in these patterns. However, one study of the stigmatization of children over the past 40 years suggests that social bias toward obese people is increasing (Latner & Stunkard, 2003).

This review focused on consequences of weight bias in dating/marital relationships, friendships/networks, and public interactions/encounters. Because stigmatization and its consequences may be situational (DeJong & Kleck, 1986), further work is needed on additional arenas where bias occurs as a social consequence of obesity, such as in groups, clubs, teams, associations, organizations, religions, neighborhoods, communities, and others. The relational dynamics for obese individuals in such other cases may present patterns similar to those identified here, or reveal greater, lesser, or different forms of bias (or lack of bias) in these other sites. For example, organizations and groups specifically oriented toward latently or manifestly helping obese individuals offer positive support for obese individuals (e.g., Allon, 1975; Sobal, 1999).

Future work on the scope of consequences of weight bias needs to extend and elaborate existing findings in several ways (DeJong & Kleck, 1986; Puhl & Brownell, 2001). Quantitative and qualitative research on these topics needs to be developed more thoroughly using (1) better conceptualization and theoretical interpretations, (2) longitudinal, comparative, and experimental research designs, (3) larger, more representative, and more diverse samples and settings, (4) more valid and reliable assessments and measures, and (5) more extensive statistical and other analytical procedures. Some existing multidimensional measures of obesity-related topics include assessments of dating, spousal, family, friend, and stranger interactions (e.g., Sobal, Nicolopoulos, & Lee, 1995). It would be useful to advance the analyses of these areas by developing more specific scales focusing on impacts of social biases regarding obesity (Sobal & Devine, 1997). Additionally, explicit comparisons need to be conducted between arenas of weight bias, including examination of additive and interactive effects of stigmatization at school, at work, in health care, with families, by friends, and in public. Further investigation of these topics should provide much needed insights and understandings of the sources, dynamics, and consequences of weight bias, stigmatization, and discrimination.

REFERENCES

Albrecht, G. L., Walker, V. G., & Levy, J. A. (1982). Social distance from the stigmatized: A test of two theories. *Social Science and Medicine, 16,* 1319–1327.

Allison, D. B., Basile, V. C., & Yuker, H. E. (1990). The measurement of attitudes toward and beliefs about obese persons. *International Journal of Eating Disorders, 10,* 599–607.

Allon, N. (1975). Latent social services in group dieting. *Social Problems, 23,* 59–69.

Allon, N. (1981). The stigma of overweight in everyday life. In B. J. Wolman (Ed.), *Psychological aspects of obesity: A handbook* (pp. 130–174). New York: Van Nostrand Rinehold.

Ball, K., Crawford, D., & Kenardy, J. (2004). Longitudinal relationships among overweight, life satisfaction, and aspirations in young women. *Obesity Research, 12,* 1019–1030.

Beck, S., & Terry, K. (1985). A comparison of obese and normal-weight families' psychological characteristics. *American Journal of Family Therapy, 13,* 55–59.

Black, D. R., Gleser, L. J., & Kooyers, K. J. (1990). A meta-analytic evaluation of couples weight loss programs. *Health Psychology, 9,* 330–347.

Brylinsky, J. A., & Moore, J. C. (1994). The identification of body build stereotypes in young children. *Journal of Research in Personality, 28,* 170–181.

Bullen, B. A., Monello, L. F., Cohen, H., & Mayer, J. (1963). Attitudes toward physical activity, food and family in obese and nonobese adolescent girls. *American Journal of Clinical Nutrition, 12,* 1–11.

Cawley, J. (2001). Body weight and the dating and sexual behaviors of young adolescents. In R. T. Michael (Ed.), *Social awakening: Adolescent behavior as adulthood approaches* (pp. 174–198). New York: Russell Sage.

Cawley, J., Joyner, K., & Sobal, J. (2006). Size matters: The influence of adolescents' weight and height on dating and sex. *Rationality and Society, 18.*

Cohen, R., Klesges, R. C., Summerville, M., & Meyers, A. W. (1989). A developmental analysis of the influence of body weight on the sociometry of children. *Addictive Behaviors, 14*, 473–476.

Cohen, S., Schwartz, J. E., Bromet, E. J., & Parkinson, D. K. (1991). Mental health, stress, and poor health behaviors in two community samples. *Preventive Medicine, 20*, 306–315.

Cohen, S., Underwood, L. G., & Gottleib, B. H. (2000). *Social support measurement and intervention: A guide for health and social scientists.* New York: Oxford University Press.

Crossrow, N. H., Jeffery, R. W., & McGuire, M. T. (2001). Understanding weight stigmatization: A focus group study. *Journal of Nutrition Education, 33*, 208–214.

Davison, K. K., & Birch, L. L. (2004). Predictors of fat stereotypes among 9–year-old girls and their parents. *Obesity Research, 12*, 86–94.

Davis-Pyles, B., Conger, J. C., & Conger, A. J. (1990). The impact of deviant weight on social competence ratings. *Behavioral Assessment, 12*, 443–455.

DeJong, W. (1980). The stigma of obesity: The consequences of naive assumptions concerning the causes of physical deviance. *Journal of Health and Social Behavior, 21*, 75–87.

DeJong, W., & Kleck, R. E. (1986). The social psychological effects of overweight. In C. P. Herman, M. P. Zanna, & E. T. Higgins (Eds.), *Physical appearance, stigma, and social behavior: The Ontario Symposium* (Vol. 3, pp. 65–87). Hillsdale, NJ: Erlbaum.

Dietz, W. H. (1990). You are what you eat—what you eat is what you are. *Journal of Adolescent Health Care, 11*, 76–81.

English, C. (1991). Food is my best friend: Self-justification and weight-loss efforts. *Research in the Sociology of Health Care, 9*, 335–345.

Falkner, N. H., French, S. A., Jeffery, R. W., Neumark-Sztainer, D., Sherwood, N. E., & Morton, N. (1999). Mistreatment due to weight: Prevalence and sources of perceived mistreatment in women and men. *Obesity Research, 7*, 572–576.

Falkner, N. H., Neumark-Sztainer, D., Story, M., Jeffery, R. W., Beuhring, T., & Resnick, M. D. (2001). Social, educational, and psychological correlates of weight status in adolescents. *Obesity Research, 9*, 32–42.

French, S. A., Perry, C. L., Leon, G. R., & Fulkerson, J. A. (1996). Self-esteem and change in body mass index over 3 years in a cohort of adolescents. *Obesity Research, 4*, 27–33.

Fu, H., & Goldman, N. (1996). Incorporating health into marriage choice models: Demographic and sociological perspectives. *Journal of Marriage and the Family, 58*, 740–758.

Gallo, L. C., Troxel, W. M., Matthews, K. A., & Kuller, L. H. (2003). Marital status and quality in middle-aged women: Associations with levels and trajectories of cardiovascular risk factors. *Health Psychology, 22*, 453–463.

Ganley, R. M. (1986). Epistemology, family patterns and psychosomatics: The case of obesity. *Family Process, 25*, 347–351.

Garn, S., Sullivan, T. V., & Hawthorne, V. M. (1989a). The education of one spouse and the fatness of the other spouse. *American Journal of Human Biology, 1*, 233–238.

Garn, S., Sullivan, T. V., & Hawthorne, V. M. (1989b). Educational level, fatness, and fatness differences between husbands and wives. *American Journal of Clinical Nutrition, 50*, 740–745.

Goffman, E. (1963). *Stigma: Notes on the management of spoiled identity.* New York: Simon & Schuster.

Gortmaker, S. L., Must, A., Perrin, J. M., Sobol, A. M., & Dietz, W. H. (1993). Social and economic consequences of overweight in adolescence and young adulthood. *New England Journal of Medicine, 329*, 1008–1012.

Halpern, C. T., Udry, J. R., Campbell, B., & Suchindran, C. (1999). Effects of body fat on weight concerns, dating, and sexual activity: A longitudinal analysis of black and white adolescent girls. *Developmental Psychology 35*, 721–736.

Hanley, C. (1951). Physique and reputation of junior high school boys. *Child Development, 22*, 247–260.

Harmatz, M. G., Gronendyke, J., & Thomas, T. (1985). The underweight male: The unrecognized problem group of body image research. *Journal of Obesity and Weight Regulation, 4*, 258–267.

Harris, M. B., Harris, R. J., & Bochner, S. (1982). Fat, four-eyed, and female: Stereotypes of obesity, glasses, and gender. *Journal of Applied Social Psychology, 12*, 503–516.

Harris, M. B., & Smith, S. D. (1983). The relationships of age, sex, ethnicity, and weight to stereotypes of obesity and self-perception. *International Journal of Obesity, 7*, 361–371.

Hayes, D., & Ross, C. E. (1987). Concern with appearance, health beliefs, and eating habits. *Journal of Health and Social Behavior, 28*, 120–130.

Hebl, M. R., & Heatherton, T. F. (1998). The stigma of obesity in women: The difference is black and white. *Personality and Social Psychology Bulletin, 24*, 417–426.

Hebl, M. R., Tickle, J., & Heatherton, T. F. (2000). Awkward moments in interactions between nonstigmatized and stigmatized individuals. In T. F. Heatherton, R. F. Kleck, M. R. Hebl, & J. G. Hull (Eds.), *The social psychology of stigma* (pp. 275–306). New York: Guilford Press.

Herpertz, S., Kielmann, R., Wolf, A. M., Langkafel, M., Senf, W., & Hebebrand, J. (2003). Does obesity surgery improve psychosocial functioning? A systematic review. *International Journal of Obesity, 27*, 1300–1314.

Hill, A. J., & Silver, E. K. (1995). Fat, friendless, and unhealthy: 9–year old children's perceptions of body shape stereotypes. *International Journal of Obesity, 19*, 423–430.

Hoerr, S. L., Kallen, D., & Kwantes, M. (1995). Peer acceptance of obese youth: A way to improve weight control efforts? *Ecology of Food and Nutrition, 33*, 203–213.

Horchner, R., Tuinebreijer, W. E., Kelder, H., & Urk, E. (2002). Coping behavior and loneliness among obese patients. *Obesity Surgery, 12*, 864–868.

Janssen, I., Craig, W. M., Boyce, W. F., & Pickett, W. (2004). Associations between overweight and obesity with bullying behaviors in school-aged children. *Pediatrics, 113*, 1187–1194.

Jarvie, G. J., Lahey, B., Graziano, W., & Framer, E. (1983). Childhood obesity: What we know and what we don't know. *Developmental Review, 2*, 237–273.

Joanisse, L., & Synnott, A. (1999). Fighting back: Reactions and resistance to the stigma of obesity. In J. Sobal & D. Maurer (Eds.), *Interpreting weight: The social management of fatness and thinness* (pp. 49–70). Hawthorne, NY: Aldine de Gruyter.

Kallen, D. J., & Doughty, A. (1984). The relationship of weight, the self-perception of weight, and self esteem with courtship behavior. *Marriage and Family Review, 7*, 93–114.

Karris, L. (1977). Prejudice against obese renters. *Journal of Social Psychology, 101*, 159–160.

Kelsey, K., Earp, J. L., & Kirkley, B. G. (1997). Is social support beneficial for dietary change? A review of the literature. *Family and Community Health, 20*, 70–82.

Kinston, W., Loader, P., & Miller, L. (1987). Emotional health of families and their members when a child is obese. *Journal of Psychosomatic Research, 31*, 583–599.

Kinston, W., Loader, P., Miller, L., & Rein, L. (1988). Interaction in families with obese children. *Journal of Psychosomatic Research, 32*, 513–532.

Klassen, M. L., Clayson, D., & Jasper, C. R. (1996). Perceived effect of a salesperson's stigmatized appearance on store image: An experimental study of students' perceptions. *International Review of Retail, Distribution, and Consumer Research, 6*, 216–224.

Klesges, R. C., Klem, M. L., & Klesges, L. M. (1992). The relationship between changes in body weight and changes in psychosocial functioning. *Appetite, 19*, 145–153.

Kolotkin, R. L., Crosby, R. D., Kosloski, K. D., & Williams, G. R. (2001). Development of a brief measure to assess quality of life in obesity. *Obesity Research, 9*, 102–111.

Kuskowska-Wolk, A., & Rossner, S. (1990). Decreased social activity in obese adults. In S. Baba & P. Zimmet (Eds.), *World data book of obesity* (pp. 265–269). New York: Elsevier.

Latner, J. D., & Stunkard, A. J. (2003). Getting worse: The stigmatization of obese children. *Obesity Research, 11*, 452–456.

Lewis, R. J., Cash, T. F., Jacobi, L., & Bubb-Lewis, C. (1997). Prejudice toward fat people: The development and validation of the antifat attitudes test. *Obesity Research, 5*, 297–307.

Margolin, L., & White, L. (1987). The continuing role of physical attractiveness in marriage. *Journal of Marriage and the Family, 49*, 21–27.

Mathews, V., & Westie, C. (1966). A preferred method for obtaining rankings: Reactions to physical handicaps. *American Sociological Review, 31*, 851–854.

McLean, N., Griffin, S., Toney, K., & Hardeman, W. (2003). Family involvement in weight control, weight maintenance, and weight-loss interventions: A systematic review of randomized trials. *International Journal of Obesity, 27,* 987–1005.

Miller, C. T., Rothblum, E. D., Brand, P. A., & Felicio, D. M. (1995). Do obese women have poorer social relationships than nonobese women? Reports by self, friends, and coworkers. *Journal of Personality, 63*, 65–85.

Millman, M. (1980). *Such a pretty face: Being fat in America.* New York: Norton.

Myers, A., & Rosen, J. C. (1999). Obesity stigmatization and coping: Relation to mental health systems, body image, and self-esteem. *International Journal of Obesity, 23*, 221–230.

Neumark-Sztainer, D., Falkner, N., Story, M., Perry, C., Hannan, P. J., & Mulert, S. (2002). Weight-teasing among adolescents: Correlations with weight status and disordered eating. *International Journal of Obesity, 26*, 123–131.

O'Hara, M. D. (1996). Please weight to be seated: Recognizing obesity as a disability to prevent discrimination in public accommodations. *Whittier Law Review, 17,* 895–954.

Parham, E. S. (1993). Enhancing social support in weight loss management groups. *Journal of the American Dietetic Association, 93*, 1152–1156.

Parham, E. S. (1999). Meanings of weight among dietitians and nutritionists. In J. Sobal & D. Maurer (Eds.), *Weighty issues: Fatness and thinness as social problems* (pp. 183–205). Hawthorne, NY: Aldine de Gruyter.

Pauley, L. L. (1989). Customer weight as a variable in salespersons' response time. *Journal of Social Psychology, 129*, 713–714.

Pearce, M., Boegers, J., & Prinstein, M. J. (2002). Adolescent obesity, overt and relational peer victimization, and romantic relationships. *Obesity Research, 10*, 386–393.

Phillips, R. G., & Hill, A. J. (1998). Fat, plain, but not friendless: Self-esteem and peer acceptance of obese pre-adolescent girls. *International Journal of Obesity, 22*, 287–293.

Puhl, R., & Brownell, K. D. (2001). Bias, discrimination, and obesity. *Obesity Research, 9,* 788–805.

Puhl, R., & Brownell, K. D. (2003). Psychosocial origins of obesity stigma: Toward changing a powerful and pervasive bias. *Obesity Reviews, 4,* 213–227.

Rand, C. W., & MacGregor, A. M. C. (1990). Morbidly obese patients' perceptions of social discrimination before and after surgery for obesity. *Southern Medical Journal, 83,* 1391–1395.

Regan, P. C. (1996). Sexual outcasts: The perceived impact of body and gender on sexuality. *Journal of Applied Social Psychology, 26,* 1803–1815.

Roberts, J. V., & Herman, C. P. (1986). The psychology of height: An empirical review. In C. P. Herman, M. P. Zanna, & E. T. Higgins (Eds.), *Physical appearance, stigma, and social behavior* (pp. 113–142). Hillsdale, NJ: Erlbaum.

Sallade, J. (1973). A comparison of psychological adjustment of obese and nonobese children. *Journal of Psychosomatic Research, 17,* 89–96.

Sarlio-Lahteenkorva, S., & Lahelma, E. (1999). The association of body mass index with social and economic disadvantage in women and men. *International Journal of Epidemiology, 28*, 445–449.

Schumaker, J. F., Krejci, R. C., Small, L., & Sargent, R. G. (1985). Experience of loneliness by obese individuals. *Psychological Reports, 57*, 1147–1154.

Sitton, S., & Blanchard, S. (1995). Men's preferences in romantic partners: Obesity vs. addiction. *Psychological Reports, 77*, 1185–1186.

Sobal, J. (1984). Marriage, obesity and dieting. *Marriage and Family Review, 7*, 115–140.

Sobal, J. (1991). Obesity and nutritional sociology: A model for coping with the stigma of obesity. *Clinical Sociology Review, 9*, 125–141.

Sobal, J. (1999). The size acceptance movement and the social construction of body weight. In J. Sobal & D. Maurer (Eds.), *Weighty issues: Fatness and thinness as social problems* (pp. 231–249). Hawthorne, NY: Aldine de Gruyter.

Sobal, J. (2004). Sociological analysis of the stigmatisation of obesity. In J. Germov & L. Williams (Eds.), *A sociology of food and nutrition: Introducing the social appetite* (2nd ed., pp 383–402). Melbourne, Australia: Oxford University Press.

Sobal, J., & Bursztyn, M. (1998). Dating people with anorexia nervosa and bulimia: Attitudes and beliefs of university students. *Women and Health, 27*, 73–88.

Sobal, J., & Devine, C. (1997). Social aspects of obesity: Influences, consequences, assessments, and interventions. In S. Dalton (Ed.), *Overweight and weight management* (pp. 289–308). Gaithersburg, MD: ASPEN.

Sobal, J., Nicolopoulos, V., & Lee, J. (1995). Attitudes about weight and dating among secondary school students. *International Journal of Obesity, 19*, 376–381.

Sobal, J., Rauschenbach, B., & Frongillo, E. (1992). Marital status, fatness, and obesity. *Social Science and Medicine, 35*, 915–923.

Sobal, J., Rauschenbach, B. S., & Frongillo, E. A. (1995). Obesity and marital quality: Analysis of weight, marital unhappiness, and marital problems in a U.S. national sample. *Journal of Family Issues, 16*, 768–786.

Sobal, J., Rauschenbach, B. S., & Frongillo, E. A. (2003). Marital status changes and body weight changes: A U.S. longitudinal analysis. *Social Science and Medicine 56*, 1543–1555.

Stack, S. (1996). The effect of physical attractiveness on video dating outcomes. *Sociological Focus, 29*, 83–85.

Staffieri, J. R. (1967). A study of social stereotype of body image in children. *Journal of Personality and Social Psychology, 7*, 101–104.

Strauss, C. C., Smith, K., Frame, C., & Forehand, R. (1985). Personal and interpersonal characteristics associated with childhood obesity. *Journal of Pediatric Psychology, 10*, 337–343.

Strauss, R. S., & Pollack, H. A. (2003). Social marginalization of overweight children. *Archives of Pediatric and Adolescent Children, 157*, 746–752.

Surtees, P. G., Wainwright, N. W. J., & Khaw, K-T. (2004). Obesity, confidant support and functional health: Cross-sectional evidence from the EPIC-Norfolk cohort. *International Journal of Obesity, 28*, 748–758.

Tiggemann, M., & Rothblum, E. D. (1988). Gender differences in social consequences of perceived overweight in the United States and Australia. *Sex Roles, 18*, 75–86.

Valtolina, G. G., & Marta, E. (1998). Family relations and psychosocial risk in families with an obese adolescent. *Psychological Reports, 83*, 251–260.

Venes, A. M., Krupka, L. R., & Gerard, R. J. (1982). Overweight/obese patients. *Practitioner, 226,* 1102–1109.

Wardle, J., Volz, C., & Golding, C. (1995). Social variation in attitudes to obesity in children. *International Journal of Obesity, 19*, 562–569.

Way, K. (1995). Never too rich . . . or too thin: The role of stigma in the social construction of anorexia nervosa. In D. Maurer & J. Sobal (Eds.), *Eating agendas: Food and nutrition as social problems* (pp. 91–113). Hawthorne, NY: Aldine de Gruyter.

Wellman, B., & Berkowitz, S. D. (Eds.). (1988). *Social structures: A network approach.* New York: Cambridge University Press.

Zdrodwski, D. (1996). Eating out: The experience of eating in public for the "overweight" woman. *Women's Studies International Forum, 19*, 665–674.

CHAPTER 12

■ ■ ■

Self-Esteem and the Stigma of Obesity

JENNIFER CROCKER
JULIE A. GARCIA

Americans are becoming increasingly overweight. Currently, 127 million (64.5%) adults in the United States are overweight, 60 million (30.5% of all adults) are obese, and 9 million (4.7% of all adults) are severely obese (American Obesity Association, 2002). Yet even as more Americans become overweight, the standard for attractiveness is thin and fit (Fallon, 1990), and overweight people are stereotyped as lazy, lacking self-discipline, and mentally slow (Allon, 1982). As the chapters in this volume document, people who are overweight face discrimination in employment, housing, and relationships. In contrast to many stigmatizing conditions, overweight persons are stigmatized by close others, including friends and family members. Even parents discriminate against their overweight children; one study found that parents of overweight daughters were willing to pay less money for their daughter's college education than parents of normal-weight daughters (Crandall, 1995). Even the overweight themselves dislike people who are overweight (Crandall, 1994).

Our goal in this chapter is to examine the implications for self-esteem of stigmatization of the overweight. In light of the harsh stereotypes and discrimination they face, it seems sensible to assume that overweight people internalize these negative views and suffer from low self-esteem. Yet studies comparing the self-esteem of overweight and normal-weight people have yielded mixed results (see Friedman & Brownell, 1995; Jarvie, Lahey, Graziano, & Framer, 1983, for reviews).

A recent meta-analysis found that, across studies, the correlation between *self-perceived weight* and self-esteem was much stronger ($r = -.34$) than the correlation between *actual* weight and self-esteem ($r = -.12$; Miller & Downey, 1999), suggesting that in some cases low self-esteem may cause people to see themselves as overweight, rather than the stigma of overweight causing them to have low self-esteem. There is considerable variability in the self-esteem of overweight people; some people are very vulnerable to the stigma of overweight, whereas others seem unfazed by it. Our first aim, then, is to explore what makes some overweight people vulnerable to low self-esteem, and how other overweight people protect their self-esteem in the face of stigma and discrimination.

Our second aim is to explore the consequences of both the beliefs and strategies that make some overweight people vulnerable to low self-esteem, and the beliefs and strategies that protect the self-esteem of other overweight people. We argue that whether or not overweight persons deflect stigma and protect self-esteem, or internalize it and damage self-esteem, there are costs for both the self and others. Essentially, we suggest that there are costs when overweight people *question* whether their weight makes them worthless, regardless of whether their ultimate resolution to this question is favorable or unfavorable to the self. Our third aim is to suggest how overweight people can respond to stigma in a way that enables them to achieve their most important goals.

VULNERABILITY AND PROTECTIVE FACTORS

Why do some overweight people have self-esteem that is vulnerable to stigma, and what makes other people resilient to this stigma? In our research, we have explored three types of beliefs that predict whether overweight people internalize stigma or deflect it: whether negative reactions from others are attributed to prejudice and discrimination, the perceived controllability of weight (and related beliefs), and beliefs about what one must be or do to have value and worth.

Attributions to Prejudice

Our first research on self-esteem and stigma of overweight was part of a broader program of research testing the hypothesis that when stigmatized people experience negative outcomes such as rejection or discrimination, their self-esteem is protected when they attribute the negative outcome to prejudice instead of to their own personal lack of deservingness (Crocker & Major, 1989). In research examining the effects of a male evaluator's criticism of an essay on women and a white student's social rejection of a black student, we found that students who could attribute the negative outcome to gender or racial prejudice had more positive affect and higher self-esteem after receiving negative feedback than those who could not attribute it to prejudice (Crocker, Voelkl, Testa, & Major, 1991). This research was consistent with our idea that attributing negative events to prejudice protects the self-esteem of stigmatized people.

When we extended this research to overweight women, however, the results suggested a more complex story (Crocker, Cornwell, & Major, 1993). When overweight women who were rejected for a potential date by a male peer attributed the rejection to their weight, their self-esteem was not protected. Specifically, overweight women who were rejected by a male evaluator were more likely to attribute their rejection to their weight, and to the man's concern with appearance, than normal-weight women who were rejected, or overweight or normal-weight women who were not rejected. However, despite recognizing the role of weight in his rejection of them, overweight women who were rejected felt more depressed and hostile, were marginally more anxious, and had lower appearance self-esteem than overweight women who were not rejected, or normal-weight women who were rejected.

Considering the pattern of results across studies, we reasoned that for black individuals and women, attributing negative outcomes to race or gender is equivalent to attributing them to the other person's sexism or racial prejudice. In fact, for black participants, attributions to "my race," "the other person's racism," and "the other's discrimination" were highly correlated and combined into a single index with good internal consistency ($\alpha = .73$). Although it may seem obvious, it is quite significant that these black students thought that someone who rejected them because of their race was racist and exhibited discrimination. Apparently, rejecting someone because of race is, on its face, illegitimate and racist (Crocker & Major, 1994), so black individuals' self-esteem does not suffer. However, overweight women do not seem to reason the same way about their weight. They believe that when they are rejected for a potential date by a man who is aware of their weight, a major cause of his response is their weight. However, they do not seem to view this response as illegitimate. Instead, they seem to think that being overweight makes them unattractive and less deserving, and therefore is a legitimate reason for rejection. Their self-esteem suffers as a result of this attribution.

Perceived Controllability of Weight

What is the difference between weight and race that accounts for this different response to rejection? Unlike race or gender, weight is seen as an attribute over which people have control (Crandall, 1994; Weiner,

Perry, & Magnusson, 1988). Despite considerable evidence that biological mechanisms make weight loss extremely difficult, overweight people are stereotyped as lazy, self-indulgent, and lacking self-discipline, and are held accountable for their weight and therefore for negative outcomes that follow from it. Rejection of an overweight person, then, is seen as justifiable, and not an instance of prejudice.

We hypothesized that if overweight women could be convinced that weight is not controllable, they would be more likely to attribute rejection to weight prejudice, and this would protect their self-esteem. Amato, Crocker, and Major (1995) tested this hypothesis in a study in which overweight and normal-weight women were rejected by a male, and their beliefs about the controllability of weight were manipulated by having them read a pseudoscientific summary of research, arguing either that the preponderance of evidence shows that weight is a function of calories consumed and calories expended (i.e., controllable), or that weight is a function of biological mechanisms such as set-points and therefore is almost impossible to change over the long-term (i.e., not controllable). As predicted, overweight women who read that weight is not controllable were more likely to attribute the rejection to weight prejudice, and had higher self-esteem, than overweight women who read that weight is controllable, or normal-weight women in either condition. Interestingly, overweight women who were told that weight is not controllable had more negative affect than any of the other three groups, perhaps because it made them hopeless about losing weight in the future. Thus, believing that weight is not controllable seems to be a double-edged sword; on one hand, it encourages overweight people to interpret rejection as revealing prejudice, instead of a personal failing, and this protects self-esteem. On the other hand, it may create a sense of powerlessness or hopelessness about the prospect of weight loss.

The Protestant Ethic

In light of evidence that beliefs about the controllability of weight are central to recognizing weight prejudice, and therefore protecting self-esteem, we examined what makes overweight people more likely to believe that weight is controllable, and therefore vulnerable to low self-esteem. Crandall and Reser (Chapter 6, this volume), show that conservative political ideologies and endorsement of the Protestant ethic are linked generally to beliefs about personal responsibility, and specifically to the belief that weight is controllable; these beliefs predict dislike of overweight people (even among the overweight themselves). In line with these findings, Quinn and Crocker (1999) found that among normal-weight and overweight women, endorsement of the Protestant ethic was significantly related to belief in the controllability of weight and dislike of the overweight. The implications of these beliefs for self-esteem depended on whether the women considered themselves to be normal weight, somewhat overweight, or very overweight. As expected, among normal-weight women, greater endorsement of the Protestant ethic predicted higher self-esteem. Among somewhat overweight women, there was no relationship between endorsement of the Protestant ethnic and self-esteem. Finally, among women who thought they were very overweight, greater endorsement of the Protestant ethic predicted lower self-esteem. Beliefs about the controllability of weight showed similar effects to Protestant ethic; beliefs about controllability predicted higher self-esteem in normal-weight women, and lower self-esteem in (self-perceived) very overweight women. To our surprise, the effects of endorsing the Protestant ethic on self-esteem were not explained by its association with controllability beliefs; to the contrary, when we examined both beliefs simultaneously, only the Protestant ethic explained self-esteem differences among overweight and normal-weight women. Perhaps the moralistic judgment inherent in endorsement of the Protestant ethic, more than controllability per se, accounts for its effects on self-esteem in overweight women.

Of course, the results of this study are correlational, so it is impossible to draw conclusions about whether endorsement of the Protestant ethic causes overweight women to have low self-esteem. We examined this issue in two studies in which we manipulated the salience of the Protestant ethic and related beliefs by having participants read essays. Ideological messages about the importance of self-discipline and the rewards of hard work hurt the self-esteem of overweight women, whereas messages that are more inclusive or encourage relaxing and savoring life have beneficial effects (Jambekar, Quinn, & Crocker, 2001). This research suggests that self-blame for weight, associated with beliefs about controllability, not recognizing weight prejudice, and Protestant ethic beliefs contribute to low self-esteem in the overweight, and that it is probably the moral judgment, and not merely the controllability beliefs per se, that account for this effect.

Externally Contingent Self-Worth

A different vulnerability factor explored in our research on stigma and self-esteem is externally contingent self-worth. As William James (1890) argued over a century ago, people differ in what they believe they must be or do to have value and worth as a person. People may base their self-esteem on a wide range of things; some people base their self-esteem on being virtuous, others on academic competence, and still others on approval and regard from others, or their physical appearance (Crocker, Luhtanen, Cooper, & Bouvrette, 2003). Crocker and Wolfe (2001) hypothesized that people with external sources of self-esteem, who depend on other people for self-worth, should be particularly vulnerable to stigma. Quinn and Crocker (1998) provided support for this hypothesis in a survey of college women; for all participants, the more they based their self-esteem on others' approval, the lower their level of self-esteem, but this effect was more pronounced for overweight than for normal-weight women.

Because weight is an important aspect of appearance, especially for women, it seems likely that basing self-esteem on one's appearance would be a particular risk factor for women. Indeed, women who base their self-esteem on their appearance, particularly those who report that their self-esteem drops when they do not look good (as opposed to rising when they look good), have lower self-esteem, more symptoms of depression, and more symptoms of disordered eating (Power & Crocker, 2004). Interestingly, men whose self-esteem was based on their appearance showed significantly fewer psychological problems than women whose self-esteem was based on appearance. Although we did not include a measure of actual or self-perceived weight in this study, other data suggest that college women, on average, believe that they are far from the cultural ideal for their gender, particularly with respect to being thin and beautiful (Sanchez & Crocker, 2005). Men in our study, on the other hand, rated themselves as meeting or exceeding the cultural ideal for men. In sum, because women (even the young, healthy, and generally affluent college freshmen in our sample) believe that their bodies fall short of the ideal, they are vulnerable to a range of psychological problems, including low self-esteem, when they base their self-esteem on appearance, and particularly when they report drops in appearance when they think they do not look good. In a subsequent study we found that the more that women based their self-esteem on appearance, the higher they scored on body shame (r = .64), body dissatisfaction (r = .54), and drive for thinness (r = .60) (Crocker, Stein, & Luhtanen, 2004).

In sum, for all women, and particularly for women who feel overweight, basing self-esteem on external sources such as appearance and others' approval appears to be a vulnerability factor for low self-esteem.

THE STIGMA OF OVERWEIGHT AND THE EGO GAP

In our view, at the heart of all of these findings on the stigma of overweight and self-esteem is something we call the "ego gap," which refers to a psychological state wherein people are focused on and concerned about their self-worth, and feel some uncertainty about whether they are worthy or worthless. When people are caught in the ego gap, they have reasons to think that they are wonderful and worthy, but they also have reasons to think that they are worthless. Thinking in the ego gap tends to be "all-or-nothing"; either I'm competent or incompetent, good or evil, worthy of love or not. As Stone, Patton, and Heen (1999) put it,

> The primary peril of all-or-nothing thinking is that it leaves our identity extremely unstable, making us hypersensitive to feedback. When faced with negative information about ourselves, all-or-nothing thinking gives us only two choices for how to manage that information, both of which cause serious problems. Either we try to deny the information that is inconsistent with our self-image, or we do the opposite: we take in the information in a way that exaggerates its importance to a crippling degree. (p. 114)

In the context of the stigma of overweight, negative stereotypes and cultural images as well as ideologies like the Protestant ethic suggest that overweight people deserve their negative outcomes because they are responsible for their weight. The stigma, when it is salient, raises questions about one's worth and value. The problem is that this binary choice—either "my weight is my fault, I deserve to be rejected, and therefore I'm worthless," or "my weight is not my fault, I don't deserve to be rejected, and therefore the other person is bad" (or bigoted or unfair)—is a limited and limiting set of options, with costs no matter which option prevails. When overweight people conclude that they are worthless, the costs in terms of psychological well-being are obvious. But there are also costs in terms of life goals and relationships that overweight persons let go of because they feel worthless, as well as costs to others, as the low self-esteem, depression, and sometimes disordered eating become burdens to others as well as the self. On the other hand, those overweight people who blame their negative outcomes on others' prejudice may protect their self-esteem, but their blaming attitude makes others feel accused and defensive, which creates conflict and separation, and ultimately has costs for the overweight person as well.

In both cases, the most important cost, in our view, is that when overweight people (or anyone, for that matter) question whether they are worthy or worthless, they are disconnected from reality and blinded to the real issues they face. They are disconnected from the reality that all human beings are flawed, nonperfect, capable of making mistakes, with strengths and weaknesses. When overweight people question their worth and value, they have difficulty recognizing that the reality is that they are human and therefore have real issues to address in their lives, some of which might concern their weight, but others of which have nothing to do with their weight. For example, perhaps the overweight person who is rejected for a job is discriminated against, but also there are almost certainly areas in which his or her job skills could be improved, because everyone has room for improvement. Perhaps the overweight woman is rejected for a date because a man is prejudiced against her, but there might also be areas in which she could improve her ability to connect with people, because strides can often be made in this domain.

To clarify, we are not suggesting that discrimination against the overweight is not a reality. Unfortunately, in our society people are inundated with messages extolling the value of beauty and thinness, and, as the chapters in this volume document, prejudice and discrimination against overweight and obese persons are very real. Rather, we suggest that when overweight people respond to stigmatization by questioning whether their weight makes them worthless (when self-esteem becomes a goal) there are already costs (Crocker & Park, 2004). Regardless of whether they blame rejection on the self or the other, or whether such attributions lead to higher or lower self-esteem, being caught in this binary choice distracts from other, more important goals.

RECOMMENDATIONS AND CONCLUSIONS

From this vantage point, we propose that the solution to the self-threat inherent in the stigma of overweight is not to vigilantly search for weight prejudice, nor is it to decide that one's weight is not controllable, nor is it to abandon ideologies about personal responsibility or the Protestant ethic. We also do not think it is realistic, in our culture, to abandon the belief that one's worth and value depends on one's physical appearance. Instead, we suggest the solution is to stop worrying about self-esteem, and to refrain from asking the question of whether being overweight makes one worthless. We recommend shifting away from a focus on "What does it mean about me?" or "What do they think about me?" or "Does my weight discredit me as a human being?" Instead, we suggest that people focus on what they need to learn about the real issues they face, and what can they do about them, as well as what they want to contribute to their relationships, to the organizations they work for, or to the world. The solution to the problem of low self-esteem may be to focus on something larger than the self, and what one wants to create or contribute.

REFERENCES

Allon, N. (1982). The stigma of overweight in everyday life. In B. Wolman (Ed.), *Psychological aspects of obesity: A handbook* (pp. 130–174). New York: Van Nostrand Reinhold.

Amato, M., Crocker, J., & Major, B. (1995, August). *The stigma of overweight and self-esteem: The role of perceived control.* Paper presented at the annual meeting of the American Psychological Association, New York.

American Obesity Association. (2002). *Obesity in the U.S.* Retrieved July 19, 2004, from www.obesity.org/subs/fastfacts/obesity_US.shtml

Crandall, C. S. (1994). Prejudice against fat people: Ideology and self-interest. *Journal of Personality and Social Psychology, 66*, 882–894.

Crandall, C. S. (1995). Do parents discriminate against their heavyweight daughters? *Personality and Social Psychology Bulletin, 21*, 724–735.

Crocker, J., Cornwell, B., & Major, B. M. (1993). The stigma of overweight: Affective consequences of attributional ambiguity. *Journal of Personality and Social Psychology, 64*, 60–70.

Crocker, J., Luhtanen, R., Cooper, M. L., & Bouvrette, S. A. (2003). Contingencies of self-worth in college students: Measurement and theory. *Journal of Personality and Social Psychology, 85*, 894–908.

Crocker, J., & Major, B. M. (1989). Social stigma and self-esteem: The self-protective properties of stigma. *Psychological Review, 96*, 608–630.

Crocker, J., & Major, B. M. (1994). Reactions to stigma: The moderating role of justifications. In M. P. Zanna & J. M. Olson (Eds.), *The psychology of prejudice: The Ontario Symposium* (Vol. 7, pp. 289–314). Hillsdale, NJ: Erlbaum.

Crocker, J., & Park, L. E. (2004). The costly pursuit of self-esteem. *Psychological Bulletin, 130*, 392–414.

Crocker, J., Stein, K. F., & Luhtanen, R. K. (2004). *Contingent self-worth, self-schemas, and symptoms of eating disorders in college women.* Unpublished manuscript, University of Michigan, Ann Arbor.

Crocker, J., Voelkl, K., Testa, M., & Major, B. M. (1991). Social stigma: Affective consequences of attributional ambiguity. *Journal of Personality and Social Psychology, 60*, 218–228.

Crocker, J., & Wolfe, C. T. (2001). Contingencies of self-worth. *Psychological Review, 108*, 593–623.

Fallon, A. (1990). Culture in the mirror: Sociocultural determinants of body image. In T. F. Cash & T. Pruzinsky (Eds.), *Body images: Development, deviance, and change* (pp. 80–109). New York: Guilford Press.

Friedman, M. A., & Brownell, K. D. (1995). Psychological correlates of obesity: Moving to the next research generation. *Psychological Bulletin, 117*, 3–20.

Jambekar, S., Quinn, D. M., & Crocker, J. (2001). The effects of feeling overweight and achievement on the self-esteem and mood of women. *Psychology of Women Quarterly, 25*, 48–56.

James, W. (1890). *The principles of psychology* (Vol. 1). Cambridge, MA: Harvard University Press.

Jarvie, G. J., Lahey, B., Graziano, W., & Framer, E. (1983). Childhood obesity and social stigma: What we know and what we don't know. *Developmental Review, 3*, 237–273.

Miller, C. T., & Downey, K. T. (1999). A meta-analysis of heavyweight and self-esteem. *Personality and Social Psychology Review, 3*, 68–84.

Power, C. M., & Crocker, J. (2004). *Ups and downs of self-esteem: Appearance contingencies and psychological well-being of male and female college students.* Unpublished manuscript, University of Michigan, Ann Arbor.

Quinn, D. M., & Crocker, J. (1998). Vulnerability to the affective consequences of the stigma of overweight. In J. S. C. Stangor (Ed.), *Prejudice: The target's perspective* (pp. 125–143). San Diego, CA: Academic Press.

Quinn, D. M., & Crocker, J. (1999). When ideology hurts: Effects of feeling fat and the Protestant ethic on the psychological well-being of women. *Journal of Personality and Social Psychology, 77*, 402–414.

Sanchez, D. M., & Crocker, J. (2005). Why investment in gender ideals affects well-being: The role of external contingencies and gender discrepancies. *Psychology of Women Quarterly, 29*, 63–77.

Stone, D., Patton, B., & Heen, S. (1999). *Difficult conversations: How to discuss what matters most.* New York: Penguin.

Weiner, B., Perry, R. P., & Magnusson, J. (1988). An attributional analysis of reactions to stigma. *Journal of Personality and Social Psychology, 55*, 738–748.

CHAPTER 13

■ ■ ■

Personal Reflections on Bias, Stigma, Discrimination, and Obesity

CAROL A. JOHNSON

> People who are affected with overweight and obesity are often victims of stigmatization and discrimination. It is time to stop blaming the victim. Many obesity researchers believe that people who struggle with their weight are pushing against thousands of years of evolution that has selected for storing energy as fat in times of plenty for use in times of scarcity. It is time to recognize their struggle, understand their challenges and support their need for lifelong efforts to achieve better health.
>
> —CENTERS FOR DISEASE CONTROL AND PREVENTION (2004)

MY WEIGHT EVOLUTION

I was a big gal upon arrival. At 6 months, I had already been pronounced "too heavy" by the medical profession. Since it is not likely for a 6-month old infant to be raiding the refrigerator at 3 A.M., or eating to numb the pain of a relationship gone sour, it seems to me that my genes were already programmed to produce a Rubenesque edition. Pictures of me as a toddler reveal a pudgy, apple-cheeked, cheerful tot. Little did I know at that point what lay in store for me, all because of numbers on a scale.

The genetic determinants of weight are evident in my family. Both of my grandmothers were large women, as was my dad. Assorted aunts, uncles, and cousins are also of the larger persuasion. Of my immediate family, only my mother escaped the "battle of the bulge."

As soon as my mother realized I was destined for grandeur of size, she monitored my food intake carefully. Let the dieting begin! The doctor recommended a 1,200-calorie diet. Feeling that he was the expert and wanting to do what was best for me, my mom went along. I began toting brown-bag lunches to school—often containing a sandwich, celery and carrot sticks, and a piece of fruit. Well-balanced, yes—but by the end of the school day I was hungry. So when my friends wanted to stop at the soda fountain for an ice cream cone, I knew I shouldn't, but it was hard to resist. I came away feeling I had done something "bad."

I got plenty of activity. As a child, I was always outside "playing," and as a teenager, my friends and I would take endless walks with our transistor radios. I liked to swim as well as play badminton and volleyball. I had a good appetite, but would not have met the criteria for binge-eating disorder. Although I did occasionally indulge in unauthorized "goodies," I was not eating excessively—no more than what my friends appeared to be eating. I just wasn't eating little enough to lose weight.

Then something new appeared: over-the-counter diet pills. The ones I wanted to try were called Regimen Tablets. You had to take a fistful several times a day. I knew my mother wouldn't approve, so I got an older friend to buy them for me. I waited for the weight to melt away, but pretty soon it became evident that I was not going to "thaw." I tossed them.

Liquid diet shakes are nothing new. We had Metrecal. Eating one meal a day seemed like a surefire way to lose weight—and it was so easy! A can for breakfast, a can for lunch, and a "balanced dinner." OK, I thought. I can do that. And I did. But, once again, I was so hungry by the end of the school day that the ice cream parlor became my oasis on the way home to my "balanced dinner."

A visit to the doctor prior to my junior year resulted in a prescription for amphetamine diet pills (something relatively new at the time). I dropped 40 pounds over the summer, and returned to school in a size 14—as opposed to a size 18—dress. I was also a sleep-deprived, nonstop talking, whirlwind of activity, subject to occasional spells of paranoia—probably because when I told the doctor the pills were losing their effect, he told me to double the dose. When I finally stopped taking the pills, I quickly reacquired the weight, as well as a bout of depression.

By the time I graduated from high school, I exceeded my chart weight by about 40 pounds. In retrospect, I wish I had been advised simply to stabilize my weight during my high school years. I think I could have handled that. Instead, I continued to ride the diet merry-go-round for many more years, and after every diet, I gained back more weight than I lost. With each of these episodes, there was the implication that I was a "failure" and my self-esteem plummeted.

EARLY LESSONS IN WEIGHT DISCRIMINATION

My earliest memories of realizing that I was "different," and in a way that would not be good, can be traced to grade school teasing. "Carol the Barrel," they called me. The difference became even more apparent when I pleaded for the same clothing styles the thinner girls were wearing, but found out no one made them in my size. The message seemed to be: "You shouldn't be the size that you are, so we won't make any cute clothes for you in that size." I often ended up in tears after a shopping trip that produced a bag of matronly looking outfits that looked more like something my grandmother would wear.

Then there was the "weigh-in" at school—which it appears is being resurrected today (or maybe it never died). I dreaded those days—and sometimes convinced my parents that I was too sick to go to school that day. We lined up behind the scales. The kids right behind me could usually see what I weighed, chuckled, and told everyone else. Generally, the teacher would advise me that I weighed too much. What I heard was "These scales tell us that there is something wrong with you." I can't imagine why schools feel the need to do this. Overweight children already *know* that they are considered too heavy. They have been told enough times, in enough ways. They don't need scales or calipers to reinforce it. It is just one more way of chipping away at the child's self-esteem and creating yet another opportunity for stigma to thrive.

By junior high school, I learned that most boys didn't want to date a larger girl. Even if they did, most wouldn't because their fends would tease them about being with "that fat girl." I sat along the wall at a lot of house parties and a lot of school dances—a "wallflower," but definitely not by choice. A boy that I liked told my cousin he would like me too—if I lost weight.

WEIGHT DISCRIMINATION: UP CLOSE AND PERSONAL

One of my dreams was to be a cheerleader. When tryouts were announced in the seventh grade, I signed up immediately and practiced night and day. After tryouts, I knew I had given a flawless performance. It was not to be, however. The physical education teacher, who was judging the competition, took me aside and gently told me that although

I was one of the best candidates, she simply could not choose me. The reason? I was too chubby. My body was unacceptable for public display.

Shortly thereafter, I became fascinated by the baton and decided to take twirling lessons. The cheerleading episode could have deterred me, but somehow it didn't. I felt awkward at first, but soon the baton seemed like an extension of my arm and I graduated to more complicated routines—such as high tosses and twirling two batons at once. I dreamed of leading the marching band down the football field. Adept as I had become, I thought maybe this time my dream would become reality. Reality did set in, but not the one I had dreamed about. Once again, I was trying to do something that chubby girls weren't supposed to do—put themselves on display. This time I didn't even try out. I was told not to bother because the uniforms wouldn't fit me. And the message pierced deeper: You're not acceptable for public viewing. The only exception to this decree occurred when the high school drama coach cast me in lead roles in all the class plays. Apparently, she believed that talent was more important than a svelte figure—and I thank Betty Jean O'Dell to this day!

I had an older cousin. We were very close. When she got married, I assumed I would be a "junior bridesmaid." It was decided by the bride's mother that this honor could be bestowed on me only if I lost weight. They wanted to be sure I would look good in the dress, of course. When I didn't lose as much weight as they thought I should, I was relegated to overseeing the guestbook. This kept me pretty much in the background and out of sight.

By the time I was a teenager, losing weight was the most important thing in my life. I truly believed, deep in my heart, that I was not as good as the thinner girls. Incidents of bias and discrimination had convinced me of that. Only by losing weight could I become their equal. Every summer vacation I vowed to lose weight by the time I returned to school in the fall. I tried my best but, except for the summer of amphetamines, it just didn't happen.

Maintaining a healthy lifestyle is not always easy for larger people due to the fact that the out of doors can be, for them, a very unfriendly, sometimes hostile environment. As a young adult, I did a lot of outdoor walking. One day some young boys rode by on their bicycles and said, "Hey, look—Twiggy of the TOPS Club!" Not long after, a carload of teenage boys saw me walking, rolled down their windows and hollered, "You'd have to walk all the way around the world to walk that off." It's easy to say "Just ignore it," but not so easy for the person who has to continually muster the courage to go out and face such verbal assaults.

College provided a bit of a breather from the constant striving for an ideal shape. As the 1960s progressed, I was able to hide under a mane of long hair, fringe, and peace jewelry. I became a sociologist, partly in an attempt to understand and unearth the sociological roots of weight discrimination. It is a more difficult quest than I ever imagined!

I have not experienced a great deal of weight discrimination in my career, but sometimes things like this can catch you by surprise, as they did during my early days as a health planner. At a public hearing on our proposed regional health plan, a woman confronted me asking: "Why don't you practice what you preach?" She assumed that my ample size signified an unhealthy lifestyle—contrary to the tenets of our health plan. I was taken aback, and curtly assured her that I did look after my health. I'm sure she didn't believe me.

Since then, my career has been relatively free of weight discrimination. Why? I believe there are a couple reasons. First, I have spent a great deal of time working in a field that continually wages its own battles against stigma—mental health. Mental health advocates and practitioners have fought the battle of stigma in their own arena, and are keenly aware of its effects and consequences. It is not difficult for them to recognize the parallels with obesity and act as allies. Second, as I studied the obesity research and enhanced my own understanding of this condition, I was gradually able to absolve myself of blame and replace it with a new sense of confidence and purpose. I do not expect to be discriminated against, and perhaps this attitude helps to deflect or neutralize it.

"SECONDARY" OR "DERIVATIVE" WEIGHT DISCRIMINATION

One does not have to be the personal target of weight discrimination to feel its effects. I was very much affected by a phenomenon I call "secondary" or "derivative" weight discrimination. What this means is that I internalized discrimination that was not aimed at me personally. For example, every time I heard a comedian tell a fat joke, I felt sad—because even though the joke was not directed toward me as an individual, it demeaned people who looked like me. It meant that if they were laughable, so was I.

Then there would be comments such as "Did you see how fat Joan has gotten? She looks terrible." And I'd want to say, "Well, I guess that means I look terrible too because I'm about the same size as Joan." How about the size 8 woman who laments, "I'm getting so fat!" Then what does that make me, at a size 22?

Society expects you to feel inferior if you are overweight, and diet ads featuring "before" and "after" photos are the perfect case in point. The "before" weight loss people never have any self-confidence or self-respect. When they lose weight and become "after" people, their self-esteem soars. If you look like one of the "before" people, the assumption is that you must not feel very good about yourself. Indeed there is research showing that "before and after" diet ads enhance weight stigma and perpetuate damaging stereotypes (Geier, Schwartz, & Brownell, 2003).

"LOSE WEIGHT AND CALL ME IN THE MORNING": EXPERIENCES WITH HEALTH PROFESSIONALS

I have always had a tendency toward hypertension, but then so did my mother—and my grandmother. A physician told me that if I lost weight, my blood pressure would go down. I said I would certainly try, but what was I supposed to do in the meantime? I did not want to walk out of his office with untreated hypertension. I asked what he would do for a thin person with a similar problem. He said he would probably prescribe medication. I asked him to do me the same courtesy.

I don't especially like to be weighed, even though I know there are times, such as prior to anesthesia, that it becomes necessary. A routine office visit usually does not fall into that category. Nurses often act as though I am being "difficult" when I tell them I do not care to be weighed. Once particular nurse huffily retorted, "I'll just have to tell the doctor you refused to be weighed!" The doctor can tell at a glance that I am overweight. The scales become a kind of "overkill."

A few years back, I went to my gynecologist for my annual exam. The paper sheet they gave me as a cover-up was too small, and I felt humiliated. It was as though I had been given a dinner napkin to cover myself. The nurse said it was the only size they had. The next time I brought a bed sheet from home. The doctor looked quite surprised when he entered the room, only to find me engulfed in a floral sheet. I told him that until he got some larger cover-ups, I would be attired in my sheet. By the next visit, he had bigger wraps.

Likewise, when I went for a mammogram, the gown I was given didn't close, and I was partially exposed in front. The technician was apologetic, and said I should write a letter to the head of the department—which I did. The next time I went in the gown was still too small. I am convinced that the underlying rationale is "We don't feel a responsibility to provide larger gowns to people who wouldn't need them if they just took control of themselves and lost weight." I have summed up my feelings about weight discrimination in a piece I call "Is There a Name for This?" in Table 13.1.

TABLE 13.1. Is There a Name for This?

- Why did they call me names? I was a nice little girl. Is there a name for this?
- Why do comedians tell jokes about fat women? And why does everyone laugh? Is there a name for this?
- Why was I rejected for cheerleading? They said I was one of the best, but too chubby to be chosen. Is there a name for this?
- Why did they tell me I couldn't be a bridesmaid until I lost weight? Is there a name for this?
- Why am I supposed to hate myself until I reach my "ideal" weight? Is there a name for this?
- Why do I rarely see anyone who looks like me in women's magazines, on TV, or in the movies? Is there a name for this?
- Why do department stores stick "Women's World" in a drab, remote area of the store? Is there a name for this?
- Why can't all large people go to the theater or ride on a plane in comfort? Is there a name for this?
- Why was a job withheld from my friend because "we can't have you out in front"? Is there a name for this?

Yes, there is a name for this—the name is discrimination. Be sure to call it by its rightful name in the future.

Note. From Johnson (2001). Copyright 2001 by Gurze Books. Reprinted by permission.

EXPERIENCES OF LARGELY POSITIVE MEMBERS

I founded the organization, Largely Positive Inc., in 1987 to promote health, well-being, and self-esteem among larger people. During my years conducting Largely Positive support groups, I have heard many stories of weight discrimination from group members. Here are just a few:

- My friend Kari told of the day she parked in a handicapped parking spot at the mall—which she was entitled to do, as she had a handicapped sticker. For years, she had been plagued by severe knee and back problems. When she returned to her car, she found a note on her windshield saying, "Other than morbid obesity, what is your handicap?" This truly illustrates the extent to which many people not only misunderstand, but abhor, obesity. It is incidents like these that keep many larger people literally "in hiding." Venturing outside leaves them continually vulnerable to this type of abuse.
- Another friend, Mary, was in the grocery store shopping for her family, when a complete stranger stopped to examine the contents of her

shopping cart and told her, "You have a lot of things in there that you certainly don't need!"

■ Our member Roger was told by a complete stranger in a fast-food restaurant that watching him eat disgusted her. She thought it would be a good idea to segregate fat people in their own restaurants.

■ Our member Bonnie was denied employment as an aide in a facility for the developmentally disabled because of her weight—despite the fact that she had performed the sought-after job flawlessly several years earlier at essentially the same weight.

■ One of our support group facilitators, Wendy, is a market researcher. Not long ago she received a call from a prospective customer who wanted her firm to assemble "five women who eat oatmeal" for an oatmeal commercial. "Of course," the man said to her, "we can't have anyone who is overweight." Trying to remain professional, she asked, "Why is that?" "Because," he replied, "we do want people who are reasonably attractive." "Are you saying that large people aren't attractive?" she shot back. At this point he might have been starting to realize that he was speaking to a large woman on the phone. "Well, no," he said. "But we need people who look fit." Wendy's turn: "Are you saying that large people don't take care of themselves?" He: "Well, not exactly, but isn't that what people think?" Bull's-eye! This is precisely why you hardly ever see a large person in a commercial.

■ When our member Lori was a young girl, she attended a friend's birthday party. She was denied the cake and ice cream served to all the other little girls; the mother of the "birthday girl" told her she was too heavy and shouldn't eat that sort of thing.

A young girl, speaking at a weight-related conference I attended, said the most painful thing about being big was not teasing from peers but the attitudes of adults, because, she said, "They should have known better and loved me for me." Remarks by children or even teenagers can be chalked up to the fact that they're immature and still have a lot to learn. But a remark by an adult is not dismissed as easily. As children, we look to adults for answers, for truth, for affirmation of our worth, and to help us make sense of the world around us and the people in it. Adults should know better.

I asked Largely Positive members one evening what makes them most angry about the weight prejudice that exists in our culture. Some of their responses follow:

- "The view that you're a failure if you can't control your weight. I sometimes think the stigma is worse than that attached to people who break ethical and legal rules."

- "The assumption that if one is overweight, one doesn't 'deserve' to actively participate in social experiences like thin people."
- "Equating fat with lazy and lack of willpower and assuming we're not fit."
- "The assumption that we *could* be thin if we just didn't 'pig out.' "
- "The idea that large people don't care about themselves."
- "The fact that large people are looked down upon and not considered as smart as thin people."
- "The blaming, the scapegoating, the heaping of all kinds of negative qualities on people just because of their weight—often by complete strangers who are presumptuous enough to set themselves up as 'judges.' "
- "People look at your size and think you are lazy, stupid and out of control. They judge you on your size and don't take the time to see what you have to offer—especially in finding employment."
- "They treat us like we have no feelings, like we're just big lumps of blubber who don't think and feel like everyone else."

THE EFFECTS OF WEIGHT DISCRIMINATION: "I AM MY WEIGHT; MY WEIGHT IS ME"

The effects of weight discrimination are pervasive and can spill over into every aspect of one's life. The following are some of the effects of weight discrimination.

Limiting Potential by "Setting the Bar Too Low"

Because larger people are constantly bombarded with messages implying they should have no self-confidence, many end up believing it and scale back their aspirations. I'm particularly distressed by weight-loss testimonials—the ones accompanied by "before" and "after" pictures. The "before" picture depicts someone who was obviously told: "Go home and find the worst possible picture of yourself. Make sure you look as pitiful as possible and that you're wearing the most unflattering outfit you've ever owned." The "after" picture is the antithesis of the "before" picture—glowing smile, attractive clothes, upbeat attitude, confident stance. And the post-weight-loss interview usually goes something like this: "Now that I've lost weight, I feel so much better about myself. I have so much more confidence and self-esteem. I can do anything!"

Putting Life on Hold

Many larger people do set goals—goals they feel can only be achieved once they lose weight. I have seen many larger people put off career advancement opportunities, educational goals, travel plans—even buying attractive clothes—until they lose the necessary amount of weight. The sad fact is that many will never achieve the ideal weight they have set for themselves, which in turn will derail many of their other dreams. Society is also very much the loser—of all of this human potential.

Acceptance of Substandard Relationships

I once saw a bumper sticker that said "No fat chicks." Because larger people do tend to have more difficulty securing romantic relationships, they may "settle" for relationships that are far from ideal. I have seen women who tolerate a mate's verbal abuse of their bodies because they are afraid that they will never find anyone else to "love" them.

Avoidance of Public Exposure

Some larger people become quite literally afraid to go out of their houses for fear of ridicule and taunting. When they do go out, they may go to great lengths to hide their bodies. As a younger person, I often wore a heavy trench coat in the heat of summer to cover up my ample outline. The fear of going out in public also makes it more difficult for larger people to get adequate exercise.

Avoidance of Health Care

Disrespect by the medical community can cause many larger people to put off or completely shun health care, including preventive care. The financial costs of obesity are said to be high, but it would be interesting to investigate how much of this is due to reluctance to seek preventive care.

MY ENLIGHTENMENT

My personal moment of truth, or "enlightenment," came after reading *The Dieter's Dilemma* by William Bennett, MD, and Joel Gurin (1982). Say the authors: "Most of what we are routinely told about how fat is gained or lost is either wrong, misleading or meaningless" (p. 4). Bennett and Gurin went on to summarize what was known at that point about the biological and physiological underpinnings of obesity. They also made the statement: "You are not to blame" (p. 4). No one had ever said that to me before—not my doctors, not my teachers, not the popular press, no one! And I couldn't figure out why. It made me very angry at first—angry because had I known about this body of research, I would not have spent half my life in a state of self-reproach for a condition scientists are still trying to unravel: "Obesity is not a moral failure—it's a disease. It's got a clear-cut biological and genetic basis," commented Richard Atkinson, MD, speaking at a conference of the North American Association for the Study of Obesity (NAASO). "We have been using a behavioral type treatment for a disease that we now all realize is much more complicated" (Atkinson, 1994).

I finally realized that weight and self-worth do *not* go hand in hand. I may still want to lose some weight for health-related reasons, but not because it would make me a better person. My weight may fluctuate, but my self-worth does not. This became crystal clear to me when, shortly after reading *The Dieter's Dilemma,* I went with a friend to a group weight-loss program. The group leader announced that "because the Fourth of July is coming up, let's make a list of all the freedoms we lose when we're overweight." I bristled: "I may want to lose some weight, but I don't feel as though I've lost any freedoms. This seems like a very negative activity." The women, of course, made that list, and went home disliking themselves even more. I went home and told my husband I was forming an organization called "Largely Positive" to promote health, self-esteem, and well-being among larger people. "Good for you!" he said.

Discrimination can't be effectively battled until those who are its victims recognize it as such and begin to fight back. Because the majority of larger people still regard excess weight as their own fault, it's tough to enlist them in the battle. Although there are some organized size-acceptance groups, they have faced a great deal of difficulty in getting their message out and often are not regarded as credible. This is all the more reason for the research community to step up to the plate and join the crusade.

PARALLELS WITH MENTAL ILLNESS

I see many parallels between public views of obesity and public perceptions of mental illness, although mental health advocates are now doing a pretty good job of battling the stigma that has long been associated with this condition. Mental illness was once thought to be caused by bad parenting, personality weakness, or character flaws. People with depression were told to just "snap out of it." We now know that genetic and biological factors strongly influence the likelihood of having mental illness, and people cannot simply "will" themselves to be rid of it. According to the National Alliance for the Mentally Ill:

- Mental illnesses can affect persons of any age, race, religion, or income. Mental illnesses are not the result of personal weakness, lack of character, or poor upbringing.
- Mental illnesses are biologically based brain disorders. They cannot be overcome through "will power" and are not related to a person's "character" or intelligence.
- Stigma erodes confidence that mental disorders are real, treatable health conditions. We have allowed stigma and a now unwarranted sense of hopelessness to erect attitudinal, structural and financial barriers to effective treatment and recovery. It is time to take these barriers down (National Alliance for the Mentally Ill, 2004).

One could easily substitute the word "obesity" for the phrase "mental illness" in the preceding statements.

DOES THE RESEARCH COMMUNITY HAVE A ROLE IN FIGHTING WEIGHT DISCRIMINATION?

Silence and a lack of protest aid discrimination. The research community has been slow to speak out in a unified voice against weight discrimination, possibly because they do not view this as part of their mission. Personally, I believe they must be in the vanguard.

Size-acceptance advocates have been waging the weight discrimination battle pretty much on their own. They have fought valiantly, but are often viewed as lacking credibility (even though many of them are quite knowledgeable about obesity and the associated research). Because the majority of larger people still regard excess weight as their own fault, it's tough to enlist them in the battle. This is all the more reason for the research community to step up and join the crusade.

Research studies on obesity seldom make it into the mainstream, and even when they are reported on the nightly news, they are soon forgotten or disregarded. Those with accurate information rarely appear on talk shows. Instead we get the self-proclaimed "gurus of girth" touting questionable and unfounded weight-loss remedies.

If the weight discrimination battle is to be won, we need the research community to become involved—to help create awareness that discrimination is, in fact, occurring and then to help disseminate accurate information to the public and to health professionals.

An encouraging sign is that NAASO has formed an Anti-Weight Discrimination Task Force to address these issues as a group. While many lauded the effort, there were those who suggested that the organization was being too "politically correct," and that stigma may serve as a motivator for people to lose weight. My response:

- There is no place for discrimination or stigma in a just, compassionate society. Discrimination in any form is reprehensible.
- Stigma may serve as a motivator for some, but it is a motivator of the cruelest kind. If stigma is regarded as a motivating force, then, taken to its logical conclusion, it should be aimed at anyone society deems less than perfect. Would we recommend that public assistance clients be enveloped by stigma to motivate them to find jobs? Would we recommend that a diabetic be subject to stigma until she brings her blood sugar into control? Would we advocate that a person with high cholesterol be stigmatized until his cholesterol is within an acceptable range? Put this way, it sounds ridiculous and mean-spirited. It is just as ridiculous and mean-spirited when applied to obese people.
- The battle against weight discrimination will not be easily won. The fact that even a few members of NAASO feel that stigma is an acceptable motivator is discouraging, given that these should be the "enlightened" folks. But hopefully those who feel this way are very much in the minority; indeed, the NAASO leadership is committed to creating a platform from which to oppose weight discrimination.

WHAT CAN BE DONE?

So how do we cope with and fight weight discrimination? Puhl and Brownell (2003) note: "Multiple means of coping have been studied, ranging from attempts to change the stigmatizing condition (losing weight) to taking pride in the condition and mobilizing social action to prevent discrimination" (p. 53). Of recent years I have committed myself to the latter coping mechanism. I believe there are a number of strategies that can be employed in the battle against weight discrimination.

Educate the Public

Crandall and Schiffhauer (1998) have suggested that "one way to reduce anti-fat prejudice is teaching them [the public] about the biological and genetic aspects of the causes of adiposity" (p. 460). While I have advocated this strategy for a long time, and still believe it is necessary, studies on the effectiveness of this strategy have been mixed. In at least one study, informing participants that obesity is mainly due to genetic factors did not result in lower bias (Teachman, Gapinski, Brownell, Rawlins, & Jeyaram, 2003).

Educate Health Professionals

It is imperative that health professionals receive accurate information about obesity and about how to treat their larger patients with respect, sensitivity, and compassion. Such information should be incorporated into all health-related curriculums in institutions of higher learning.

Educate Parents

Given the increased emphasis on childhood obesity, it is critical for parents to have an accurate and realistic understanding of the determinants of weight. More than anything, the homes of overweight children must be "safe havens." Given the discrimination, bias, and stigma they will face in the outside world, they must have one place where they are guaranteed to have unconditional love, support, and understanding.

Teach Acceptance to Children

Discrimination must be derailed at a very early age. Adults must teach children that it's wrong to make cruel remarks about large people, and that a person's size, like the color of one's skin, is simply another element of the diversity that makes each of us unique, special, and interesting. And it's not just the responsibility of parents. Teachers can integrate lessons in size acceptance into an ongoing dialogue about the importance of respecting human diversity. One Largely Positive member told me how she deals with curiosity about her size in the children she works with:

> "Working in child care, I deal with children of all ages. We do everything together—dance, tell jokes, dig in the sandbox—all kinds of things. But one thing that almost always occurs is that a bright, curious 3-year-old will call to my attention that I am 'fat.' They never 'attack' me with this news, but they are noticing the difference between themselves, their parents, friends, and, of course, myself. I never take offense or become embarrassed. I simply state that isn't it wonderful that everyone is so different and interesting, and what a boring place

this world would be if it were any different. Their eyes light up and you can see the excitement in their expressions of newfound knowledge—then my eyes light up as I confirm the planting of some very positive seeds!"

Allies Come in All Sizes!

The army battling weight discrimination can include people of all shapes and sizes. There are those who feel you have to be fat to truly understand what larger people go through, and this may be true. But compassion and empathy are size-neutral, and can be brought to bear on discrimination by people of all shapes and sizes.

Protest Negative Portrayals of Larger People

There must be an organized way of protesting negative and biased portrayals of larger people in the media, perhaps through a Media Watch campaign. I asked Largely Positive members to name the one thing they would do to improve the way large people are portrayed in the media. Here are some of their responses:

- "Show them having fun and enjoying life just like thin people—because they do!"
- "Show them walking and playing sports. I walk a lot with my dog, and a lot of my thin friends can't walk as long as I can."
- "Create a show that portrays large people in a sexy way."
- "Give them more credible roles."
- "Cease the portrayal of the fat person as being slovenly, ever jovial, putting themselves down, being unattractive to the opposite sex and uninvolved in athletics."
- "Have TV shows and movies portray large people in flattering roles—no fat jokes or derogatory remarks."
- "I would portray heavy people as people with no reference to their weight. Story lines would be exactly the same as they are now with thin people—filled with love, excitement, and just normal everyday problems."
- "Large people should be shown in about the same numbers as they actually occur in real life. To look at most forms of the media now, you'd never know society contained any large people!"
- "Stop cartoons and jokes about large-size people."
- "Portray us as attractive, energetic, intelligent, confident, and caring people with a lot of talent to give to the world."

To this list I would add, stop portraying "The Headless People." My dear mother, Bernice, who passed away as I was finishing this chapter, had become increasingly irritated by TV news segments on obesity in which cameras are trained on the stomachs of larger people as they walk down the street. She used to call them "the headless people," and she felt that this was a dehumanizing, disrespectful practice. It made the people seem like nothing more than stomachs, she said. It also implies that the condition of obesity relates only to the stomach, which we know is not true. I concur with my mother. It is time to retire "the headless people" as the visual representation of obesity.

Employ a Positive, Confident Attitude to Repel Discrimination

Are there actions that can be taken by larger people themselves to repel discrimination? Possibly. When I became more confident, donned a positive attitude, and shed weight-related guilt, I sensed a change in the reaction I was getting from others. As I came to believe in myself and my abilities, others did too. I no longer *expected* discrimination. A lackluster attitude, downbeat body language, self-deprecation, lack of self-confidence, all may help to create a fertile environment for discrimination, while a confident, upbeat, positive demeanor may help to inhibit it. I am not suggesting that weight discrimination will be brought to its knees by a positive attitude—only that it is one way for larger people themselves to start fighting back and reject the stereotypes.

CONCLUSION

Weight discrimination can have a omnipresent and lasting impact on the life of an overweight person. It can be much more limiting on that person's life than the excess weight itself. A major problem is that weight discrimination is often not recognized as such, especially by larger people themselves. The fight to end it must include those who study it, as well as those who are affected by it.

REFERENCES

Atkinson, R. (1993). Paper presented at the annual meeting of the North American Association for the Study of Obesity, Milwaukee, WI.

Atkinson, R. (1994). Genetic factors influence the response of energy metabolism, body weight, and body composition. *Obesity Research, 2*, 470–471.

Bennett, W., & Gurin, J. (1982). *The dieter's dilemma*. New York: Basic Books.

Centers for Disease Control and Prevention. (2004). *Public health perspectives on obesity and genetics: What we know, what we don't know and what it means*. Retrieved December 15, 2004, from www.cdc.gov/genomics/info/perspectives/files/obesknow.htm

Crandall, C. S., & Schiffhauer, K. L. (1998). Anti-fat prejudice: Beliefs, values, and American culture. *Obesity Research, 6*, 458–460.

Geier, A. B., Schwartz, M. B., & Brownell, K. D. (2003). "Before and after" diet advertisements escalate weight stigma. *Eating and Weight Disorders, 8*, 282–288.

Johnson, C. (2001). *Self esteem comes in all sizes*. Carlsbad, CA: Gurze Books.

National Alliance for the Mentally Ill. (2004). *Inform yourself about mental illness*. Retrieved December 14, 2004, from www.nami.org

Puhl, R., & Brownell, K. D. (2003). Ways of coping with obesity stigma: Review and conceptual analysis. *Eating Behaviors, 4*, 53–78.

Teachman, B. A., Gapinski, K. D., Brownell, K. D., Rawlins, M., & Jeyaram, S. (2003). Demonstrations of implicit anti-fat bias: The impact of providing causal information and evoking empathy. *Health Psychology, 22*, 68–78.

PART IV

■ ■ ■ ■

Remedies

CHAPTER 14

■ ■ ■

Legal Theory on Weight Discrimination

ELIZABETH E. THERAN

As a subject of legal concern in the United States, weight discrimination is a relatively new field. Only in the last 15 years or so have people who believe they have been discriminated against on the basis of their weight—whether they were denied a job, demoted, fired, or denied access to a restaurant or theater—begun to seek redress regularly in the courts. These lawsuits have enjoyed, at best, a mixed reception. While some courts have been amenable to claims of weight discrimination under existing laws, others have shown themselves to be outright hostile to the notion of legally actionable weight discrimination, and various media outlets have been quick to echo and amplify that hostility in the press. This chapter sets forth the different kinds of claims weight-discrimination plaintiffs bring in court, identifies some of the types of claims that have succeeded, and highlights some of the obstacles these plaintiffs face. The ultimate conclusion to be drawn is that the existing structure of U.S. anti-discrimination law condemns many weight-discrimination claims to failure because, with very few exceptions, we lack laws that specifically prohibit discrimination on the basis of weight.

EXISTING ANTI-DISCRIMINATION LAWS

There are currently no federal laws, and only a handful of state and local laws, that expressly prohibit discrimination on the basis of weight or, more generally, appearance. Thus, people who feel that they have been the victims of weight discrimination and want to seek redress in court usually must bring suit under laws prohibiting discrimination based on other characteristics: most commonly disability, sex, or race. The following section describes briefly the existing federal, state, and local anti-discrimination laws most often used by plaintiffs claiming weight discrimination, with a particular eye to how weight claims fit into the frameworks of those laws.

The Equal Employment Opportunity Commission (EEOC) is the federal agency charged with enforcing many anti-discrimination statutes, including the Americans with Disabilities Act, the Rehabilitation Act (as to claims by federal employees), Title VII of the Civil Rights Act of 1964, and the Age Discrimination in Employment Act, discussed later. As a general matter, when an agency with this kind of authority issues an interpretation of a statutory provision, unless that interpretation plainly conflicts with the language of the law itself, courts accord some level of deference to the agency's interpretation (*United States v. Mead Corp.*, 2001). However, for various reasons, courts do not always defer to the EEOC's interpretation of a statute—for example, because Congress did not confer formal "rule-making authority" on the agency (*General Electric Co. v. Gilbert*, 1976), or because a given court simply thinks the EEOC's interpretation is wrong (*General Dynamics Land Systems, Inc. v. Cline*, 2004). In the section that follows, then, the reader will note that the EEOC's interpretation of a given provision will not always agree with the approach a court, or multiple courts, may take. In the context of a lawsuit, the court's approach governs, but in jurisdictions that have not yet addressed the question, the issue is open for argument.

Weight as Disability: The Americans with Disabilities Act and the Rehabilitation Act

The Americans with Disabilities Act (ADA) of 1990, 42 U.S.C. §§ 12101 *et seq.*, and the Rehabilitation Act of 1973, 29 U.S.C. §§ 791 *et seq.*, prohibit discrimination against individuals with physical and mental disabilities. The Rehabilitation Act governs discrimination by the federal government, federal contractors, and programs receiving federal financial assistance, while the ADA governs discrimination by the private sector and by state and local governments. The two statutes tend to be interpreted together, and employ the same legal standards and analysis in assessing claims of discrimination (e.g., 29 U.S.C. §§ 791(g), 793(d), 794(d) (2001) [providing that the ADA standards apply to claims under the Rehabilitation Act]; 29 C.F.R. app. § 1630.2(g) (2001) [noting that Congress intended all Rehabilitation Act case law on defining "disability" to apply to the ADA]). Accordingly, in the section that follows, any reference to the ADA may also be taken to apply to the Rehabilitation Act, unless otherwise specified.

The ADA offers broad protection against disability discrimination in employment (Title I),[1] public services (Title II),[2] and privately owned public accommodations (Title III). Weight-discrimination plaintiffs can seek relief in any of the three categories, although the greatest number of weight-discrimination lawsuits under the ADA are probably Title I employment discrimination cases. Other plaintiffs have sued under Title III, claiming they were denied access to restaurants or other public accommodations on the basis of their weight. Each section of the ADA presents its own challenges for weight-discrimination plaintiffs and implicates the larger question of whether a given instance of weight discrimination is really discrimination on the basis of a "disability," or whether it is in fact discrimination on the basis of something else.

With regard to employment discrimination claims, the question of what constitutes a "disability" within the meaning of Title I of the ADA is of particular significance for victims of weight discrimination who are contemplating filing suit. Title I generally prohibits discrimination "against a qualified individual with a disability because of the disability of such individual in regard to job application procedures, the hiring, advancement, or discharge of employees, employee compensation, job training, and other terms, conditions, and privileges of employment" (42 U.S.C. § 12112(a)). A "qualified individual with a disability," according to the statute, is "an individual with a disability who, with or without reasonable accommodation, can perform the essential functions of the employment position that such individual holds or desires" (42 U.S.C. § 12111(8)). "Disability," in turn, has a three-part statutory definition: "(A) a physical or mental impairment that substantially limits one or more of the major life activities of such individual; (B) a record of such an impairment; or (C) being regarded as having such an impairment" (42 U.S.C. § 12102(2)). Finally, although the statute does not define "impairment," the administrative regulation promulgated by the EEOC (29 C.F.R. § 1630.2(h)), which applies to all titles of the ADA, defines it as follows:

> (1) Any physiological disorder, or condition, cosmetic disfigurement, or anatomical loss affecting one or more of the following body systems: neurological, musculoskeletal, special sense organs, respiratory (including speech organs), cardiovascular, reproductive, digestive, genito-urinary, hemic and lymphatic, skin, and endocrine; or (2) Any mental or psychological disorder. . . .

More or less every authority to consider the question has concluded that overweight or obesity, standing alone, is not considered a "disability" within the meaning of the ADA (e.g., 29 C.F.R. app. § 1630.2(j); *Francis v. City of Meriden*, 2d Cir. 1997; *Andrews v. Ohio*, 6th Cir. 1997).[3] The only generally recognized exception is for "morbid" obesity, generally defined as a body weight of either 100% or 100 pounds over one's ideal weight. Some courts have held that even morbid obesity does not itself constitute an impairment within the meaning of the ADA; these courts require proof that a plaintiff's obesity stems from another, underlying physiological condition, like diabetes or a genetic disorder, in order to constitute the basis for a suit under the ADA (e.g., *Fredregill v. Nationwide Agribusiness Insurance Co.*, S.D. Iowa 1997; *Francis*, 2d Cir. 1997). Others have held that morbid obesity, standing by itself, may qualify so long as it substantially limits the person in a major life activity (e.g., *Cook v. Rhode Island Department of Mental Health, Retardation, and Hospitals,* 1st Cir. 1993); *Gaddis v. Oregon*, 9th Cir. 2001; *Connor v. McDonald's Restaurant*, D. Conn. 2003).

For victims of weight discrimination who do not regard their weight as an actual impairment, the ADA's protections for those who are "regarded as" disabled may be of particular relevance. In its Interpretive Guidance on Title I of the ADA (29 C.F.R. app. § 1630.2(l)), the EEOC lists three different ways in which an individual may be "regarded as" disabled under the statute:

> (1) The individual may have an impairment which is not substantially limiting but is perceived by the employer or other covered entity as constituting a substantially limiting impairment;
>
> (2) The individual may have an impairment which is only substantially limiting because of the attitudes of others toward the impairment; or
>
> (3) The individual may have no impairment at all but is regarded by the employer or other covered entity as having a substantially limiting impairment.[4]

The EEOC further notes in its discussion of perceived disabilities that "an individual rejected from a job because of the 'myths, fears and stereotypes' associated with disabilities would be covered under this part of the definition of disability, whether or not the employer's . . . perception were shared by others in the field and whether or not the individual's actual physical or mental condition would be considered a disability under the first or second part of this definition."

Although most courts have accepted, or purport to accept, the EEOC's definition of "regarded as" disabled, the courts' reception of claims involving obesity has been mixed. In *Cook v. Rhode Island Department of Mental Health, Retardation, and Hospitals* (1st Cir. 1993), the first major federal decision to address the issue, the First Circuit Court of Appeals upheld a jury verdict in favor of the plaintiff, Bonnie Cook, who claimed under the Rehabilitation Act that her employer had discriminated against her because it regarded her as disabled. Cook was rejected when she reapplied for a position she had held previously—with a "spotless" work record—as an institutional attendant at a state facility for the mentally handicapped. At 5′2″ tall and 320 pounds, Cook passed her prehire physical, but the state refused to rehire her on the grounds that her weight "compromised her ability to evacuate patients in case of an emergency and put her at greater risk of developing serious ailments . . . [that] would promote absenteeism and increase the likelihood of workers' compensation claims" (p. 21).

After a jury trial that resulted in a verdict for Cook, the state appealed. On appeal, the state argued that (1) Cook was not "disabled" under the law because her morbid obesity was both "mutable" and voluntary; (2) Cook's rejection from this one job did not prove that her employer regarded her as "substantially limited"; and (3) Cook was not "qualified" for the position she sought because her obesity in fact rendered her incapable of performing the job. The First Circuit disagreed, finding that morbid obesity could itself constitute a disabling impairment under the statute and that the state's rationale for refusing to hire Cook made it clear that the state regarded her as "substantially limited" in the life activity of working:

> If the rationale proffered by an employer in the context of a single refusal to hire adequately evinces that the employer treats a particular condition as a disqualifier for a wide range of employment opportunities, proof of a far-flung pattern of rejections may not be necessary. Put in slightly more concrete terms, denying an applicant even a single job that requires no unique physical skills, due solely to the perception that the applicant suffers from a physical limitation that would keep her from qualifying for a broad spectrum of jobs, can constitute treating an applicant as if her condition substantially limited a major life activity, *viz.*, working. (p. 26)

The court explicitly rejected the state's arguments that Cook was not entitled to the protection of the Rehabilitation Act because her weight was "mutable" or "voluntary," noting that neither the Rehabilitation Act nor its regulations contain any language excluding physiological impairments that might not be constant or that may be affected by voluntary behavior on the part of the affected individual.[5]

Another successful "perceived disability" case involving obesity was *EEOC v. Texas Bus Lines* (S.D. Tex. 1996). The claimant in that case, Arazella Manuel, was a morbidly obese woman who applied for a job as a bus driver with the defendant, but was not hired. Manuel had a very strong interview and passed the driver's test, but failed the prehire physical because the examining physician felt that she "would not be able to move swiftly in the event of an accident." However, both the doctor's report and his deposition testimony revealed that "inability to move swiftly" was not on the Department of Transportation's list of disqualifying conditions for drivers. Accordingly, the court concluded, echoing the language of the EEOC's Interpretive Guidance, "Texas Bus Lines made the decision not to hire Manuel because of a perception of disability based on 'myth, fear or stereotype.' . . . Texas Bus Lines regarded Manuel as disabled and, therefore, unable to work as a driver based on her alleged impaired mobility without the benefit of objective medical testing or findings" (p. 979).

In the years since *Cook* and *Texas Bus Lines* were decided, the Supreme Court has issued several important decisions interpreting, and effectively narrowing, the "regarded as" prong of the ADA. In *Sutton v. United Air Lines* (1999), the Court ruled that "regarded as" plaintiffs must establish that their employer believes that they have a substantially limiting impairment within the meaning of the ADA, when they either have no impairment or have an impairment that is not substantially limiting. The Court in *Sutton* also emphasized that disability determinations under the ADA are to be made on an individual basis, rather than by per se categorization of different conditions as "disabilities" or not. Nonetheless, some courts (e.g., *Francis*, 2d Cir. 1997; *Rinehimer v. CemcoLift, Inc.*, 3d Cir. 2002) have imposed an additional hurdle on disability plaintiffs by holding that the condition the plaintiff is "regarded as" having must be one that, if the plaintiff indeed had it, would constitute a disability under the ADA.[6] Thus, for example, if an employee alleged that his employer regarded him as disabled because he was fifty pounds overweight, he could not bring a successful "regarded as" claim in these courts—regardless of the effect of those fifty pounds on his functioning or his employer's perception thereof—because being fifty pounds overweight is not itself considered an ADA disability (*Andrews*, 6th Cir. 1997). This position stands in stark contrast to the EEOC's view in its guidance that nondisabling conditions may nonetheless be "regarded as" disabling by employers. Courts have also taken an ever-narrowing view of what constitutes being "substantially limited in a major life activity," which makes it increasingly difficult for all plaintiffs, including those alleging weight discrimination, to prevail. For example, employers' views that employees were substantially limited with respect to classifications such as "police officer," "senior management positions," and "active law enforcement jobs" have all been rejected as too narrow to be actionable (*Rossbach v. City of Miami*, 11th Cir. 2004; *Fredregill*, S.D. Iowa 1997; *Smaw v. Virginia Department of State Police*, E.D. Va. 1994). Several courts (*Andrews*, 6th Cir. 1997; *Forrisi v. Bowen*, 4th Cir. 1986; *Francis*, 2d Cir. 1997; *Fredregill*, S.D. Iowa 1997) have even expressed the view that allowing weight-discrimination claims to be brought under the ADA dilutes or debases the statute's purpose and trivializes the suffering of "truly" disabled individuals.

For people who feel that they have been discriminated against on the basis of their weight, disability-based anti-discrimination statutes like the ADA and the Rehabilitation Act are, at best, only partial avenues of relief. Insofar as courts are willing to view obesity as a disability—or a perceived disability—at all, they tend to draw the line at "morbid" obesity or at obesity that stems from an independent physiological disorder, like a metabolic disorder or diabetes. In any case, there are potentially far bigger problems with classifying weight as a disability than the low probability of success in litigation. One of the most serious problems may be the potential for backlash both against the disability rights movement and against overweight people themselves (Krieger, 2000). As the other chapters in this volume make clear, the cultural perception of weight as a controllable stigma, however inaccurate, is a strong one in this country. In the legal field, one need only consider the hysterical public reaction to *Pelman v. McDonald's Corp.* (S.D.N.Y. 2003), the tort suit filed against McDonald's in 2002 by parents of children claiming that McDonald's was negligent in its marketing of fast food, for confirmation that, in this country, one's weight is more or less considered to be one's own fault.[7] Another disadvantage may be obscuring the real issue in many instances of weight discrimination, particularly for individuals who are less than morbidly obese—discrimination based on negative stereotypes associated with appearance. Some of these claims have succeeded under other statutes, as shall be seen below, but under very limited circumstances.

Weight and Race, Gender, or National Origin: Title VII of the Civil Rights Act of 1964

Unlike the ADA and the Rehabilitation Act, Title VII of the Civil Rights Act of 1964 deals exclusively with discrimination in employment. With regard to employers, Title VII prohibits both discrimination against employees and retaliation against them for filing a charge of discrimination. Its principal anti-discrimination provision (42 U.S.C. § 2000e-2(a)) reads as follows:

> It shall be an unlawful employment practice for an employer—
>
> (1) to fail or refuse to hire or to discharge any individual, or otherwise to discriminate against any individual with respect to his compensation, terms, conditions, or privileges of employment, because of such individual's race, color, religion, sex, or national origin; or
>
> (2) to limit, segregate, or classify his employees or applicants for employment in any way which would deprive or tend to deprive any individual of employment opportunities or otherwise adversely affect his status as an employee, because of such individual's race, color, religion, sex, or national origin.

The categories of discrimination listed in the statute—race, color, religion, sex, and national origin—do not include weight or appearance. As a result, weight-discrimination cases cannot be brought under Title VII if they involve discrimination *only* on the basis of weight and not one of the protected characteristics listed in the statute. However, courts have recognized a type of claim called a "plus" claim—most commonly race-plus or sex-plus—in which the plaintiff alleges discrimination based on one or more of the enumerated Title VII categories plus another characteristic, like weight or age (*Phillips v. Martin Marietta Corp.*, 1971). For example, employees in the airline industry have successfully challenged their employers' use of different weight standards for male and female flight attendants (*Frank v. United Airlines, Inc.*, 9th Cir. 2000; *Gerdom v. Continental Airlines, Inc.*, 9th Cir. 1982; *Air Line Pilots Association, International v. United Airlines, Inc.*, E.D.N.Y. 1979; *Laffey v. Northwest Airlines, Inc.*, D.D.C. 1973). In these cases, the courts did not invalidate employers' weight standards generally, nor did they hold that a man and a woman of the same height must be permitted to weigh the same number of pounds; rather, they held that employers could not have a weight standard in place for only one sex, or entirely different standards based on sex (e.g., women must comply with "light-boned" height–weight tables while men need only comply with "heavy-boned"). Flight attendants and female police officers have also successfully challenged their employers' disparate enforcement of facially neutral weight policies—for example, disciplining or terminating overweight women but not overweight men (e.g., *Donoghue v. Orange County*, 9th Cir. 1987; *Air Line Pilots Association, International v. United Airlines, Inc.*, E.D.N.Y. 1979).[8]

As with the ADA, however, not all courts employ the same legal standard for Title VII "plus" claims. One particularly troubling development has been that some courts, like the Fifth Circuit Court of Appeals, have limited viable "plus" claims to those in which the "plus" characteristic is "immutable," based on the exercise of a "fundamental right," or independently protected by law (*Jefferies v. Harris County Community Action Association*, 5th Cir. 1980; *Schmittou v. Wal-Mart Stores, Inc.*, D. Minn. 2003; *Arnett v. Aspin*, E.D. Pa. 1994; *Judge v. Marsh*, D.D.C. 1986). Thus, for example, claims based on sex-plus-race (an immutable trait protected by Title VII), sex-plus-marital status (exercise of a "fundamental right"), or sex-plus-age (a trait protected by the Age Discrimination in Employment Act), would be viable, but sex-plus-weight would not. Other courts, however, have taken a broader view, holding that the purpose of "plus" claims is to preclude discrimination against virtually all subgroups of protected groups (*Brown v. Henderson,* 2d Cir. 2001; *Back v. Hastings on Hudson Union Free School District*, 2d Cir. 2004; *Marks v. National Communications Association, Inc.*, S.D.N.Y. 1999). Most jurisdictions simply have not decided the issue.

Ultimately, then, whether one may raise a viable claim of weight discrimination as a "plus" under Title VII depends on two main factors: whether the discriminatory acts may be characterized as involving a prohibited trait under Title VII and whether one's jurisdiction requires "immutability" or fundamental-right status for the "plus" characteristic. Title VII cannot be used to reach weight discrimination by "equal-opportunity" discriminators who treat all overweight employees, regardless of race, sex, national origin, ethnicity or religion, equally badly. One court has even held that an employer's firing an African American employee on the basis of obesity constitutes a "legitimate nondiscriminatory reason" for firing the plaintiff sufficient to defeat his Title VII claim of race discrimination *(Hilliard v. Morton Buildings, Inc.*, D. Del. 2002).

Weight and Age: The Age Discrimination in Employment Act of 1967

The Age Discrimination in Employment Act (ADEA) of 1967 prohibits age-based discrimination in employment in exactly the same terms as Title VII (29 U.S.C. § 623(a); *Lorillard v. Pons*, 1978). In theory, "plus" claims are also viable under the ADEA as part of a showing that an employer discriminated against a subgroup of older[9] workers. However, a significant limitation was imposed by the Supreme Court in *Hazen Paper Co. v. Biggins* (1993), where the Court held that "there is no disparate treatment under the ADEA when the factor motivating the employer is some feature other than the employee's age." Since *Hazen Paper*, courts (e.g., *Frank*, 9th Cir. 2000) have rejected ADEA claims based on "a factor that is merely correlated with age." Accordingly, the few ADEA claims brought by plaintiffs alleging age discrimination on the basis of increasing weight with age have not been successful (e.g., *Frank*, 9th Cir. 2000; *Ellis v. United Airlines, Inc.*, 10th Cir. 1996).

Weight and the Federal Constitution: 42 U.S.C. § 1983

42 U.S.C. § 1983, most commonly referred to as Section 1983, gives private individuals the right to sue governmental or quasi-governmental entities that may have violated their constitutional rights. The statute authorizes suits against the federal government (*The Civil Rights Cases* [1883]), state governments (42 U.S.C. § 1983), and private entities (for example, privately run prisons or private companies that provide medical services to prison inmates) that satisfy the legal requirement of "state action." It does not allow for suits against purely private individuals or entities (*Burton v. Wilmington Parking Authority*, 1961).

With regard to constitutional claims, the level of scrutiny that a court will apply—and therefore the likelihood that a court will find a constitutional violation—depends on whether the plaintiff's claim implicates the exercise of a "fundamental right" or discrimination against a "suspect class." It is by now well established in American constitutional law that there are a total of two "suspect classes," race and national origin, that receive the most intense form of scrutiny, and two "quasi-suspect classes," gender and illegitimacy, that receive a heightened level of review (*City of Cleburne v. Cleburne Living Center*, 1985; *Clark v. Jeter*, 1988). Discrimination based on other characteristics receives rational basis review, the most deferential form of review, which asks only whether the challenged action is "rationally related to a legitimate state interest"(*Cleburne*, 1985; *Schroeder v. Hamilton School District*, 7th Cir. 2002 [observing that "discrimination against . . . the elderly, overweight, undersized, and disfigured, will only constitute a violation of equal protection if it lacks a rational basis"]). As a practical matter, very few governmental actions fail rational basis review unless, as Justice O'Connor has noted, they evidence "a bare . . . desire to harm a politically unpopular group" or "inhibit personal relationships" (*Lawrence v. Texas*, 2003 (O'Connor, J., concurring)).

Although some victims of weight discrimination have attempted to bring legal claims against a governmental entity under Section 1983, these claims have generally been unsuccessful. For example, in *United States v. Santiago-Martinez* (9th Cir. 1995), the Ninth Circuit rejected the plaintiff's claim that the prosecution's striking of obese jurors from his trial on drug charges violated the Equal Protection Clause. The court rested its ruling on the application of rational basis review to constitutional claims involving obesity. This kind of categorical approach to constitutional claims of discrimination makes it very unlikely that future weight-discrimination claims will meet with a different reception.

Weight as Appearance Discrimination: State and Local Laws

There are two states, Michigan and the District of Columbia, and two cities, San Francisco and Santa Cruz, California, that have their own laws prohibiting discrimination on the basis of weight. Michigan's statute, the Elliott–Larsen Civil Rights Act (2000), provides that "the opportunity to obtain employment, housing and other real estate, and the full and equal utilization of public accommodations, public service, and educational facilities without discrimination because of religion, race, color, national origin, age, sex, height, weight, familial status, or marital status as prohibited by this act, is recognized and declared to be a civil right." The District of Columbia's human rights law (2001) prohibits discrimination based on, *inter alia*, "personal appearance," which the statute defines as "the outward appearance of any person, irrespective of sex, with regard to bodily condition or characteristics, manner or style of dress, and manner or style of personal grooming, including, but not limited to, hair style and beards." The law includes an exception, however, for "the requirement of cleanliness, uniforms, or prescribed standards, when uniformly applied for admittance to a public accommodation, or when uniformly applied to a class of employees for a reasonable business purpose; or when such bodily conditions or characteristics, style or manner of dress or personal grooming presents a danger to the health, welfare or safety of any individual." Neither statute appears to have resulted in much litigation, although it is impossible to know or quantify the effect of the statutes on employers, governments, or owners of public accommodations in drafting their policies.

The same is mostly true of the city ordinances in San Francisco, passed in 2000, and Santa Cruz, passed in 1992. However, the ordinances have resulted in a few notable legal successes—not through litigation in the courts, but through mediation and negotiation. In San Francisco, Jennifer Portnick, an aerobics instructor who weighs 240 pounds, filed a discrimination complaint after Jazzercise refused to hire her as a certified instructor. Jazzercise had told Portnick that it could not hire her, even though she was in excellent cardiovascular shape, because she needed to develop a "more fit appearance" in order to be a "role model[s] for Jazzercise enthusiasts" (Fernandez, 2002b). After mediation through the San Francisco Human Rights Commission, the case settled and Jazzercise agreed to change its company policy (Fernandez, 2002a). In Santa Cruz, a group called the Body Image Task Force used the city's weight discrimination ordinance to negotiate with two movie theater companies over the installation of a few extra-wide seats in newly constructed theaters (Garchik, 1995).

Plaintiffs have also brought weight-discrimination suits under state law in states that do not have specific laws prohibiting weight or appearance discrimination. Most of these cases, which usually claim disability discrimination, run into the same problems as federal suits under the ADA: while a few state courts have embraced obesity, or morbid obesity, as a disability (*Gimello v. Agency Rent-A-Car Systems*, N.J. Super. Ct. App. Div. 1991; *State Division of Human Rights v. Xerox Corp.*, N.Y. App. Div. 1985), most others do not absent a separate underlying physiological cause (e.g., *Greene v. Union Pacific Railroad Co.*, W.D. Wash. 1981; *Cassista v. Community Foods, Inc.*, Cal. 1993; *Krein v. Marian Manor Nursing Home*, N.D. 1987; *Civil Service Commission v. Commonwealth*, Pa. 1991). While some state courts have resisted stereotyped views of overweight and obese people (e.g., *Parolisi v. Board of Examiners of New York*, N.Y. Sup. Ct. 1967), others have embraced them (e.g., *Greene*, W.D. Wash. 1981; *Metropolitan Dade County v. Wolf*, Fla. Dist. Ct. App. 1973). And weight plaintiffs in state court are just as likely as those in federal court to fall into the dreaded "disability gap" of being either too disabled to be qualified for their jobs or insufficiently disabled to merit statutory protection (e.g., *Gregg v. National League of Professional Baseball Clubs*, E.D. Pa. 2002; *Cassista*, Cal. 1993; *Philadelphia Electric Co. v. Commonwealth*, Pa. Commw. Ct. 1982). In short, most non-weight-specific state anti-discrimination laws add little or nothing to the relatively bleak landscape of federal protections against weight-based discrimination.

THE NEED FOR LEGISLATION

As the preceding discussion has aimed to make clear, weight is not one of the categories that most American anti-discrimination statutes seek to protect. With the exception of the few jurisdictions that prohibit discrimination on the basis of weight or appearance, victims of weight discrimination and their advocates are forced to attempt to shoehorn their claims into these other statutory frameworks if they want to seek relief in court. As a result, certain groups of weight-discrimination victims—those who cannot fit their claims into the statutory categories—are systematically left without recourse. Individuals who are overweight but not morbidly obese forgo many of the few legal opportunities out there by not being "disabled" under the ADA. Those who work for employers who systematically discriminate against overweight people without regard to sex, race, or national origin cannot make use of Title VII. Under most circumstances, Title VII will usually be of little use to male victims of weight discrimination unless there is a nexus to race, because experience suggests that overweight female employees are even more likely to be subject to weight discrimination than overweight male employees. (This is not to minimize the very real discrimination that exists against overweight males; rather, the point is simply that there will be fewer situations in which a given employer demonstrably treats overweight males *worse* than it does overweight females.)

At the same time, based on current public perceptions of weight and obesity, it would be highly unrealistic to expect widespread legislation targeting weight discrimination anytime soon. The chapters in this volume paint a very clear picture of the state of weight bias and discrimination in the United States today. Ultimately, the best hope for obtaining support for new legislation will probably lie in educating the general public about the etiology of weight and weight discrimination and overcoming the perception of stigma controllability, which continues to play a very strong role in the opposition to civil rights protections based on weight. Until the general public can understand and accept the distinction between weight and grooming or other purely voluntary physical conditions like hair length, tattoos, or piercings, legislators and activists will have an uphill battle to fight. Another important message to convey is that even if one views a condition like weight as undesirable, unhealthy, unfortunate, unattractive, or any other "un," the answer to a "weight problem" is not employment discrimination or any other kind of discrimination. Denying a person a job, a seat in a restaurant, or access to a movie theater is not going to make him or her, or anyone else, any thinner or healthier, or improve us as a society. The sooner people begin to understand this notion, the sooner a meaningful legal remedy for weight discrimination will be possible.

NOTES

1. In 2001, the Supreme Court issued a significant decision on the scope of Title I of the ADA. In *Board of Trustees of the University of Alabama v. Garrett*, the Court held that private suits for money damages under Title I of the ADA, which prohibits discrimination in employment, are unconstitutional as against state governments. The *Garrett* ruling did not affect the rights of individuals to file suit against private sector employers and local governments. With regard to state governments, as the *Garrett* Court observed, Title I still applies in full; although individuals cannot sue for money damages, the United States may still do so, and individuals may sue for injunctive relief. As

a practical matter, the Court's ruling in *Garrett* is likely to limit the number of claims against the states, because the federal government has traditionally filed few cases, and aggrieved individuals seldom have the money to fund a lawsuit without any prospect of monetary damages.

2. In *Tennessee v. Lane* (2004), the state raised the same argument against Title II of the ADA that the state of Alabama raised in *Garrett*: that it was unconstitutional as applied to state governments. With regard to Title II, however, the Supreme Court rejected this constitutional challenge—at least as applied to the question of access to the state courts—but declined to consider whether Title II was constitutional as applied to other public services, such as state-owned hockey rinks.
3. Interestingly, however, in the context of Medicare benefits, the Department of Health and Human Services recently removed language from its Medicare Coverage Issues Manual that declared obesity not to be an "illness," thereby paving the way for Medicare coverage of obesity and obesity-related conditions (United States Department of Health and Human Services, 2004).
4. But see *Sutton v. United Air Lines, Inc.* (1999) (listing "two apparent ways in which individuals may fall within [the definition of 'regarded as' disabled]: (1) a covered entity mistakenly believes that a person has a physical impairment that substantially limits one or more major life activities, or (2) a covered entity mistakenly believes that an actual, nonlimiting impairment substantially limits one or more major life activities"). It is something of an open question whether prong (2) of the *Sutton* Court's definition incorporates prong (2) of the EEOC's definition.
5. See also *Mendez v. Brown* (D. Mass. 2004) (morbidly obese plaintiffs stated a valid disability and/or perceived disability claim under Title II of the ADA when they alleged that the state denied morbidly obese women medically recommended breast reduction surgery under the Medicaid Act).
6. Compare, for example, *Rossbach v. City of Miami* (11th Cir. 2004) (in order to prevail under "regarded as" theory, plaintiff must show "(1) that the perceived disability involves a major life activity; and (2) that the perceived disability is 'substantially limiting' and significant"); *McInnis v. Alamo Community College District* (5th Cir. 2000) ("The plaintiff . . . must establish that the impairment, if it existed as perceived, would be substantially limiting.").
7. The court granted McDonald's' motion to dismiss the lawsuit, finding principally that McDonald's had no duty to warn the plaintiffs, or the public, about the dangers of its food because the nutritional content of McDonald's fare was or should have been well known to consumers. The decision is currently on appeal before the U.S. Court of Appeals for the Second Circuit.
8. But see *Jones v. City of Mount Vernon* (S.D.N.Y. 2000) (finding no violation despite fact that female, nonobese plaintiff rejected for exceeding weight maximum demonstrated that overweight and even obese men were not rejected).
9. The Supreme Court recently held that the ADEA's protections were limited to discrimination only on the basis of relative old age, not youth (*General Dynamics Land Systems, Inc. v. Cline*, 2004).

REFERENCES

Federal Cases

Air Line Pilots Association, International v. United Airlines, Inc., No. 73 C 1082, 1979 U.S. Dist. LEXIS 11790 (E.D.N.Y. 1979)
Andrews v. Ohio, 104 F.3d 803 (6th Cir. 1997)
Arnett v. Aspin, 846 F. Supp. 1234 (E.D. Pa. 1994)
Back v. Hastings on Hudson Union Free School District, 365 F.3d 107 (2d Cir. 2004)
Board of Trustees of the University of Alabama v. Garrett, 531 U.S. 356 (2001)
Brown v. Henderson, 257 F.3d 246 (2d Cir. 2001)
Burton v. Wilmington Parking Authority, 365 U.S. 715 (1961)
City of Cleburne v. Cleburne Living Center, 473 U.S. 432 (1985)
Clark v. Jeter, 486 U.S. 456 (1988)
Cook v. Rhode Island Department of Mental Health, Retardation, and Hospitals, 10 F.3d 17 (1st Cir. 1993)
Connor v. McDonald's Restaurant, No. 3:02 CV 382 SRU, 2003 WL 1343259 (D. Conn. Mar. 19, 2003)
Donoghue v. Orange County, 848 F.2d 926 (9th Cir. 1987)
EEOC v. Texas Bus Lines, 923 F. Supp. 965 (S.D. Tex. 1996)
Ellis v. United Airlines, Inc., 73 F.3d 999 (10th Cir. 1996)
Forrisi v. Bowen, 794 F.2d 931 (4th Cir. 1986)
Francis v. City of Meriden, 129 F.3d 281 (2d Cir. 1997)
Frank v. United Airlines, Inc., 216 F.3d 845 (9th Cir. 2000)
Fredregill v. Nationwide Agribusiness Insurance Co., 992 F. Supp. 1082 (S.D. Iowa 1997)
Gaddis v. Oregon, 21 Fed. Appx. 642 (9th Cir. Oct. 19, 2001) (unpublished)
General Dynamics Land Systems, Inc. v. Cline, 540 U.S. 581 (2004)
General Electric Co. v. Gilbert, 429 U.S. 125 (1976)
Gerdom v. Continental Airlines, Inc., 692 F.2d 602 (9th Cir. 1982) (en banc)
Greene v. Union Pacific Railroad Co., 548 F. Supp. 3 (W.D. Wash. 1981)
Gregg v. National League of Professional Baseball Clubs, No. Civ.A. 01-1867, 2002 WL 32348274 (E.D. Pa. Mar. 13, 2002)
Hazen Paper Co. v. Biggins, 507 U.S. 604 (1993)
Hilliard v. Morton Buildings, Inc., 195 F. Supp. 2d 582 (D. Del. 2002)
Jefferies v. Harris County Community Action Association, 615 F.2d 1025 (5th Cir. 1980)
Jones v. City of Mt. Vernon, 114 F. Supp. 2d 274 (S.D.N.Y. 2000)
Judge v. Marsh, 649 F. Supp. 770 (D.D.C. 1986)
Laffey v. Northwest Airlines, Inc., 366 F. Supp. 763 (D.D.C. 1973), *aff'd in relevant part*, 567 F.2d 429 (D.C. Cir. 1977)
Lawrence v. Texas, 539 U.S. 558 (2003)
Lorillard v. Pons, 434 U.S. 575 (1978)
Marks v. National Communications Association, Inc., 72 F. Supp. 2d 322 (S.D. N.Y. 1999)
McInnis v. Alamo Community College District, 207 F.3d 276 (5th Cir. 2000)
Mendez v. Brown, 311 F. Supp. 2d 134 (D. Mass. 2004)

Pelman v. McDonald's Corp., 237 F. Supp. 2d 512 (S.D.N.Y. 2003)
Phillips v. Martin Marietta Corp., 400 U.S. 542 (1971) (per curiam)
Rinehimer v. CemcoLift, Inc., 292 F.3d 375 (3d Cir. 2002)
Rossbach v. City of Miami, 371 F.3d 1354 (11th Cir. 2004)
Schmittou v. Wal-Mart Stores, Inc., No. Civ.011763, 2003 WL 22075763 (D. Minn. Aug. 22, 2003)
Schroeder v. Hamilton School District, 282 F.3d 946 (7th Cir. 2002)
Smaw v. Virginia Department of State Police, 862 F. Supp. 1469 (E.D. Va. 1994)
Sutton v. United Air Lines, Inc., 527 U.S. 471 (1999)
Tennessee v. Lane, 541 U.S. 509 (2004)
The Civil Rights Cases, 109 U.S. 3 (1883)
United States v. Mead Corp., 533 U.S. 218 (2001)
United States v. Santiago-Martinez, 58 F.3d 422 (9th Cir. 1995) (per curiam)

State Cases

Cassista v. Community Foods, Inc., 856 P.2d 1143 (Cal. 1993)
Civil Service Commission v. Commonwealth, 591 A.2d 281 (Pa. 1991)
Gimello v. Agency Rent-A-Car Systems, 594 A.2d 264 (N.J. Super. Ct. App. Div. 1991)
Krein v. Marian Manor Nursing Home, 415 N.W.2d 793 (N.D. 1987)
Metropolitan Dade County v. Wolf, 274 So.2d 584 (Fla. Dist. Ct. App. 1973)
Parolisi v. Board of Examiners of New York, 285 N.Y.S.2d 936 (N.Y. Sup. Ct. 1967)
Philadelphia Electric Co. v. Commonwealth, 448 A.2d 701 (Pa. Commw. Ct. 1982)
State Division of Human Rights v. Xerox Corp., 491 N.Y.S.2d 106 (NY. App. Div. 1985)

Federal Statutes and Regulations

Age Discrimination in Employment Act of 1967, 29 U.S.C. §§ 621 *et seq.*
Rehabilitation Act of 1973, 29 U.S.C. §§ 791 *et seq.*
Civil Action for Deprivation of Rights, 42 U.S.C. § 1983
Title VII of the Civil Rights Act of 1964, 42 U.S.C. §§ 2000e *et seq.*
The Americans with Disabilities Act of 1990, 42 U.S.C. §§ 12101 *et seq.*
Regulation to Implement the Equal Employment Provisions of the Americans with Disabilities Act: Definitions, 29 C.F.R. § 1630.2 (2004)
United States Equal Employment Opportunity Commission, Interpretive Guidance on Title I of the Americans with Disabilities Act, 29 C.F.R. app. § 1630.2 (2001)

State and Local Statutes

D.C. CODE ANN. § 2-1401.02 (2001)
MICH. STAT. ANN. § 3.548(102) (Michie 2000)
SAN FRANCISCO, CA., POLICE CODE art. 33 (2000)
SANTA CRUZ, CA., MUNICIPAL CODE ch. 9.83 (1995)

Secondary Sources

Fernandez, E. (2002a, May 7). Exercising her right to work. *San Francisco Chronicle*. Retrieved November 16, 2004, from sfgate.com

Fernandez, E. (2002b, February 24). Pursuing fat chances in a slim world. *San Francisco Chronicle*. Retrieved November 16, 2004, from www.naafa.org/news/fatfitness.html

Garchik, L. (1995, February 8). Room with a view. *San Francisco Chronicle*. Retrieved November 16, 2004, from sfgate.com.

Krieger, L. H. (2000). Afterword: Socio-legal backlash. *Berkeley Journal of Employment and Labor Law, 21*, 476–520.

United States Department of Health and Human Services. (2004, July 15). Press release: HHS announces revised Medicare obesity coverage policy. Retrieved November 16, 2004, from www.hhs.gov/news/press/2004pres/20040715.html

CHAPTER 15

■ ■ ■

Remedies for Weight-Based Discrimination

SONDRA SOLOVAY

> Employment problems of the overweight have been sorely neglected. . . . Viewed as less desirable colleagues by coworkers and as less motivated by personnel managers, overweight individuals suffer from employment discrimination. . . . Further complicating the problem is the fact that poor and black women comprise a disproportionate percentage of these victims. . . . Employment discrimination is not the only form of weight-based discrimination. The overweight must also face discrimination in accommodations and education, as well as biased treatment by the medical profession, life insurance companies, and retailers. . . .
>
> —MASON (1982)

Nearly a quarter of a century after Mason's observations, equality for fat people remains elusive, while prejudice flourishes.[1] Make no mistake about it—weight discrimination is a civil rights issue. If mainstream civil rights advocates continue to ignore it, we will find ourselves repeating our cultural history: Decades of civil rights violations lead to the need for affirmative actions to address the resulting systemic inequities.

In addition to discrimination in employment, jury service, accommodations, education, the medical profession, insurance (especially health insurance, which is unavailable to most fat people as individual purchasers), retailers, service providers, interstate travel (via airplane, train, car, and bus), and social settings, families with fat people now face a formidable hurdle: an increase in affirmative discrimination by the government and court systems. In 1982 and 1988 two mentally disabled adults were forcibly removed from home settings and committed to institutions because of their weight (*Pope v. Western Center, Department of Public Welfare, Commonwealth of Pennsylvania,* 1982, and *McPherson v. Court of Appeals of Minnesota*, 1991).

Today the United States government, its agencies, and the courts exuberantly declare a "war on fat." They launch media campaigns that increase the stigma faced by fat people, remove children from their homes and from the legal custody of their parents based on the child's weight, prosecute a woman for felony child endangerment when her child died at a high weight, and remove three aspiring foster children from their home of 6 years based on their new father's weight (Jones, personal communications, 2001–2004; Vogel, 2001). Government campaigns and custody-type cases involving weight often pit doctor against patient or parent and raise serious ethical and legal issues.

Despite the tremendous prejudice fat people encounter, many fat people not only survive, but thrive. This chapter examines legal remedies and strategies that may be available to fat people who are victims of discrimination and celebrates the extraordinary efforts of fat people, attorneys, and size-rights activists who share their skills and time in the pursuit of justice, fairness, and equality.

LEGAL PROTECTION FROM DISCRIMINATION IN THE UNITED STATES

Everyone talks about the "epidemic of obesity," when it is weight discrimination that has reached epidemic proportions. Although the problem of weight prejudice is severe, the remedies available to victims are meager and inconsistent. No federal law exists that specifically prohibits weight-related discrimination. There is no portion of the United States Constitution that expressly forbids this discrimination. While the Constitution might reasonably be interpreted to disallow unequal treatment based on this characteristic/condition, that constitutional question has not yet been litigated meaningfully in a court of law. As discrimination increases in severity and threatens rights Americans consider basic and fundamental, such as the sanctity of the family unit and the ability to travel between the states, Constitutional arguments will be made.

The Rehabilitation Act of 1973 and the Americans with Disabilities Act are federal laws that prohibit disability discrimination. The Rehabilitation Act of 1973 focuses on federal agencies and groups that are federally funded, while the Americans with Disabilities Act provides broader protections that focus on the nongovernment actors. Airlines are excluded from the Americans with Disabilities Act and are governed instead by the Air Carrier Access Act. Using disability laws to address weight matters is complex and somewhat controversial, but is the most promising of the federal remedies (see Chapter 14, this volume, for more discussion of these laws). Unfortunately, few fat people and distressingly few attorneys realize this.

Occasionally, federal laws prohibiting discrimination based on race or sex may be helpful in fighting weight-based discrimination. Oppressions of all types are intimately linked. It is impossible to effectively explore weight discrimination without considering the ways bias based on race, sex, physical ability, heterosexism, gender expression, class, ethnicity, and religion function in American culture and how they impact weight issues. First, because there are more fat women than men, more fat black and Latina women than white women, and more fat people in lower socioeconomic classes than in higher ones, people in those traditionally disadvantaged groups are poised to receive disproportionately more discriminatory treatment based on their weight. Second, the further away a person moves from the mainstream ideal, the more discrimination they face. For instance, while an employer might be willing to hire a fat white woman or a thin Latina woman, the fat Latina faces a double whammy of discrimination. Other characteristics, like age over 55 and lesbian status, become a quadruple whammy.

When women are subjected to weight-related discrimination, while their male counterparts are not similarly discriminated against, Title VII of the Civil Rights Act of 1964 may provide a remedy (42 U.S.C. §2000e-2, 1994). Similarly, when people face discrimination based on their weight *because* of their race, this federal remedy should be applicable. Nevertheless, successfully pursuing even these cases can be tricky.

In 1992, Mr. Hill was fired after 3 years on the job. He was told he was being fired for his failure to comply with body-fat standards. On his complaint with the Department of Labor he checked the box marked "race—black" as the type of discrimination he experienced and explained in the narrative that he was singled out for weight discrimination because of his race. When Hill attempted to bring a claim under the Americans with Disabilities Act (discussed later) the court wrote: "Hill's EEOC charge alleged race discrimination. His district court complaint, in contrast, alleged discrimination on the basis of disability. Hill contends that his disability discrimination claim is one that could reasonably be expected to grow out of the allegation of his EEOC charge. The Court cannot agree" (*Hill v Johnson Controls World Services, Inc.*, 1994). Unable to amend his earlier complaint due to time restrictions, Mr. Hill lost his case.

In addition to the few protections at the federal level, individual states and cities may have laws that protect people from weight prejudice. Weight or appearance discrimination is expressly outlawed in only a handful of places in the country. Most notably these include the state of Michigan; Washington, DC; and the cities of San Francisco and Santa Cruz in California. Other United States cities are currently considering such legislation.

Conceivably, weight discrimination could be illegal under individual state constitutions, but in practice, state and local disability laws are often the only legal tools available to victims of bias. Frequently, coverage as a disability is decided by individual judicial interpretation, jury decisions, and case law, resulting in decisions that vary widely even between neighboring towns.

THE COURT OF PUBLIC OPINION

Frequently finding little relief from the court of law, people who face discrimination and the attorneys and activists trying to help often turn to another court—the court of public opinion.

In San Francisco a fitness company erected a billboard. The face of a space alien hovered over the freeway with a caption that read, "When they come, they'll eat the fat ones first." Led by *Fat!So?* author Marilyn Wann (1998), a diverse group of local activists converged on the sidewalk outside the gym. Dressed in alien costumes they carried signs like "Bite Me!" and "I'm Yummy!" The activists included plus-sized aerobics teachers who led the protesters in movement, singing as they worked out. Several gym members joined the demonstration, including one man in a wheelchair who recounted his experiences with discrimination at the fitness club.

The good-natured protest caught the attention of the public and of the San Francisco Human Rights Commission. Local attorneys, educators, and activists of all sizes organized a hearing on weight discrimination, inviting city residents to talk about the discrimination they faced in employment, housing, and health care. On June 10, 1999, the Commission resolved:

> *Whereas* people experience discrimination based on their body size in employment, resulting in failure to be hired, unfair termination, denial of promotions, and on-the-job harassment; and *Whereas* people experience discrimination based on their body size in housing and real estate transactions, resulting in denial of rental opportunities by landlords, harassment by landlords and co-tenants, and disadvantages in home-buying and business opportunities; and *Whereas* people experience discrimination based on body size in public accommodations, resulting in denial of services by public and nonprofit agencies, being ignored by commercial retailers, verbal harassment by

> employees of public and private organizations and businesses, and denial of reasonable accommodation for various body sizes; and *Whereas* discrimination based on body size is a serious social problem in San Francisco and elsewhere, resulting in verbal and physical violence, lack of self-esteem, eating disorders, psychological problems, depression, poor health care, and suicide; and *Whereas* discrimination based on body size robs San Francisco of the talents and skills of many people who otherwise would participate more fully in improving the lives of all San Franciscans; and *Whereas* the Human Rights Commission works to eliminate unfair discrimination against all people; *Therefore, Be It Resolved*, that the San Francisco Human Rights Commission encourages the Board of Supervisors and the Mayor to enact legislation adding "body size" or a comparable phrase to San Francisco's antidiscrimination ordinance.

As a result, the Board of Supervisors held further hearings and, in May, 2000, voted unanimously to add "height and weight" to the list of protected categories in the city's anti-discrimination ordinances.

On July 26, 2001, the San Francisco Human Rights Commission issued Compliance Guidelines to Prohibit Height and Weight Discrimination.[2] The guidelines outline rights and responsibilities and have the full force of law. Weight is defined therein as:

> A numerical measurement of total body weight, the ratio of a person's weight in relation to height or an individual's unique physical composition of weight through body size, shape, and proportions. "Weight" encompasses, but is not limited to, an impression of a person as fat or thin regardless of the numerical measurement. An individual's body size, shape, proportions, and composition may make them appear fat or thin regardless of numerical weight.

The careful crafting of the definition takes into account the fact that in our diet-obsessed society even thin people can face discrimination for being too fat. For example, a slender woman who wears a size 6 may be denied employment at a fashion magazine because of her weight when the magazine staff wears size 0 or 2 and a muscular police candidate may exceed weight minimums despite being physically fit to handle the job.

The Guidelines further recommend diversity training in height/weight issues for workers in San Francisco and require equitable accommodations: "Fixed seats are often too small for large or tall people. Businesses, such as theaters with fixed seating, will provide an adequate amount of seating without arms and with extra leg room" (Compliance Guidelines to Prohibit Weight and Height Discrimination, 2001, Section IV (A) Example 1). Importantly, the Guidelines also address access and equal treatment in the medical profession instructing, "Medical providers must not deny treatment based on a person's weight or height. Further, medical providers must not make weight loss or weight gain related intervention a condition for treatment" (Compliance Guidelines to Prohibit Weight and Height Discrimination, 2001, Section IV (B)). Rather than being victimized by a nasty gym advertising campaign, San Franciscans utilized the court of public opinion to create a legal remedy where none existed before.

FAT AND FIT: THE JENNIFER PORTNICK STORY

While San Francisco was holding hearings and passing the height/weight ordinance, 38-year-old vegetarian Jennifer Portnick was busy attending Jazzercise classes. Jennifer often took back-to-back classes, and worked out 6 times a week. Because she was both wonderfully fit and fabulously perky, her teacher frequently asked her to demonstrate moves in front of the class and later encouraged her to apply for Jazzercise teacher certification. Though she had the needed skills, Jennifer weighed 240 pounds. Jazzercise officials rejected her saying, "Jazzercise sells fitness . . . a Jazzercise applicant must have a higher muscle-fat ratio and look leaner than the public. People must believe Jazzercise will help them improve, not just maintain their level of fitness."

It was an honor to represent Jennifer in her complaint against Jazzercise—the first to be concluded using the San Francisco law. A lawsuit was avoided and the complaint was dropped through successful mediation with the San Francisco Human Rights Commission. Jazzercise agreed to a global policy change whereby weight would no longer be an issue in the certification/continuing-certification process of instructors/franchisees. In the court of public opinion the verdict was virtually unanimous: Jennifer should be judged by her merits, not her measurements!

BUSINESS AND EMPLOYMENT DISCRIMINATION

Workplace issues are the most frequently litigated weight-related matters and receive the bulk of attention from scholars focusing on civil rights for fat people. When people ask whether it is legal to discriminate against people because of their weight on the job, they expect a simple "yes" or "no." Actually, it depends.

The Americans with Disabilities Act

The Americans with Disabilities Act (ADA) is a federal law that may provide certain fat people with redress for discrimination, either because they have a disability or because they are perceived as having a disability. Many state disability laws are similar, though some are more liberal. In the absence of a state or local law specifically prohibiting discrimination, there is little legal alternative but disability law. Sometimes state law on employment discrimination "occupies the field" of employment regulation, making the validity of local ordinances that add additional protected categories to anti-discrimination employment law uncertain. In California, where two cities have already enacted weight-based protections and a third city is expected to do so shortly, the question is unresolved.

The vast majority of legal scholars who have examined weight discrimination and disability laws in detail agree. In her article "Fat," Law Professor Jane Korn accurately summarizes the current opinion, "I conclude that the law should consider obesity to be either an actual or a perceived disability" (Korn, 1997). Nevertheless, whether weight is covered under the ADA remains a question. Some courts are open to this argument, while others are not. Whether weight discrimination is illegal may depend not on the discriminatory act or on the impact on the victim, but rather on the jurisdiction in which it occurred. In addition, for purposes of the ADA and similar disability laws, protection may hinge on the size of the person, with super-size ("morbidly obese") people protected more easily than moderately fat ("obese") people.

Applying disability law to weight issues is complex. Many fat people do not consider themselves disabled, may be ableist themselves, and are loathe to add more stigma to their load. Similarly, many traditionally disabled people share bias against fat people and fear that the few rights they have will be diluted when fat people use disability law. Then again, many people who are considered disabled by the mainstream society do not consider themselves disabled. Rather than labeling or "othering" a segment of our community, it is important to understand that when a building is constructed with stairs instead of a ramp, the architecture is disabling for those people who cannot use stairs (for an intriguing discussion about weight and modern constructions of disability, see Cooper, 1998). Many in the Deaf community do not consider themselves disabled, but rather members of a linguistic minority, despite the fact that the ADA expressly labels deaf people as disabled. In fact, the legal definition of disability and the lay definition of disability are substantially different.

The sticking point for fat people trying to use the ADA is most often the threshold question of whether the fat person is a "qualified individual with a disability" where "disability" has a three-part test: "(a) a physical or mental impairment that substantially limits one or more of the major life activities of such individual; (b) a record of such impairment; or (c) being regarded as having such an impairment" (42 U.S.C. § 12112(8) (1995) and 42 U.S.C. § 12102(2) (1995)). Physical or mental impairment is defined as: "(1) Any physiological disorder, or condition, cosmetic disfigurement, or anatomical loss affecting one or more of the following body systems: neurological, musculoskeletal . . . respiratory . . . cardiovascular, reproductive, digestive . . . skin, and endocrine," though weight "within 'normal' range is specifically excluded unless the result of a physiological disorder" (29 C.F.R. § 1630.2(h) (2001)).

One of the most egregious errors in judicial interpretation of disability law arises in this question of who counts as "disabled." It is disingenuous for the legislative and judicial branches of the government to attempt to limit fat people's use of disability remedies while simultaneously engaging in campaigns directly, or via the Surgeon General, that label fat people as diseased and therefore a dangerous drain on the nation's economy and a major threat to the nation's health. When fat people, even merely moderately fat people, encounter medical personnel, they are treated as having a physiological disorder, a condition, and even a disfigurement. In medical files a fat person with no health concerns at all will be described as "obese" or "morbidly obese" even absent a measurement of weight or presence of any health problem. It makes no sense that a fat person is treated as impaired in the doctor's office or by health insurance companies, but treated as able-bodied in the courtroom. Further, current policy has a strange result. A fat person is protected from discrimination brought on by the unsubstantiated perception that they cannot do the job because of their weight, but utterly without protection if they are passed over due to the pure bigotry of an employer who simply hates fat people and does not want to hire one.

CHILD CUSTODY

I spent my 30th birthday in Albuquerque, New Mexico, waist deep in documents, trying to help bring 3-year-old Anamarie Martinez-Regino back home. The child, who was receiving medical care, was removed from her parents' custody abruptly. Doctors requested the child be brought in for an exam. When the mother brought her child in for the medical appointment, security was poised to seize the child. Though laws vary by state, normally a child is only removed prior to a court proceeding if there are exigent circumstances. Anamarie was removed due to her weight under the guise that her weight was a threat to her life. In reality, her weight was not an emergency; if there are any effects of weight they are seen over time. If there was a threat to her life, and this is indeed a controversial assertion, that threat was not imminent. A month or two spent preserving the basic fundamental rights of the family to stay together by going to court before seizing Anamarie would not have hurt her. In fact, in the unlikely event that the parents were deemed unfit by a court, the child could have been relocated to other relatives or to foster parents in a manner that was significantly less traumatic than being snatched, screaming, from the arms of mother in a medical setting that is supposed to be a place of care and trust. Here, to justify this suspicious seizure of the child with no notice or chance for a hearing, a racist rationale was used: because the family was of Mexican descent they were deemed a "flight risk." Racism and weight discrimination frequently go hand in hand. This family was lucky. Local attorney Troy Pritchard and his wife volunteered to help them with their case, and numerous activists and experts from the National Association to Advance Fat Acceptance and the International Size Acceptance Association launched campaigns and even flew in at their own expense to help. The family was eventually reunited.

Despite the fact that state custody abuse based on weight generally targets poor people of color and single parents of all races, the progressive legal community has been largely silent on the topic. It is simply inappropriate for the state to put the force of law behind the regulation of weight during childhood, absent actual abuse like forced feeding or forced starvation. Most fat children are in need of state protection to ensure that they receive equal education opportunities and are not targeted for stigma and violence in their schools or homes. That is clearly where state energies should flow.

Fat children may even need protection from their own medical providers when those providers emphasize weight loss rather than fitness and criticism rather than self-esteem. Sometimes members of the medical establishment prescribe dangerous medications, procedures, and diets for children because of their own prejudices about fat, and sometimes they do it out of parental pressure. Even well-meaning doctors have been manipulated into testifying against their own patients when child welfare agencies become involved. Parents of fat children are in a difficult bind—on one hand, they need to protect their children from bias in the doctor's office while on the other hand they must make sure their children receive health care. Because of the potential for state intervention, parents of fat children should approach the choice of practitioner carefully, especially if the family is a member of a racial minority, poor, or a single parent. Bias on the part of the medical staff can lead to a desperate, expensive struggle to keep the family together. Expensive, time-consuming civil lawsuits will result.

Unfortunately, things will likely get worse before they get better. Parents may be coerced into getting gastric bypass surgery for their children at the peril of losing them to the state should the children remain fat (Wilde, 2004). The mortality risks of these surgeries mean parents who subject children to surgery may lose them on the operating table instead, or even after the procedure if there are serious complications. It is important to realize that the bariatric surgeons are not neutral medical providers; they have a significant monetary interest in selling surgeries that cost tens of thousands of dollars. Follow-up cosmetic surgery is frequently needed, adding tens of thousands more to the total cost. There are also substantial ethical implications to condemning a child to the lifetime of abnormal eating that follows these procedures, with few safeguards in place to protect the child's ability to decide his or her own fate when the child reaches an age to do so. Doctors and nutritionists who become involved in contested cases (or cases that become contested when the child ages) are at significant malpractice risk themselves from both the parents and the young subjects of the medical interventions.

CONCLUSION

Remedies for weight-based discrimination are as varied as the discrimination itself. While courts are inconsistent in dispensing justice, people all sizes of large are consistently the recipients of weight-related bigotry. It is imperative that the government, medical professionals, and attorneys work together to combat this tenacious prejudice and that victims of discrimination continue to stand up for their rights in all available forums, including the court of public opinion.

NOTES

1. Language choices are important. Biodiversity is normal. People come in a wide range of shapes and sizes. In this article I avoid the use of the word "overweight" because this word assumes there is a correct, ideal weight. Similarly, I avoid use of the words "obesity" and "morbid obesity" whenever possible. These words assume the validity of a medical diagnosis while obscuring the underlying, highly controversial assertion that fat is, in and of itself, an abnormal and negative condition. In solidarity with fat activists and size-acceptance civil rights organizations, I reclaim and use the "F-word": Fat.
2. See www.ci.sf.ca.us/site/sfhumanrights_page.asp?id=5911.

REFERENCES

Cooper, C. (1998). *Fat and proud: The politics of size* (pp. 117–124). London: Women's Press.

Hill v. Johnson Controls World Services, Inc. 1994 WL 562583 (S.D.GA.), 3 A.D. Cases 805 (1994), at 2 as quoted in Solovay, S. (2000). *Tipping the scales of justice: Fighting weight-based discrimination* (pp. 124–125). Amherst, NY: Prometheus Books.

Korn, J. B. (1997, February). Fat. *Boston University Law Review, 77*(1), p. 27.

Mason, K. V. (1982). Note. *Employment Discrimination against the Overweight*, 15 U. Mich. J.L. Ref.337, 338.

McPherson v. Court of Appeals of Minnesota 476 N.W.2d 520 (Court of Appeals of Minnesota, 1991).

Pope v. Western Center, Department of Public Welfare, Commonwealth of Pennsylvania, 69 PA.CMWLTH 572, 452 A.2d 581 (1982).

Vogel, C. (2001, August 25). At 500 pounds, dad may lose foster sons. *The Buffalo News*, 25 A1, final edition.

Wann, M. (1998). Why I encourage you to use the F-word. In *Fat!so?: Because you don't have to apologize for your size* (p. 18). Berkeley, CA: 10 Speed Press.

Wilde, M. (2004). *Bioethical and legal implications of pediatric bypass surgery*, 40 Willamette L. Rev. 575.

CHAPTER 16

■ ■ ■

Improving Medical Practice

JAMES L. EARLY
JUDY A. JOHNSTON

The issues of bias and stigma have always been and may always be problematic for the health care profession. It is in our nature to live by comparison. We judge everything from colors to marriage partners by comparing the options. This becomes a problem, however, when we begin to ascribe moral equivalents to human characteristics. We may personally wish to be at an "ideal" weight, but does that make 20, 50, or 100 additional pounds morally wrong? Does my preference for green make blue a lesser or tainted color? The health care system holds in its hands the welfare of a very diverse group of patients. They come in all colors, ethnicities, sexual preferences, religions, and beliefs. They also come in all sizes and shapes. The purpose of this chapter is to examine how we can best and most inclusively serve these overweight and obese patients with understanding and with quality outcomes.

In order to evaluate barriers to the diagnosis and treatment of overweight and obesity in the health care system, we first examine our own attitudes. We then proceed through an accepted methodology to successfully integrate the prevention and treatment of obesity into the practice of medicine.

OBESITY AS A TREATABLE DISEASE

There is evidence of uncertainty among health care practitioners when it comes to their role in the prevention and treatment of obesity. A growing body of literature examines both explicit and implicit attitudes of health care professionals regarding obesity. When assessing the attitudes of medical students, residents, practicing physicians, nurses, and other health care professionals, one theme is clear—ambivalence. (Ablah, Early, Wetta-Hall, Burdal, & Zayat, 2004; Campbell & Crawford, 2000; Chambliss, Finley, & Blair, 2004; Hoppe & Ogden, 1997; Kristeller & Hoerr, 1997; Weise, Wilson, Jones, & Neises, 1992). This ambivalence among health care practitioners regarding their role in obesity management is not unlike their feelings regarding other lifestyle issues such as smoking and alcoholism (Aira, Kauhanen, Larivaara, & Rautio, 2003; Harvey & Hill, 2001). These attitudes involve beliefs regarding the degree to which the patient's obesity represents a personal failure of willpower and an uncertainty about their own responsibility to diagnose and treat.

The Implicit Associations Test (IAT) is a method used to examine automatic associations a person has toward a social group (Greenwald, McGhee, & Schwartz, 1998). Using the IAT, researchers have illustrated the deep-seated nature of our unconscious negative attitudes toward obesity across all groups examined, including those health professionals that specifically treat and research obesity (Teachman & Brownell, 2001). These negative feelings are also present in the treatment of conditions where a substantial component of the problem is thought to be psychological or seen as a matter of choice. In one study, physicians spent less time and ordered more tests on their obese patients with migraine headache than on normal-weight patients with the same problem (Hebl & Xu, 2001). Illnesses such as fibromyalgia, headache, chronic fatigue, and attention-deficit/hyperactivity disorder are often viewed through such a bias by health care professionals (Asbring & Narvanen, 2003; Shaw, Wagner, Eastwood, & Mitchell, 2003; Weber et al., 2002). While some of these conditions are seen as more or less a matter of personal control, each has eventually either been classified as a disease or been included in payment systems along with other diseases.

Obesity has not fared as well in either acceptance as a disease or as a condition worthy of reimbursement (Downey, 2002). However, two recent policy changes at the federal level recognize the importance of obesity. First, on April 2, 2002, the Internal Revenue Service determined that obesity is indeed a disease and issued a ruling (Internal Revenue Service Internal Revenue Bulletin, 2002) which allows taxpayers to deduct the cost of weight loss programs as medical expenses from their adjusted gross income if the individual is diagnosed as obese by a physician. The second policy change came with the Health and Human Services announcement that the Center for Medicare and Medicaid Services will remove the language in the Medicare Coverage Issue Manual stating that "obesity is not an illness" (Health and Human Services Press Release: Revised Medicare Obesity Coverage Policy, July 15, 2004).

The importance of these changes is that they place obesity and its treatment in the same category as other chronic illnesses, such as diabetes, hypertension, and cardiovascular disease. Now scientific evidence can be legitimately generated, reviewed, and brought to the table to determine which interventions may improve outcomes. While these policy statements do not guarantee immediate inclusion of obesity in the mainstream of American medicine, they do change the landscape and open the debate, removing barriers to future research and treatment. These policy changes occurred at the same time as initiatives such as Senator Harkin's Healthy Lifestyles and Prevention (HeLP) America Act of 2004. This initiative was designed to impact how we view obesity in every facet of our lives, from prevention and treatment to the places where we live, learn, work, and play. Such initiatives allow the application of models of care to have much greater impact on the design of both practice-based and public health approaches to obesity prevention and treatment (Office of the Federal Register, 2003).

ATTITUDES, KNOWLEDGE, AND SKILLS IN MEDICAL PRACTICE

Despite the uncertainty of our attitudes, there is general consensus that obesity is both a public and private health concern that must be addressed. Never before has the environment been so difficult to navigate, with fast food in every nook and cranny and physical activity being supplanted by computer screens and videogames. Looking back through history, our efforts in this field have been characterized by a lack of structure and consistency. In order to provide a framework for our discussion of these efforts, we have selected Bloom's taxonomy as a guide. In 1956, Benjamin Bloom developed a classification of levels of intellectual behavior in learning, called Bloom's Taxonomy. Using terms appropriate to the higher education setting in which he worked, Bloom named three domains of educational activities: cognitive, affective, and psychomotor. These domains or categories are commonly referred to as knowledge, attitudes, and skills (Bloom, 1956). This approach has long been used in academic medicine to help outline reasonable approaches to disease management.

Cognitive Domain, the category most used, refers to knowledge. Knowing the facts is the bottom level in the sequence of progressive contextualization of information. Affective Domain, or attitude, is less intuitive than knowledge. Attitude either limits or expands the ability of individuals and organizations to place information in the proper context. Attitude is concerned with values and perception of values. It ranges from simple awareness through being able to distinguish implicit values through analysis. Psychomotor Domain describes skill development. As with the other categories, skill development takes place through a series of experiences and internalizations of those experiences until the skill becomes habit. Knowledge and attitude are necessary, but not sufficient, for skill development.

Using this model, let us examine traditional clinical approaches to the treatment of obesity. Because bias, stigma, and discrimination have been barriers to development of a comprehensive approach to obesity prevention and treatment, we address attitudes first. It is of critical importance to understand how patients have viewed health care providers' attitudes toward obesity. In one study involving over 250 women in an outpatient setting, investigators assessed the perceptions of these patients regarding their obesity treatment at the hands of their primary physicians. Although participants, in general, were satisfied with the knowledge of their physicians and the care they received, they were less satisfied with the skill and expertise of their physicians regarding obesity. It is of concern that 50% said their physician had not suggested any of the most common methods for weight loss and 75% seldom, if ever, looked to their physician for help with weight management (Wadden et al., 2000). In another study using focus groups of obese patients, researchers discovered that the traditional approaches to weight loss therapy including exercise and eating habits counseling were generally not viewed as useful by patients. This may be because physicians frequently failed to credit the patient with life experience or a prior knowledge base (Murphree, 1994). These findings suggest that the therapeutic relationship is often strained when it comes to the topic of obesity.

More evidence of this disconnect between providers and patients can be found in an examination of the traditional medical office. The physical environment is often challenging, with chairs that defy comfort and safety, and narrow doors leading to small or poorly arranged restrooms and exam rooms (Kushner, 2002). During the intake process, the patient again encounters an apparent lack of concern for their special needs. Due to the lack of adequately sized equipment, height and weight measurements, needed for accurate body mass index (BMI) calculations, are frequently determined by patient report. One wonders if the office would also accept patient self-report for his or her blood pressure reading or cholesterol level. The message, conveyed by lack of attention to the physical environment, is often reinforced by insensitivity to the emotional stresses of semi-public weighing and the use of gowns totally inadequate to avoid embarrassment. At best, these deficiencies lead to inaccuracy in diagnosing the degree of the patient's problem. At worst, they send a clear message that measurement and treatment of obesity is not valued by the practitioner and his or her team. The attitudes of the staff and the conduciveness of the physical environment either enhance or form a barrier to the next step in Bloom's Taxonomy—the exchange of knowledge.

Obesity, by virtue of its rather unique status as a "semi-disease," has long been treated by anecdote and untested methods. In a publication of the National Heart, Lung, and Blood Institute (NHLBI) and the North American Association for the Study of Obesity (2000) titled *The Practical Guide to Evaluation and Treatment of Overweight and Obesity in Adults,* the authors state, "Overweight and obesity, serious and growing health problems, are not receiving the attention they deserve from primary care practitioners. Among the reasons cited for not treating overweight and obesity is the lack of authoritative information to guide treatment" (p. vi). The treatment of most medical conditions rests on knowledge derived from a solid research base. Unlike obesity, the treatment of everything, from urinary tract infections to depression, is backed up by randomized clinical trials, an expanding base of pharmacological therapy, and an internationally accepted code for reimbursement. Without this base of science and knowledge, medical school curricula have avoided the topic and, consequently, sidestepped the issue of weight and obesity management (Banasiak & Murr, 2001). Not surprisingly, then, the general public has looked to family, friends, and the media to guide its decisions regarding treatment. This also opens the door to the availability and promotion of diets, supplements, and nutritional advice of unproven quality and questionable safety. With the publication of the NHLBI guidelines, we see an attempt to form an expert consensus around a body of knowledge.

Skills, the third category of Bloom's Taxonomy, spring from a solid base of knowledge worked into a usable form. As our knowledge of the etiology of obesity expands to include environmental, psychosocial, genetic, and other factors, we are beginning to understand why traditional medical practice has struggled to incorporate obesity management into their skill set. Physicians have generally lacked specific skills in the diagnosis and treatment of obesity and in the effective utilization of multidisciplinary teams, both of which are critical to the treatment of this disease. Additionally, treatment skills and team involvement support the cost-effective use of the practitioner's time. Having identified deficits in the areas of attitudes, knowledge, and skills we now discuss how these elements can be addressed across the continuum of patient care in order to increase the consistency and structure in the medical treatment of obesity.

BUILDING A BETTER MODEL

Office visits progress through a sequence of chronological events that start with the patient's entrance into the medical environment. The use of a five-step model can help us to better systematize the treatment of obesity in the clinical setting (Early, 2000). Step 1 is the *intention to treat*. Each practicing physician must decide whether he or she seriously intends to treat obesity and then announce that intention through the practice environment. This environment extends from the curbside and parking lot, through the building, to the waiting room, and on to the doctor's examining room. All along this continuum, the attitude of the practice is expressed by the accessibility or inaccessibility of the physical environment. Care needs to be taken to assure that all facilities are not only handicapped friendly, but are also adequate in size to comfortably accommodate obese patients. For example, the waiting room needs to welcome the obese patient with sturdy, armless, or wide chairs and adequate space to assure comfort and safety.

Step 2 in this model is the *intake process*. This includes both the interactions with staff and the procedures that prepare the patient for the provider encounter. The practice needs to foster positive staff attitudes, as well as to develop and adopt routine policies, procedures, and forms for use in the intake process. Front-desk staff should be friendly and welcoming to all patients. To accomplish this it is critical that the practice facilitate a discussion among staff regarding bias and discrimination and how discriminatory attitudes can damage the patient's experience. Procedures used to collect measurement data should ensure patient privacy and respect. The intake should include the BMI and severity classification, a waist measurement on appropriate patients, accurate blood pressure determinations, and recording of this information on a well-organized chart or flow sheet. This will require the availability of appropriate equipment such as scales that weigh to at least 500 pounds, spring-loaded tape measures for accurate waist measures, a stadiometer for accurate height measurement, and large-size blood pressure cuffs. These measurements should be conducted in the privacy of an exam room rather than in the middle of a busy hallway. Forms should reflect a logical sequence of data collection and facilitate the use of that data. Important information should be positioned in the chart through the use of preprinted forms or of a stamp that supports easy access to vital information over multiple visits (Kushner, 2002).

Step 3 is the *physician–patient encounter*. This is where the provider and the patient come face to face and directly address the patient's concerns and the clinical information that has been collected. Steps 1 and 2 set the stage for and inform a discussion of the patient's overweight or obesity. However, the physical environment can again present a barrier even before the practitioner enters the room. The comfort and modesty of the obese patient can be compromised if gowns are not available in XXL or larger sizes. The examining table can provide another challenge if it is not sturdy. In addition, a solid stepping stool that can be placed at varying distances from the examining table is often needed in place of the standard pullout steps.

A review of past history and data collected during the intake can begin the process. This often leads to a conversation regarding the chronic nature of the disease and the role of inheritance, physiology, and genetics in its cause. This approach emphasizes that it is not simply a personal behavioral failure on the patient's part that leads to obesity, but rather a complex process that involves the patient and his or her interaction with his or her environment (Wadden & Foster, 2000). Attitudes, knowledge, and skills, as described in Bloom's Taxonomy, are all very important during this third step. The provider must listen to the patient's concerns with a nonjudgmental attitude, keeping in mind that most obese patients have been on countless diets and have been judged and suffered under the medical system and society for years. An empathetic, not sympathetic, understanding of the patient's struggle in today's "toxic" environment will go a long way toward forming a trusting relationship.

The physician who is successful in treating obesity has a belief in the potential of patients to change. A working knowledge of behavioral theory will help providers understand how behaviors develop and change over time, as well as how skill development can increase the patient's self-confidence and performance. An understanding of the physiology of obesity and pharmacological and surgical treatment options is, of course, a critical dimension of quality treatment. At this point, it should be clear to the patient that the practice is serious about obesity treatment. This awareness creates the potential for a long-term partnership. In order to cement such a partnership, it is important to determine and support the patient's motivation through the course of treatment and the process of altering his or her behavior.

Step 4 is use of *office systems* to provide continued reinforcement to the patient. Office systems include the consistent use of a knowledgeable team, educational materials, skill development tools, and follow-up procedures and practices. Patient change can be supported through the use of self-help tools, plans for accountability, counseling by office team members, phone support systems, group sessions, and so on. Printed materials that use appropriate lay language can also be valuable additions to the office toolbox. Diet diaries and exercise logs can be used for self-monitoring and for patient self-report. One-page descriptive handouts on fruit and vegetable selection and simple preparation ideas can also be useful, and one-page stretching and flexibility guides and walking charts listing calories burned can be provided. Tailored diets, meal-replacement strategies, and recipe modifications can also be used effectively. The careful and coordinated use of any number of these aids can strengthen the likelihood of success once a solid treatment partnership has been established.

Follow-up must be systematic and must go beyond the personal advice of the provider. Techniques for follow-up can include the use of phone scripts that instruct patients on how to report progress to an answering machine or dedicated line. Staff can return calls at the patient's request or if they sense the need for intervention or reinforcement. Use of the skills of the entire treatment team is critical to the success of this step. While it is helpful to have the expertise of dietitians and exercise specialists in the practice, all members of the office team can and should expand their knowledge of obesity and chronic-illness treatment in order to broaden the quality and intensity of follow-up. Group visits can offer a way to educate patients in an efficient and cost-effective manner. Members of the team, especially those with professional credentials, may be able to bill individually for their services, or their inclusion in the office visit can allow enhanced billing.

Step 5 is *outcomes*. Outcomes refer to the technical achievement of measurable goals such as weight loss, improvement of laboratory values, and the like. But outcomes also include improved patient satisfaction, skill development and application, and the achievement of other patient-selected goals. Without tracking outcomes, the practice has no way of accurately measuring success or of systematically improving its quality of practice. Some of the most important outcomes to track are the simple outcome measures that are most valued by both the provider and the patient. At this level, outcomes related to specific behaviors, such as walking a set number of minutes or steps, eating a designated number of servings of fruit and vegetables or meal replacements, or meal planning can be monitored and reinforced by the team. More comprehensive, office-based outcomes may then include tracking of weight, BMI, fitness levels, and other physical measurements. In addition, many practices will value the ability to track the impact of obesity management on other chronic illnesses, such as hypertension and diabetes, medication use, or costs. Such outcomes may be beyond the scope of an individual practice but may be tracked by larger systems or managed care organizations and provide research projects for academic clinical practices. In the future, there will be more and more impetus to gather data for the purpose of accreditation, for justifying reimbursement, and for providing an evidence base for treatment.

In the end, this entire process will be deeply affected by our view of obesity as a chronic disease. In a well-constructed office treatment system, the patient is neither a victim nor a perpetrator, but rather a patient with a disease that demands management. We believe that knowledge and skills are necessary to provide the best care. However, without an empathetic and nonjudgmental attitude toward the patients and their disease, it is unlikely that the practitioner's knowledge and skills will be adequate for long-term success. Today, we have safe and scientifically effective drug therapies, new methods for classifying obesity, and new treatment guidelines, along with increased dollars for obesity research. We have an improved understanding of nutrition and exercise and better models for applying behavioral theory to practical treatment of the disease. Now we have to do a better job of integrating these advances with our understanding of how beliefs and attitudes pave the way to the development of excellent systems of obesity management.

REFERENCES

Ablah, E., Early, J., Wetta-Hall, R., Burdal, C. A., & Zayat, J. (2004). *Medical residents' beliefs and attitudes regarding obesity.* Paper presented at the annual meeting of the Southwest Psychological Association, San Antonio, TX.

Aira, M., Kauhanen, J., Larivaara, P., & Rautio, P. (2003). Factors influencing inquiry about patients' alcohol by primary care physicians: Qualitative semi-structured interview study. *Family Practice, 20*(3), 270–275.

Asbring, P., & Narvanen, A. L. (2003). Ideal versus reality: Physicians' perspectives on patients with chronic fatigue syndrome (CFS) and fibromyalgia. *Social Science and Medicine, 57*(4), 711–720.

Banasiak, M., & Murr, M. M. (2001). Medical school curricula do not address obesity as a disease. *Obesity Surgery, 11*(6), 677–679.

Bloom, B. S. (Ed.). (1956). *Taxonomy of educational objectives: The classification of educational goals.* New York: Longmans.

Campbell, K., & Crawford, D. (2000). Management of obesity: Attitudes and practices of Australian dietitians. *International Journal of Obesity, 24,* 701–710.

Chambliss, H. O., Finley, C. E., & Blair, S. N. (2004). Attitudes toward obese individuals among exercise science students. *Medicine and Science in Sports and Exercise*, *36*(3), 468–474.

Downey, M. (2002). Insurance coverage for obesity treatments. In D. H. Bessesen & R. Kushner (Eds.), *Evaluation and management of obesity* (pp. 139–144). Philadelphia, PA: Hanley & Belfus.

Early, J. (2000). *Practical approaches to managing obesity in clinical practice*. Presentation at the American Association of Clinical Endocrinologists 9th annual meeting and clinical congress, Atlanta, GA.

Greenwald, A. G., McGhee, D. E., & Schwartz, J. L. K. (1998). Measuring individual differences in implicit cognition: The implicit association test. *Journal of Personality and Social Psychology 74*, 1464–1480.

Harvey, E. L., & Hill, A. J. (2001). Health professionals' views of overweight people and smokers. *International Journal of Obesity, 25*, 1253–1261.

Hebl, M. R., & Xu, J. (2001). Weighing the care: Physicians' reactions to the size of a patient. *International Journal of Obesity Related Disorders*, *25*(8), 1246–1252.

Hoppe, R., & Ogden, J. (1997). Practice nurses' beliefs about obesity and weight related interventions in primary care. *International Journal of Obesity Related Metabolic Disorders, 21,* 141–146.

Internal Revenue Service Internal Revenue Bulletin 2002-16. (2002, April 22). *Part 1, Section 213. Medical, Dental, etc., Expenses Rev. Rul. 2002-19.* Washington, DC: Author.

Kristeller, J. L., & Hoerr, R. A. (1997). Physician attitudes toward managing obesity: Differences among six specialty groups. *Preventive Medicine, 26*, 542–549.

Kushner, R. (2002). Office-based obesity care: Setting up the office environment. In D. H. Bessesen & R. Kushner (Eds.), *Evaluation and management of obesity.* Philadelphia: Hanley & Belfus.

Murphree, D. (1994). Patient attitudes toward physician treatment of obesity. *Journal of Family Practice*, *38*(1), 45–48.

National Heart, Lung, and Blood Institute (NHLBI) & North American Association for the Study of Obesity (NAASO). (2000). *Practical guide to the identification, evaluation, and treatment of overweight and obesity in adults* (NIH Publication No.00-4084). Bethesda, MD: National Institutes of Health.

Office of the Federal Register, National Archives and Records Administration. (2003, October 22). Federal Register, 68(204). Retrieved July 22, 2004, from www. access.gpo.gov.su_docs/fedreg/a031022c.html

Shaw, K., Wagner, I., Eastwood, H., & Mitchell, G. (2003). A qualitative study of Australian GPs' attitudes and practices in the diagnosis and management of attention-deficit/hyperactivity disorder (ADHD). *Family Practice*, *20*(2), 129–134.

Teachman, B. A., & Brownell, K. D. (2001). Implicit anti-fat bias among health professionals: Is anyone immune? *International Journal of Obesity, 25*, 1525–1531.

Wadden, T. A., Anderson, D. A., Foster, G. D., Bennet, A., Steinberg, C., & Sarwer,

D. B. (2000). Obese women's perceptions of their physicians' weight management attitudes and practices. *Archives of Family Medicine*, *9*, 854–860.

Wadden, T. A., & Foster, G. D. (2000). Behavioral treatment of obesity. In M. D. Jensen (Ed.), *The medical clinics of North America: Obesity* (pp. 441–461). Philadelphia, PA: Saunders.

Weber, M., Daures, J. P., Fabre, N., Druais, P. L., Dardenne, J., Slama, A., et al. (2002). Influence of general practitioners' personal knowledge on migraine in medical attitudes towards their patients suffering from migraine. *Revue Neurologique (Paris)*, *158*(4), 439–445.

Wiese, H. J., Wilson, J. F., Jones, R. A., & Neises, M. (1992). Obesity stigma reduction in medical students. *International Journal of Obesity Related Metabolic Disorders*, *16*, 859–868.

CHAPTER 17

■ ■ ■

Improving the Health Care System

CHRISTINA C. WEE
SUSAN Z. YANOVSKI

Increasingly, health is viewed as encompassing not only a person's physical well-being but also his or her emotional and psychological well-being. As discussed in preceding chapters, obesity, more than any other common medical condition, affects health on multiple levels. Hence, providing quality health care to persons who are overweight or obese includes addressing these different health domains.

Because of widespread societal bias and stigma, persons with obesity may have low self-esteem and poor self-image; consequently, addressing the health care needs of this population requires sensitivity and patience on the part of health providers. This is particularly challenging in the wake of the obesity epidemic, in which clinicians are called to address the issue of weight and weight control on a routine basis with their patients. This comes at some risk if providers interact with patients in an insensitive manner or at an inopportune time. Moreover, not all obese patients are motivated to attempt weight loss; many have made such attempts numerous times, only to regain the lost weight. Repeated discussions about losing weight with patients who are not currently motivated or able to attempt weight loss treatment may alienate and deter them from seeking care for other important health issues.

Unfortunately, the social bias and discrimination encountered by obese persons extends to the health care arena and has important implications for the health of persons with obesity. As described in Chapter 2 (this volume), anti-fat bias in health professionals can lead to impaired clinical judgment, disrespectful treatment of obese patients, and reluctance by health professionals to treat patients who are obese (Hebl &

Xu, 2001, Puhl & Brownell, 2001). This in turn may cause people who are obese to avoid seeking health care. Given the strong association between obesity and medical and psychological conditions, avoidance of medical care among obese persons can have dire consequences. Obese women are less likely to undergo cancer screening for breast, cervical, and colorectal cancer (Rosen & Schneider, 2004; Wee, McCarthy, Davis, & Phillips, 2000, 2004). While the mechanisms for such disparities are unclear, barriers to screening may include transportation difficulties, greater discomfort with screening procedures, restrictions in weight capacity of the equipment used in screening, and greater embarrassment and reticence on the part of the patients as well as provider bias. Interestingly, studies suggest that obese Caucasian women are less likely than Caucasian men or African American women or men to undergo preventive screening (Rosen & Schneider, 2004; Wee et al., 2000, 2004). Studies show that obese Caucasian women are less likely to report breast and cervical cancer screening than normal-weight women; in contrast, screening is similar between obese and normal-weight black women (Wee et al., 2000, 2004). One recent study comparing colon cancer screening by body weight found no difference in screening according to weight in men; however, women who were moderately and extremely obese were less likely to report screening (Rosen & Schneider, 2004). Although not as systematically documented, disparities in other areas of health may occur.

Hence, improving the health care system to better address the needs of obesity requires more comprehensive efforts in addition to changing clinicians' attitudes and biases. It also includes structuring the system to provide a safe, accessible, and comfortable environment. Unfortunately, health care bias against obese persons is systemic and institutionalized. To achieve meaningful improvement in the quality of care delivered to persons with obesity requires change at several levels. In this chapter, we discuss three major areas within health care that we believe contribute to the suboptimal care of people who are obese and suggest potential approaches to rectify these deficiencies. These three areas include infrastructure, attitudes of health providers, and reimbursement systems for health care.

IMPROVING HEALTH CARE INFRASTRUCTURE TO BETTER SERVE PATIENTS WITH OBESITY

Addressing the Basic Care Needs of Patients with Obesity

The increasing cost of health care in recent decades has resulted in an infrastructure aimed at reducing cost and maximizing efficiency. Much of the health care infrastructure was designed prior to the obesity epidemic, and even state of the art facilities and equipment do not always consider the growing size of the average patient. Inadequate facilities and equipment not only offend obese patients but act as physical barriers to quality and appropriate care. Fortunately, the recent explosion in weight loss surgeries (Mitka, 2003) has focused attention on these deficiencies in health care infrastructure for caring for patients with obesity. In addition to the inadequacies discussed in Chapter 16 (this volume), obese patients face many difficulties when they are hospitalized. Standard-sized stretchers and wheelchairs often do not have adequate weight capacity (Hahler, 2002) and when used to transport extremely obese patients can result in injury to both patient and medical personnel. Inadequately sized beds can pose similar hazards. Basic needs such as patient transfers and accomplishing activities of daily living become major challenges. Many tasks that are usually accomplished by one or two medical personnel may require six or seven. Therefore, hospitals need to invest in appropriate equipment and higher staffing levels to ensure patient and staff safety and adequate patient care.

Because nurses and other front-line personnel encounter most of the physical challenges related to caring for obese patients, a growing literature has emerged that identifies problem areas and the need to adapt standard practices to accommodate the needs of obese patients. For example, medical facilities should have appropriately sized equipment for large patients, including large gowns in several different sizes, blood pressure cuffs (including thigh cuffs), scales that can weigh patients of 400 pounds or more, and adequately sized beds and examinations tables (Hahler, 2002). In addition, toilets and commodes should be of appropriate size and securely bolted to the ground. Physical examination procedures may also need to be adapted to accommodate patients' weight and size (Hahler, 2002). For example, obese persons may have compromised respiratory status, which impacts positioning. Staff must be trained on proper body mechanics when transferring patients. Severely obese patients may require special attention to enhancing their mobility, both in the hospital and at home, which may require a multidisciplinary team that includes physical and occupational therapists (Hahler, 2002). Finally, special consideration needs to be paid to the home environment and the social support needs of patients who are obese.

Holland and colleagues (Holland, Krulish, Reich, & Roche, 2001) at the Mayo Clinic describe one model for addressing the basic care needs of their severely obese patients. To preserve patient dignity and privacy, the authors advocate that special rooms and supplies be prepared prior to the arrival of the patient. They have also developed an intranet equipment checklist that catalogs their hospital's expanded capacity equipment and personal care items, their current availability, and physical properties and considerations based on body weight and body habitus. They additionally schedule advanced multidisciplinary care planning meetings shortly after patients are admitted, including members from the nutrition department, social work, transfer/safety team, nursing education, and physical and occupational therapy to address the specific needs previously described.

Addressing Deficiencies in Diagnostic Evaluations

Another major deficiency in health care infrastructure relates to the inadequacy of current diagnostic technology and practices. These deficiencies are ubiquitous and can lead to disparities in care and in adverse health outcomes for persons with obesity. To illustrate this point, we discuss the diagnostic challenges for patients with obesity in three aspects of care: emergency care, diagnostic evaluation in heart disease, and screening for breast cancer.

Managing Trauma Patients with Severe Obesity

Perhaps the most dramatic example of how ill-equipped the health care infrastructure can be for patients with severe obesity occurs in emergency situations and when patients are critically ill. Trauma, for example, is the fifth leading cause of death in the United States. The mortality rate among severely obese persons suffering from trauma, however, is 8 times that of normal-weight individuals (body mass index of less than 25 kg/m^2) (Smith-Choban, Weireter, & Maynes, 1991).

There are several potential contributors to this higher mortality rate (Bushard, 2002). In the care of trauma patients, efficient assessment and maintenance of airway, breathing, and circulation are crucial. Persons with obesity are physiologically more vulnerable in these situations because the airway and breathing mechanisms are compromised due to excess adipose tissue, which causes an increase in workload. In addition, obese patients may have higher baseline oxygen requirements and carbon dioxide production, reduced cardiac compliance or reserve, and low residual lung capacity (Bushard, 2002). Standard protocols to evaluate and manage such critically ill patients often rely on identification of bony landmarks that are less apparent in obese patients. Furthermore, standard diagnostic tools such as ultrasounds and computed tomography (CT) scans are often unhelpful; in obese patients, ultrasounds may not be able to penetrate the patient's adipose tissue or body fat to obtain diagnostic information, and standard CT scans are usually only able to accommodate patients weighing less than 250–350 lbs. (although scans with larger capacities are available at a higher cost). Diagnostic peritoneal lavage, an invasive procedure to diagnose internal bleeding, is contraindicated in extremely obese patients because catheters and trocars are too short and anatomical landmarks may not be available (Bushard, 2002). Adequately sized cervical collars and splints that stabilize fractures are also not routinely available in emergency rooms or ambulances, increasing the risk of further tissue injury or neurological damage. While some of the challenges of evaluating obese patients in the emergency setting cannot be easily overcome, others, such as ensuring the availability of appropriate equipment are achievable, and would clearly be beneficial for managing trauma in emergency situations.

Diagnosing Heart Disease in Obese Patients

Limitations in diagnostic technology also affect the quality of care in non-urgent settings. For example, obese men and women are substantially more likely to develop heart disease (Shaper, Wannamethee, & Walker, 1997; Willett et al., 1995). However, common diagnostic tests are often unreliable or inaccurate in obese patients. Electrocardiograms in cases of severe obesity, for example, contain nonspecific abnormalities and are not as sensitive in capturing conditions such as ventricular hypertrophy (enlargement of the heart muscle), which can occur commonly with obesity (Alpert et al., 2000).

Other noninvasive tests such as nuclear perfusion studies and echocardiography also have limitations (Gottdiener, 2001; Hansen, Woodhouse, & Kramer, 2000). Because of their chest wall thickness, severely obese patients are ill-suited for echocardiography, an ultrasound of the heart muscle. An alternative of using tranesophageal echocardiography provides better images but may result in higher risk of complications (Garimella, Longaker, & Stoddard, 2002). In contrast, nuclear perfusion imaging of the heart results in an overdiagnosis of heart disease. Hansen and colleagues (2000) propose methods that potentially improve the problem of overdiagnosis in obese patients with nuclear imaging; however, these adaptations introduce a greater element of subjectivity in estimating whether a potential finding is a reflection of pathology or an artifact of adipose tissue.

The "gold standard" for the diagnosis of heart disease among obese and normal weight patients is through cardiac catheterization. However, as with many other diagnostic studies, standard cardiac catheterization tables typically have a weight limit of 300–350 pounds. In addition, many cardiologists may be hesitant to perform this procedure in severely obese patients because of concerns about its technical difficulty and potential procedural complications. In a retrospective study, McNulty et al. (2002) found that severely obese patients had the same complication rate as those who weighed less. The investigators made special accommodations to minimize complications in obese patients, including attention to physical positioning and sedation of patients, and making adaptations to X-ray techniques. Their work suggests that although obese patients are at higher risk of complications from traditional cardiac catherization, these risks can be minimized by modifying standard techniques. Hence, routine avoidance of these procedures in severely obese patients with clinical indications for evaluation may not be warranted when appropriate protocols are instituted to accommodate patients' size and medical risk.

Although the limitations of many diagnostic modalities are troubling, there is also evidence many of these modalities can be adapted or improved upon so that they can be applied safely and accurately to patients with obesity (Laslett & Rozema, 1991). Nevertheless, greater innovation and research are needed to both adapt existing technologies and develop new methodologies to improve diagnostic accuracy in patients with obesity. Moreover, promising results need to be disseminated more widely so that they are implemented and made available in all communities.

Breast Cancer Screening in Women with Obesity

As discussed previously, cancer is a leading cause of death among patients with obesity. Many cancers, such as breast and colon cancer, are detectable early through screening, and yet, despite the higher risk for these cancers among persons with obesity, screening rates are lower in obese women than among normal-weight women (Rosen & Schneider, 2004; Wee et al., 2000, 2004). Many factors likely contribute to this lower rate. In Chapter 16 (this volume), Early and Johnston discuss some of the barriers and deficiencies in the infrastructure at physician offices. These barriers may contribute to lower rates of Pap testing to screen for cervical cancer for patients with obesity. These barriers also apply to other forms of cancer screening, including that for colorectal and breast cancer. Screening for these cancers require that the patient disrobe, a source of embarrassment for many patients, but especially for patients who are obese. This experience is worsened if adequately sized gowns are not available or if examination tables are inadequate and patients risk injury.

In addition to these barriers, there are technical difficulties unique to cancer screening in obese patients. With breast cancer, screening mammography is potentially less accurate and more physically uncomfortable for obese women (Kerlikowske, Grady, Barclay, Sickles, & Ernster, 1996). Breast tissue in obese women on average tends to be thicker, which causes a dispersion in radiation that produces a less sharp image (Guest et al., 2000). Several studies demonstrate that mammography images are less optimal in obese women compared to their normal-weight counterparts (Elmore et al., 2004; Guest et al., 2000; Hunt & Sickles, 2000). In addition, the mammogram plates used to compress and image breast tissue may not be adequate for very large breasts, resulting in the need for additional images and compression, which are often uncomfortable or painful for women. The impact of these technical differences between obese and normal-weight women is not completely clear. However, recent research has found that obese women are more likely to have larger and more advanced breast cancers when diagnosed by mammography even after accounting for the frequency of screening (Hunt & Sickles, 2000). Moreover, there is a higher rate of false positives in obese women due to normal breast tissue appearing abnormal on mammograms (Elmore et al., 2004; Hunt & Sickles, 2000), resulting in a higher number of unnecessary follow-up procedures and greater anxiety.

Thus, improvements are needed in screening technology to improve quality and accuracy in patients with obesity, as well as to reduce discomfort in women with large breasts. In addition to improving the current capabilities of mammography technology, researchers and developers should also explore the potential of other approaches. There is growing interest in using magnetic resonance imaging (MRI) technology for breast cancer screening, generally because of its improved image quality, which may be potentially more accurate than conventional mammography for detecting breast cancer in obese women.

IMPROVING PROVIDER SKILLS AND ATTITUDES

Previous chapters in this volume (Chapters 2 and 16) have described the presence of weight bias in medical practice and its impact on patient health and well-being. Many studies have documented the discomfort health care providers feel when treating patients with obesity (Foster et al., 2003). Physicians and nurses rarely receive formal training in the management of obese patients, and many find encounters with their obese patients to be a source of frustration (Frank, 1993). Although there is some indication that patient perceptions regarding their physician's weight-management attitudes are improving (Wadden et al., 2000), patients continue to report weight-related reasons for delaying or avoiding health care (Drury & Louis, 2002).

There is evidence, however, that increasing efforts are being made to address the gap in knowledge, skills, and attitudes of health care professionals in treating patients who are obese. Governmental agencies such as the National Institutes of Health have developed guidelines for the evaluation and management of overweight and obesity in adults (Clinical Guidelines, 1998) and children (Barlow & Dietz, 1998), and professional societies have also worked to develop continuing medical educational materials on obesity, generally with a focus on weight management.

Although there are not currently any specific recommendations for medical training in the care and management of patients with obesity (Accreditation Council for Graduate Medical Education, 1999; Association of American Medical Colleges Task Force, 1998), the first medical school course in obesity management has just been established at Duke School of Medicine (Croasdale, 2004), with an aim of teaching future physicians to effectively treat and counsel obese patients. In addition to providing didactic information regarding the causes, consequences, and treatment of obesity, the course aims to help physicians approach obese patients in a nonjudgmental manner, to assess motivation and readiness for change, and to identify barriers to weight loss.

Although the focus of most of these efforts is on weight management, these strategies can help increase the knowledge and skills of health professionals to address special health care needs of obese patients, including needs that are independent of weight loss. For example, hospitals are developing in-service training sessions for health care personnel to provide appropriate medical care for patients with obesity. Such training may include attention to issues of safety, access to care, enhancing provider attitudes, and adapting practice procedures for patients who may have limited mobility. Professional literature is also increasingly addressing special health care needs of patients with obesity, including the need for sensitive and respectful care (Ahmed, Lemkau, & Birt, 2002; National Task Force on the Prevention and Treatment of Obesity, 2002). Online resources are also becoming more available. For example, the VHA Patient Safety Center, Department of Veteran's Affairs, in Florida, has developed an online bariatric resources guide to offer technological solutions that can assist in the care of obese patients, such as making decisions whether to buy or rent bariatric equipment, lists of ambulatory mobility aids, and equipment safety checklists (Baptiste et al., 2003). A manufacturer of bariatric medical equipment has recently developed an Internet-based initiative to provide information to hospitals on the treatment of bariatric patients, including ergonomics and sensitive treatment of patients (Yu, 2004).

Thus, while much work is needed to improve provider skills and attitudes toward providing respectful and sensitive medical care for large patients, it is an area of active interest in professional education, industry, and health care settings. Specific attention to the impact of stigma and bias on the health care of persons who are obese should be an integral part of the specialized curricula that are developed.

RESTRUCTURING FINANCIAL REIMBURSEMENT AND INCENTIVES IN HEALTH CARE

Thus far, we have proposed several areas within health care that require improvements to allow for sensitive and appropriate care for patients who are obese. Many of these accommodations will result in additional costs to the health care system, at least in the short term. Unfortunately, the current health care payment system places high value on efficiency and cost-containment, at times at the expense of the physician–patient relationship and access to quality care.

Cost-control programs take many forms and include restrictions on choice of physicians, utilization review, limited access to specialists, use of nonphysician providers, shorter appointment times, and financial incentives for physicians (Gallagher & Levinson, 2004) to limit health care use and maximize efficiency. Physician financial incentives to contain cost can take various forms and may lead providers to feel uncomfortable because of a financial conflict of interest whereby physicians, the traditional advocates of patients' health interests, are being rewarded to limit care. Under the current system, clinicians are under great pressure to see a large volume of patients, which almost always translates into less time spent with individual patients. Keating et al. (Keating, Landon, Ayanian, Borbas, & Guadagnoli, 2004) found that 62% of physicians in California felt pressured to see large numbers of patients, even though 32% of them believed that this would compromise patient care.

The current health care payment system and pressures to contain cost can negatively affect the health and care of obese patients in several ways. Obese patients tend to be more sick, have more medical conditions, and have higher health care utilization (Fontaine, Faith, Allison, & Cheskin, 1998; Wee et al., 2005). Hence, obese patients are more likely to encounter systems barriers to care and become more frustrated, which in turn may discourage patients from obtaining needed care and interfere with the physician–patient relationship. Evidence suggests that higher utilizers in plans that "manage" or contain care are more likely to switch primary care providers (Sorbero, Dick, Zwanziger, Mukamel, & Weyl, 2003).

The current system also affects the way that physicians practice. Physicians may try to avoid patients who are more sick or who are higher health care utilizers (and disproportionately obese), especially if they have capitated insurance plans (Shen et al., 2004). Whether current health care reimbursement directly leads to disparities in the care of obese patients is not clear. However, at least one study (Hebl & Xu, 2001) found in a hypothetical scenario that while physicians would prescribe more tests to an obese patient relative to a thinner patient, they were also more likely to spend less time with the obese patient. Moreover, physicians reported that treating obese patients was a waste of time, and that they would enjoy their work less the heavier their patients were. Physicians also reported being more annoyed and having less patience with patients who were heavier. Whether physicians' treatment of patients would improve if physicians were remunerated based on care provided and time spent rather than capitated forms of payment is unclear, but worthy of study.

Less time spent between physician and patients, discontinuity of care, and reductions in discretionary care have a disproportionately adverse effect on obese patients. Because physicians may harbor biases against obese patients, the quality of physician–patient interactions is especially important in order for physicians to get to know their patients and overcome these biases. Similarly, increased contact with physicians may be required before obese patients feel comfortable or develop trust in their provider. Patients' relationships with their physicians are especially important in the context of cancer screening and other preventive services since patients are more likely to follow recommendations about screening if they trust and respect their doctor (Gallagher & Levinson, 2004). Finally, because of the uncertainty regarding the effectiveness of weight-loss interventions, as well as the added costs, many aspects of managing weight are still considered discretionary and not reimbursed by many health care payers. A recent survey by Novation found that cost estimates reach as high as $500,000 each year per institution to make improvements to accommodate more severely obese individuals (Hospitals Feel the Weight, 2003). These improvements are important and necessary and will have a positive impact on not only the care of obese patients, but also the safety and professional satisfaction of health providers and staff. Hence, it is imperative that health care payers recognize these efforts.

CONCLUSION

Persons with obesity, particularly those with severe obesity, are often poorly served by the health care system. Difficulties in performing physical examinations, as well as limitations in diagnostic equipment, may impede prompt diagnosis and treatment. The increasing time pressures on health care providers may serve to limit the time spent with patients whose medical problems or physical condition require additional staff time or attention. In addition, despite the increasing prevalence of obesity, the attitudes of health care personnel continue to reflect bias against obese persons, leading to suboptimal provider–patient interactions, and consequent patient avoidance of necessary medical care. The combination of decreased screening and difficulty in accurate diagnosis may contribute to the increased morbidity and mortality seen in obese persons.

Fortunately, the increase in the prevalence of severe obesity as well as the increasing popularity of bariatric surgery has spurred manufacturers of medical and diagnostic equipment to develop and market an increasing range of appropriately sized offerings. Offices, clinics, and hospitals are increasingly devoting attention to accommodating severely obese patients with specialized equipment and supplies, leading to improved comfort and safety for both patients and staff. Advances in understanding of the strong biological underpinnings of obesity are helping medical professionals to view obesity as a complex and multifactorial medical condition rather than a weakness of will; nevertheless, substantial prejudices remain. Increased attention to confronting and overcoming these prejudices can be incorporated in medical training and continuing education.

Research is needed to identify the most effective ways to improve diagnostic accuracy and treatment in patients with obesity, both through enhancing physical examination and modifications of existing technologies. Although investments in capital equipment, supplies, and the increased time spent in sensitively caring for obese patients may result in an increase in health care costs over the short term, improving access to the health care system should enhance prevention, early detection, and treatment, ultimately benefiting the health of obese patients.

AUTHOR NOTE

The opinions expressed herein are those of the authors and do not necessarily reflect the views of the National Institute of Diabetes and Digestive and Kidney Diseases, the National Institutes of Health, or the U.S. Department of Health and Human Services.

REFERENCES

Accreditation Council for Graduate Medical Education (ACGME). (1999). *ACGME Outcome Project: General competencies*. Retrieved August 2, 2004, from www.acgme.org/outcome/comp/compFull.asp.

Ahmed, S. M., Lemkau, J. P., & Birt, S. L. (2002). Toward sensitive treatment of obese patients. *Family Practice Management, 9,* 25–28.

Alpert, M. A., Terry, B. E., Cohen, M. V., Fan, T. M., Painter, J. A., & Massey, C. V. (2000). The electrocardiogram in morbid obesity. *American Journal of Cardiology, 85,* 908–910.

Association of American Medical Colleges Task Force. (1998). *Report I: Learning Objectives for Medical Student Education. Guidelines for Medical Schools (MSOP Report).* Washington, DC: Association of American Medical Colleges.

Baptiste, A., Kelleher, V., Nelson, A., Fragala, G., Chance, R., Carver, M., & et al. (2003). *Bariatric Resource Guide.* VISN8 Patient Safety Center, Department of Veterans Affairs, James A. Haley Veterans Hospital, Tampa, FL. Retrieved August 2, 2004, from www.patientsafetycenter.com/techResGuide/summary-02new.htm

Barlow, S. E., & Dietz, W. H. (1998). Obesity evaluation and treatment: Expert Committee recommendations. The Maternal and Child Health Bureau, Health Resources and Services Administration and the Department of Health and Human Services. *Pediatrics, 102,* E29.

Bushard, S. (2002). Trauma in patients who are morbidly obese. *AORN Journal, 76,* 585–589.

Clinical guidelines on the identification, evaluation, and treatment of overweight and obesity in adults—The evidence report. National Institutes of Health. (1998). *Obesity Research, 6,* 51S–209S.

Croasdale, M. (2004, May 24). New course at Duke focuses on obesity. Retrieved August 2, 2004, from www.ama-assn.org/amednews/2004/05/24/prse0524.htm

Drury, C. A., & Louis, M. (2002). Exploring the association between body weight, stigma of obesity, and health care avoidance. *Journal of the American Academy of Nurse Practitioners, 14,* 554–561.

Elmore, J. G., Carney, P. A., Abraham, L. A., Barlow, W. E., Egger, J. R., Fosse, J. S., et al. (2004). The association between obesity and screening mammography accuracy. *Archives of Internal Medicine, 164,* 1140–1147.

Fontaine, K. R., Faith, M. S., Allison, D. B., & Cheskin, L. J. (1998). Body weight and health care among women in the general population. *Archives of Family Medicine*, 7, 381–384.

Foster, G. D., Wadden, T. A., Makris, A. P., Davidson, D., Sanderson, R. S., Allison, D. B., et al. (2003). Primary care physicians' attitudes about obesity and its treatment. *Obesity Research, 11,* 1168–1177.

Frank, A. (1993). Futility and avoidance. Medical professionals in the treatment of obesity. *Journal of the American Medical Association, 269,* 2132–2133.

Gallagher, T. H., & Levinson, W. (2004). A prescription for protecting the doctor-patient relationship. *American Journal of Managed Care, 10,* 61–68.

Garimella, S., Longaker, R. A., & Stoddard, M. F. (2002). Safety of transesophageal echocardiography in patients who are obese. *Journal of the American Society of Echocardiography, 15,* 1396–1400.

Gottdiener, J. S. (2001). Overview of stress echocardiography: Uses, advantages, and limitations. *Progress in Cardiovascular Disease, 43,* 315–334.

Guest, A. R., Helvie, M. A., Chan, H. P., Hadjiiski, L. M., Bailey, J. E., & Roubidoux, M. A. (2000). Adverse effects of increased body weight on quantitative measures of mammographic image quality. *American Journal of Roentgenology, 175,* 805–810.

Hahler, B. (2002). Morbid obesity: A nursing care challenge. *Dermatology Nursing, 14,* 249–252, 255–256.

Hansen, C. L., Woodhouse, S., & Kramer, M. (2000). Effect of patient obesity on the accuracy of thallium-201 myocardial perfusion imaging. *American Journal of Cardiology, 85,* 749–752.

Hebl, M. R., & Xu, J. (2001). Weighing the care: Physicians' reactions to the size of a patient. *International Journal of Obesity Related Metabolic Disorders, 25,* 1246–1252.

Holland, D. E., Krulish, Y. A., Reich, H. K., & Roche, J. D. (2001). How to creatively meet care needs of the morbidly obese. *Nursing Management, 32,* 39–41.

Hospitals feel the weight of treating the severely obese. (2003). Retrieved July 20, 2004, from www.novationco.com/pressroom/pr_news031216.asp

Hunt, K. A., & Sickles, E. A. (2000). Effect of obesity on screening mammography: Outcomes analysis of 88,346 consecutive examinations. *American Journal of Roentgenology, 174,* 1251–1255.

Keating, N. L., Landon, B. E., Ayanian, J. Z., Borbas, C., & Guadagnoli, E. (2004). Practice, clinical management, and financial arrangements of practicing generalists. *Journal of General Internal Medicine, 19,* 410–418.

Kerlikowske, K., Grady, D., Barclay, J., Sickles, E. A., & Ernster, V. (1996). Effect of age, breast density, and family history on the sensitivity of first screening mammography. *Journal of the American Medical Association, 276,* 33–38.

Laslett, L., & Rozema, R. (1991). Method to allow safe catheterization of extremely obese patients. *Catheterization and Cardiovascular Diagnosis, 24,* 135–136.

McNulty, P. H., Ettinger, S. M., Field, J. M., Gilchrist, I. C., Kozak, M., Chambers, C. E., et al. (2002). Cardiac catheterization in morbidly obese patients. *Catheterization and Cardiovascular Interventions, 56,* 174–177.

Mitka, M. (2003). Surgery for obesity: Demand soars amid scientific, ethical questions. *Journal of the American Medical Association, 289,* 1761–1762.

National Task Force on the Prevention and Treatment of Obesity. (2002). Medical care for obese patients: Advice for health care professionals. *American Family Physician, 65,* 81–88.

Puhl, R., & Brownell, K. D. (2001). Bias, discrimination, and obesity. *Obesity Research, 9,* 788–805.

Rosen, A. B., & Schneider, E. C. (2004). Colorectal cancer screening disparities related to obesity and gender. *Journal of General Internal Medicine, 19,* 332–338.

Shaper, A. G., Wannamethee, S. G., & Walker, M. (1997). Body weight: Implications for the prevention of coronary heart disease, stroke, and diabetes mellitus in a cohort study of middle aged men. *British Medical Journal, 314,* 1311–1317.

Shen, J., Andersen, R., Brook, R., Kominski, G., Albert, P. S., & Wenger, N. (2004).

The effects of payment method on clinical decision-making: Physician responses to clinical scenarios. *Medical Care, 42,* 297–302.

Smith-Choban, P., Weireter, L. J., Jr., & Maynes, C. (1991). Obesity and increased mortality in blunt trauma. *Journal of Trauma, 31,* 1253–1257.

Sorbero, M. E., Dick, A. W., Zwanziger, J., Mukamel, D., & Weyl, N. (2003). The effect of capitation on switching primary care physicians. *Health Services Research, 38,* 191–209.

Wadden, T,A., Anderson, D. A., Foster, G. D., Bennett, A., Steinberg, C., & Sarwer, D. B. (2000). Obese women's perceptions of their physicians' weight management attitudes and practices. *Archives of Family Medicine, 9,* 854–860.

Wee, C. C., McCarthy, E. P., Davis, R. B., & Phillips, R. S. (2000). Screening for cervical and breast cancer: Is obesity an unrecognized barrier to preventive care? *Annals of Internal Medicine, 132,* 697–704.

Wee, C. C., McCarthy, E. P., Davis, R. B., & Phillips, R. S. (2004). Obesity and breast cancer screening. *Journal of General Internal Medicine, 19,* 324–331.

Wee, C. C., Phillips, R. S., Legedza, A. T. R., Davis, R. B., Soukup, J. R., Colditz, G. A., & Hamel, M. B. (2005). Health care expenditures associated with overweight and obesity among U.S. adults: The importance of age and race. *American Journal of Public Health, 95,* 159–165.

Willett, W. C., Manson, J. E., Stampfer, M. J., Colditz, G. A., Rosner, B., Speizer, F. E., et al. (1995). Weight, weight change, and coronary heart disease in women. Risk within the "normal" weight range. *Journal of the American Medical Association, 273,* 461–465.

Yu, R. (2004, March 16). Obesity epidemic brings business to area hospitals, but at a price. *Dallas Morning News*, p. A1.

CHAPTER 18

Improving the Fitness Landscape

HEATHER O. CHAMBLISS
STEVEN N. BLAIR

The fitness industry is booming, with products and promotions promising easy weight loss simply by joining a gym or using the latest exercise gadget. At the same time, public health guidelines recommending physical activity for general health benefits and weight management are widely publicized. However, physical activity participation among the population is low, and increasing physical activity levels among children and adults is a major public health initiative (U.S. Department of Health and Human Services, 2000).

Common barriers to physical activity include socioenvironmental factors such as safety concerns, lack of affordable or convenient facilities, and competing sedentary interests as well as personal factors such as lack of time, low self-efficacy, and dislike of exercise (Napolitano & Marcus, 2000). Individuals who are overweight or obese often face additional barriers for physical activity, including fears of embarrassment, health problems, limited access to facilities and equipment, and weight bias and discrimination by health and fitness professionals (Ball, Crawford, & Owen, 2000; Faith, Leone, Ayers, Heo, & Pietrobelli, 2002; Lyons & Miller, 1999).

Bias, discrimination, and stigma may limit the accessibility and appeal of exercise for many overweight and obese individuals. Because physical activity is a key component for achieving and maintaining good health and a healthy body weight, these are timely and important issues for the fitness field. In this chapter, we will discuss the major sources of obesity bias and discrimination within fitness settings, identify consequences of bias, present possible solutions, and suggest directions for research.

SOURCES OF OBESITY BIAS WITHIN THE FITNESS LANDSCAPE

Prejudicial Attitudes

Stigma and negative stereotypes toward obese individuals are common throughout modern culture, and obesity has been named one of the last socially acceptable forms of prejudice (Puhl & Brownell, 2001). Many obese individuals report experiencing disparaging remarks and mistreatment in various areas of daily living including employment practices, educational opportunities, and interpersonal relationships (Puhl & Brownell, 2001). Further, negative attitudes and stereotypes directed toward obese patients have been documented among diverse groups of health professionals, including physicians (Loomis, Connolly, Clinch, & Djuric, 2001), nurses (Maroney & Golub, 1992), dietitians (Oberrieder, Walker, Monroe, & Adeyanju, 1995), medical students (Wigton & McGaghie, 2001), and obesity specialists (Schwartz, Chambliss, Brownell, Blair, & Billington, 2003; Teachman & Brownell, 2001). For example, in a survey of family practice physicians, a significant number endorsed negative beliefs toward obese patients, describing them as lacking self-control, lazy, and sad (Loomis et al., 2001).

Prejudicial attitudes toward obese individuals have also been observed among exercise and fitness professionals. For example, undergraduate and graduate students majoring in exercise science have exhibited implicit negative associations toward obese individuals, automatically associating obese individuals with words meaning "bad" and "lazy" (Chambliss, Finley, & Blair, 2004), an effect that has been observed among other groups of health professionals (Schwartz et al., 2003; Teachman & Brownell, 2001). In addition, students endorsed certain anti-fat beliefs and stereotypes, most often in the areas of physical unattractiveness and weight blame. Of particular importance to health promotion are negative attitudes observed for lifestyle behaviors among obese persons, including assumptions regarding eating junk food, control of weight loss, and physical coordination (Chambliss et al., 2004).

Erroneous Assumptions: Fitness, Fatness, and Health

Perhaps one of the most harmful negative assumptions pertains to external evaluations of health and fitness. A common misperception equates weight with health, such that individuals who are of normal weight are perceived as healthy and individuals who are obese are always unhealthy. We advocate that a person with a body mass index (BMI) in the overweight or obese category who exercises regularly, eats a healthful diet, does not smoke, has normal blood pressure, and has no metabolic abnormalities such as blood lipids, inflammatory markers, and fasting plasma glucose can properly be labeled as healthy. However, size often overshadows all other health indicators, including physical activity level and fitness.

It is widely known that exercise is effective in both the prevention and treatment of many conditions commonly associated with obesity, including cardiovascular disease, diabetes, and osteoarthritis. Current public health recommendations encourage all adults to engage in at least 30 minutes daily of moderate intensity physical activity for health benefits (U.S. Department of Health and Human Services, 1996). Individuals engaging in the recommended amount of physical activity will likely achieve at least a moderate level of physical fitness, and research has demonstrated that fitness is an important determinant of health and longevity, regardless of body weight (Farrell, Braun, Barlow, Cheng, & Blair, 2002; Wei et al., 1999). The idea that a person can be "fit and fat" is difficult for many people to accept, particularly given that a common reason for participating in exercise is to control weight and improve appearance. Despite evidence that fitness is more important than body weight in influencing health, many health professionals continue to focus primarily on weight, often making inappropriate assumptions regarding a person's health status. In a pilot study of graduate exercise science students, participants rated profiles of overweight and obese individuals significantly worse on physical fitness, physical activity, and health, even though the health information presented was the same as for the normal-weight profiles (unpublished data). In another survey of fitness professionals, approximately 70% believed that normal weight was very important to a person's health (Hare, Price, Flynn, & King, 2000). As with assumptions regarding character, it is likely that obese individuals encounter prejudgment of their health and fitness status based strictly on their size.

Facility and Equipment Access

Individuals who are obese report limited access to facilities and equipment in various settings; this includes health care settings, where equipment such as wheelchairs, hospital gowns, and examination tables may not accommodate larger-sized individuals. Although awareness of these issues seems to have increased in medical settings (National Task Force on the Prevention and Treatment of Obesity, 2002), relatively little attention has been given to limitations in facility and equipment access in fitness settings. Assessment equipment such as standard blood pressure cuffs, skinfold calipers, and scales may not give accurate readings for larger individuals. Fitness center facilities such as shower and changing stalls may not comfortably accommodate patrons who are obese. Often fitness equipment is not designed for individuals who are obese, and upper weight limits and narrow bench seats or handrails may prevent use of this equipment by obese clients. In addition, cardiovascular and weight training equipment is often arranged to save space, hindering easy passage among equipment. Finally, clothing and exercise accessories are often difficult to find in larger sizes, particularly specialized articles such as biking shorts and sports equipment. These difficulties encountered by obese individuals can be a strong deterrent to physical activity participation.

Employment Opportunities

Although limited data are available, there is evidence of hiring discrimination within the fitness industry. Perhaps most well known is the case involving Jennifer Portnick, a fitness instructor who was denied Jazzercise certification until she achieved "a more fit appearance" (Fernandez, 2002; see also Chapter 15, this volume). This type of discrimination is not unique to the fitness field. For example, in a study involving a mock employment interview for a sales or systems analyst position, participants recommended overweight "applicants" less often than normal-weight applicants (Pingitore, Dugoni, Tindale, & Spring, 1994). Given the focus on body shape, it is likely that hiring biases are even more common in fitness fields than in the general population. This area warrants further study, as the images portrayed as the fitness ideal are often unattainable and could further contribute to feelings of alienation toward physical activity for individuals who are overweight or obese.

CONSEQUENCES OF OBESITY BIAS AND DISCRIMINATION

Avoidance of Physical Activity

Underutilization of fitness facilities and services and avoidance of exercise are perhaps the most obvious consequences of obesity bias within fitness settings. Anticipation of prejudicial attitudes may cause obese individuals to avoid physical activity due to fears of embarrassment or ridicule. For many adults who were overweight as children, such fears have a long history. Faith and colleagues (2002) found that children who reported greater weight criticism also reported less sports enjoyment compared with peers. When fitness professionals communicate negative attitudes, there is a strong potential for obese clients to feel alienated by these judgments and resist seeking wellness services. In health care settings, obese women have been found to be less likely to seek preventive medical services, including breast and gynecological screening and exams, relative to normal-weight women (Fontaine, Faith, Allison, & Cheskin, 1998; Wee, McCarthy, Davis, & Phillips, 2000). Although this effect has not been systematically documented in fitness settings, it is likely that many obese individuals similarly avoid participating in physical activity.

Reduced Quality of Care and Increased Risk of Injury

Failure to seek assistance from fitness professionals may have the potential to increase risk of injury during exercise participation. Medical comorbidities associated with obesity such as hypertension, diabetes, and osteoarthritis are additional concerns. While physical activity is recommended in the treatment of these conditions, special accommodations and monitoring may be indicated. Because fitness equipment and traditional exercises are often not designed for larger-sized individuals, well-trained professionals can further assist clients by modifying exercises and devising a tailored physical activity program to meet individual needs and goals. However, inaccurate assumptions by fitness professionals regarding a person's health and fitness status can result in mismatched exercise prescriptions and erroneous health information. These misperceptions may also inhibit the rapport between professional and client, limiting the effectiveness of lifestyle counseling and wellness activities. Thus, training in special populations such as those who are obese should be an important part of the education and certification process for fitness professionals.

Fewer Employment Opportunities

Employees within the fitness industry are often hired to present an ideal body image. While it can be argued that clients may perceive a professional with a lean and muscular body as an expert, a lack of variability in body types among fitness professionals results in few role models projecting the message of "health and fitness at any size." Without observable role models of overweight and obese individuals living a healthy lifestyle, "fit and fat" remains a remote idea, perpetuating stereotypes and reinforcing unrealistic weight loss and fitness goals.

COMBATING OBESITY BIAS WITHIN THE FITNESS INDUSTRY

Professional Education

One of the most important steps needed to improve the fitness landscape for obese individuals is to enhance the training of fitness and health professionals. Given the prevalence of obesity, it seems reasonable that obesity and physical activity would be a primary topic in degree programs and professional courses. However, few opportunities for specialized continuing education or certification currently exist, and obesity is often addressed sporadically in traditional coursework. Despite a lack of training in obesity, fitness professionals often report feeling competent and having adequate knowledge in working with obese individuals. Yet, misperceptions regarding obesity persist even among trained and confident professionals. For example, in a recent survey, psychological problems were rated as equally important to the etiology of obesity as genetics (Hare et al., 2000). Thus, fitness and health professionals should be encouraged to critically evaluate their skills and experience in working with persons who are obese and to seek further training and professional development in the area.

Ideally, professional education regarding physical activity and obesity would be multifaceted, focusing on empathy and communication skills as well as learning to tailor programs to meet the physical and psychosocial needs of obese clients. An emphasis on understanding and sensitivity is especially important, as professional training often focuses on the health risks of obesity, and individuals working in the field who are lean and fit may not understand the barriers to exercise that obesity presents. In addition, physical educators and fitness professionals working with children must learn to effectively address teasing and mistreatment of obese children by their peers and present physical activities in a fun and inclusive way. This is particularly important given that the stigmatization of children by their peers appears to have worsened over the past 40 years (Latner & Stunkard, 2003).

Although cultural stigma and an environment promoting ideal physique and physical performance create challenges in combating negative attitudes and obesity stereotypes within fitness settings, evidence from recent research suggests that educational interventions and experience may be helpful in addressing the problem. For example, perceptions of greater personal responsibility for obesity have been associated with stronger associations with a "lazy" stereotype (Chambliss et al., 2004); thus, education regarding the complex etiology of obesity may help combat negative attitudes. In addition, evidence supports that personal experience with friends and family who are obese may lessen negative attitudes (Chambliss et al., 2004; Schwartz et al., 2003), suggesting that efforts to enhance empathy among health and fitness professionals through training and hands-on experience (e.g., weighted suits, focused internships, educational workshops) may help reduce bias and stigma toward obese individuals.

Specialized training is also needed to assist fitness professionals in developing expertise in adapting physical activity programs for overweight and obese individuals. Before prescribing an exercise or wellness program, a complete health and lifestyle assessment should be administered to avoid inaccurate assumptions regarding current health status and lifestyle behaviors and to assist in tailoring the program to meet the individual needs of the client. Certification courses offered through major professional organizations are needed to ensure that fitness professionals are capable of monitoring health risks and making appropriate recommendations for lifestyle change.

Equipment Design and Availability

Within the fitness industry, more attention should be given to meeting the needs of larger-sized individuals. While progress has been made in certain special populations such as the elderly and persons with disabilities, few accommodations have been implemented for obese individuals. Upper weight limits of equipment, for example, should be reasonable and well communicated, as this information is often difficult to find in the user's manual or on the equipment itself. While commercial-grade fitness equipment, such as treadmills and stationary bicycles, has weight limits of 300 lbs. or more, limits of home fitness equipment are often considerably less. Seats and platforms should be wide and sturdy, and positions of handles and controls should allow for easy access by individuals of different body sizes and shapes. Fitness facilities should make certain that available fitness equipment is appropriate for a variety of body shapes and sizes, that equipment is positioned for safety and ease of maneuvering, and that staff are trained in the specifications of equipment and possibilities for exercise modification when appropriate.

Advocacy by Professional Organizations

In order to promote change within the fitness industry and academic settings, major professional organizations within fitness, health, and exercise science must identify and call for needed changes. However, advocacy efforts in the area of obesity bias and discrimination have been notably absent from major professional organizations. For example, a recent position stand from the American College of Sports Medicine (ACSM) focused on intervention strategies for weight loss, yet issues of professional training and certification recommendations for program modification were not addressed (Jakicic et al., 2001). Similarly, the *Guidelines for Exercise Testing and Prescription* published by ACSM address in detail the special populations of children, the elderly, and pregnant women, as well as cardiac and pulmonary patients. However, obesity is primarily discussed in the context of weight loss and body composition, with little attention given to the special needs of exercisers who are overweight or obese (American College of Sports Medicine, 2000). Similarly, the primary certifying organizations for fitness professionals consider obesity in the context of coursework but do not offer special certification to credential professionals for working with obese clients.

The lack of organizational advocacy in the area of physical activity and obesity is surprising given the current public health focus on obesity and the creation of outlets to meet the needs of other special populations. One excellent example is the International Council on Active Aging (ICAA), an organization "dedicated to changing the way we age by uniting professionals in the retirement, assisted living, fitness, rehabilitation, and wellness fields to help dispel society's myths about aging. We will also help these professionals to empower aging baby boomers and older adults to improve their quality of life and maintain their dignity" (www.icaa.cc/About_us/ICAAstory_files/frame.htm). The ICAA recently published a checklist to assist consumers in evaluating age-friendly fitness facilities to serve as a resource for professionals and consumers (www.icaa.cc/PressInfo/facilitychecklist.htm). Similar advocacy steps are needed to promote physical activity and fitness among persons who are overweight and obese, and a checklist for weight-friendly fitness facilities adapted from the ICAA version is presented as an appendix to this chapter. (See Appendix 18.1.)

Future Research

Finally, further research is needed to document the effects of obesity bias and discrimination on the adoption and maintenance of physical activity. In addition, studies are needed to determine the effectiveness of interventions to reduce negative attitudes and improve the services provided by fitness professionals. Methods such as consciousness raising, empathy training through the use of weighted suits, and continuing education and specialized certification have been suggested to combat this problem, but most programs are in the pilot stages and have limited data to allow evaluation of effectiveness.

CONCLUSION

The fitness landscape is an area where little has been done to address obesity bias and discrimination. Increased awareness, specialized education, and improvements in fitness facilities and services are simple ways to make physical activity more accessible and acceptable to individuals of all body shapes and sizes. Improving the fitness landscape to reduce bias and discrimination, thereby more effectively promoting physical activity, can have a significant public health impact and enhance the well being and quality of life of many individuals who are overweight or obese.

ACKNOWLEDGMENTS

We thank the Rudd Institute for its support of research in this area. We also acknowledge our colleagues, Carrie Finley, Christy Greenleaf, and Scott Martin, who have contributed their insight and expertise to our work. We thank Colin Milner and the International Council on Active Aging for allowing us to adapt their fitness facility checklist. Finally, we extend our appreciation to the university students, fitness professionals, and clients of The Cooper Institute's Clinical Weight Management Program who have participated in our research and helped us learn about issues regarding physical activity and obesity.

SUGGESTED RESOURCES

International Council on Active Aging. 1-866-335-9777 or www.icaa.cc/

Irwin, C. C., Symons, C. W., & Kerr, D. L. (2003). The dilemmas of obesity: How can physical educators help? *Journal of Physical Education, Recreation and Dance, 74*(6), 33–39.

REFERENCES

American College of Sports Medicine. (2000). *ACSM's guidelines for exercise testing and prescription* (6th ed). Philadelphia, PA: Lippincott Williams & Wilkins.

Ball, K., Crawford, D., & Owen, N. (2000). Too fat to exercise? Obesity as a barrier to physical activity. *Australian and New Zealand Journal of Public Health, 24*(3), 331–333.

Chambliss, H. O., Finley, C. E., & Blair, S. N. (2004). Attitudes toward obese individuals among exercise science students. *Medicine and Science in Sports and Exercise, 36*(3), 468–474.

Faith, M. S., Leone, M. A., Ayers, T. S., Heo, M., & Pietrobelli, A. (2002). Weight criticism during physical activity, coping skills, and reported physical activity in children. *Pediatrics, 110*(2), e23.

Farrell, S. W., Braun, L., Barlow, C. E., Cheng, Y. J., & Blair, S. N. (2002). The relation of body mass index, cardiorespiratory fitness, and all-cause mortality in women. *Obesity Research, 10*(6), 417–423.

Fernandez, E. (2002, February 24). Teacher says fat, fitness can mix. *San Francisco Chronicle,* p. A21.

Fontaine, K. R., Faith, M. S., Allison, D. B., & Cheskin, L. J. (1998). Body weight and health care among women in the general population. *Archives of Family Medicine, 7,* 381–384.

Hare, S. W., Price, J. H., Flynn, M. G., & King, K. A. (2000). Attitudes and perceptions of fitness professionals regarding obesity. *Journal of Community Health, 25*(1), 5–21.

Jakicic, J. M., Clark, K., Coleman E., Donnelly, J. E., Foreyt, J., Melanson, E., et al. (2001). Appropriate intervention strategies for weight loss and prevention of weight regain for adults. *Medicine and Science in Sports and Exercise, 33*(12), 2145–2156.

Latner, J. D., & Stunkard, A. J. (2003). Getting worse: The stigmatization of obese children. *Obesity Research, 11*(3), 452–456.

Loomis, G. A., Connolly, K. P., Clinch, C. R., & Djuric, D. A. (2001). Attitudes and practices of military family physicians regarding obesity. *Military Medicine, 166,* 121–125.

Lyons, P., & Miller, W. C. (1999). Effective health promotion and clinical care for large people. *Medicine and Science in Sports and Exercise, 31*(8), 1141–1146.

Maroney, D., & Golub, S. (1992). Nurses' attitudes toward obese persons and certain ethnic groups. *Perceptual and Motor Skills, 75,* 387–391.

Napolitano, M. A., & Marcus, B. H. (2000). Breaking barriers to increased physical activity. *Physician and Sportsmedicine, 28*(10), 88–93.

National Task Force on the Prevention and Treatment of Obesity. (2002). Medical care for obese patients: Advice for health care professionals. *American Family Physician, 65*(1), 81–88.

Oberrieder, H., Walker, R., Monroe, D., & Adeyanju, M. (1995). Attitude of dietetics students and registered dieticians toward obesity. *Journal of the American Dietetic Association, 95,* 914–916.

Pingitore, R., Dugoni, B. L., Tindale, R. S., & Spring, B. (1994). *Journal of Applied Psychology, 79*(6), 909–917.

Puhl, R., & Brownell, K. D. (2001). Bias, discrimination and obesity. *Obesity Research, 9,* 788–805.

Schwartz, M. B., Chambliss, H. O., Brownell, K. D., Blair, S. N., & Billington, C. (2003). Weight bias among health professionals specializing in obesity. *Obesity Research, 11*(9), 1033–1039.

Teachman, B. A., & Brownell, K. D. (2001). Implicit anti-fat bias among health professionals: Is anyone immune? *International Journal of Obesity, 25,* 1525–1531.

U.S. Department of Health and Human Services. (1996). *Physical activity and health: A report of the Surgeon General.* Atlanta, GA: U.S. Department of

Health and Human Services, Centers for Disease Control and Prevention, National Center for Chronic Disease Prevention and Health Promotion.

U.S. Department of Health and Human Services. (2000). *Healthy people 2010*. Washington, DC: Department of Health and Human Services.

Wee, C. C., McCarthy, E. P., Davis, R. B., & Phillips, R. S. (2000). Screening for cervical and breast cancer: Is obesity an unrecognized barrier to preventive care? *Annals of Internal Medicine, 132,* 697–704.

Wei, M., Kampert, J. B., Barlow, C. E., Nichaman, M. Z., Gibbons, L. W., Paffenbarger, R. S., Jr., et al. (1999). Relationship between low cardiorespiratory fitness and mortality in normal-weight, overweight, and obese men. *Journal of the American Medical Association, 282*(16), 1547–1553.

Wigton, R. S., & McGaghie, W. C. (2001). The effect of obesity on medical students' approach to patients with abdominal pain. *Journal of General Internal Medicine*, *16*, 262–265.

APPENDIX 18.1. Weight-Friendly Fitness Facility Evaluation

This survey is to be used by people interested in selecting a weight-friendly fitness facility or by health and fitness professionals when evaluating a facility. Complete this evaluation by answering each question to indicate *no*, *yes*, or *not applicable*.

	NO	YES	N/A	Notes
Facility and operations				
1. Is the parking lot and pathway to the center:				
a. Accessible?				
b. Level and smooth?				
c. Close to the entrance?				
2. Does the facility have power door openers at exterior and interior entrances?				
3. Are the exterior and interior doors wide enough to allow easy passage?				
4. Is there elevator access to other areas of the center?				
5. Are all areas of the facility accessible to wheelchairs?				
6. Is the facility's atmosphere one you feel comfortable in?				
7. Are the locker rooms and showers able to accommodate larger-sized individuals?				
a. Locker sizes?				
b. Shower privacy?				
c. Adequate circulation space?				
8. Does the organization belong to a professional fitness association that specializes in fitness for overweight and obese clients?				
9. Does the facility offer a stretching area or stations off the floor?				
10. Does the facility have a lap pool with:				
a. Built-in steps or stairs to accommodate larger-sized individuals and persons with disabilities?				
b. A lift to accommodate larger-sized individuals and persons with disabilities?				

(continued)

	NO	YES	N/A	Notes
11. Does the facility have a group exercise pool with:				
a. Built-in steps or stairs to accommodate larger-sized individuals and persons with disabilities?				
b. A lift to accommodate larger-sized individuals and persons with disabilities?				
12. Are chairs in waiting areas able to accommodate larger-sized individuals?				
13. Are there dedicated areas for weight management classes?				
a. Lecture and group activity room?				
b. Cooking and food preparation?				
c. Exercise room?				
Equipment				
14. Does the facility's cardiovascular equipment include:				
a. Treadmills?				
b. Cycles and rowers?				
c. Steppers?				
d. Cross-trainers?				
e. Ellipticals?				
15. Do the treadmills have the following weight-friendly features?				
a. Upper weight limit able to safely accommodate larger-sized individuals (*defined* as 350 pounds or above)?				
b. Easily entered and exited by larger-sized individuals or persons with a variety of functional abilities and disabilities?				
c. A slow starting speed, ideally 0.5 miles per hour?				
d. A "coasting" feature when stopped?				
e. Supportive handrails?				
f. Emergency lanyard with belt clip?				
g. Wide and stable platform?				
h. Keypad within easy reach?				
i. Low impact?				

(continued)

j. Adequate space to move easily between equipment?				
k. Adequate space to move easily behind the equipment?				
16. Do the cycles and rowers have the following weight-friendly features?				
a. Upper weight limit able to safely accommodate larger-sized individuals?				
b. Easily entered and exited by larger-sized individuals or persons with a variety of functional abilities and disabilities?				
c. Wide and comfortable seat?				
d. Keypad within easy reach?				
e. Seat and arm adjustments that are easy to access and easy to adjust?				
f. Adequate space to move easily between equipment?				
g. Adequate space to move easily behind the equipment?				
17. Do the steppers have the following weight-friendly features?				
a. Upper weight limit able to safely accommodate larger-sized individuals?				
b. Easily entered and exited by larger-sized individuals or persons with a variety of functional abilities and disabilities?				
c. Keypad within easy reach?				
d. Adequate space to move easily between equipment?				
e. Adequate space to move easily behind the equipment?				
18. Do the cross-trainers have the following weight-friendly features?				
a. Upper weight limit able to safely accommodate larger-sized individuals?				
b. Easily entered and exited by larger-sized individuals or persons with a variety of functional abilities and disabilities?				
c. Keypad within easy reach?				

(continued)

d. Supportive handrails?				
e. Adequate space to move easily between equipment?				
f. Adequate space to move easily behind the equipment?				
19. Do the ellipticals have the following weight-friendly features?				
a. Upper weight limit able to safely accommodate larger-sized individuals?				
b. Easily entered and exited by larger-sized individuals or persons with a variety of functional abilities and disabilities?				
c. Keypad within easy reach?				
d. Supportive handrails?				
e. Adequate space to move easily between equipment?				
f. Adequate space to move easily behind the equipment?				
20. Does the facility's strength equipment (free weights or weight machines) have the following weight-friendly features?				
a. Easily entered and exited by larger-sized individuals or persons with a variety of functional abilities and disabilities?				
b. Range-of-motion adjustments that allow larger-sized individuals and those with functional limitations to be in the proper position while exercising?				
c. Easily adjustable hand, seat, and pad positions?				
d. Ability to change resistance from a seated position?				
e. Small increments in the:				
i. Selectorized weight stacks?				
ii. Dumbbells?				
iii. Barbells?				
f. Adequate space to move easily between equipment?				
g. Wider seats and benches for people who need extra surface for support and balance?				

(continued)

Programming				
21. Does the facility offer programs designed to meet the needs of those with a variety of chronic conditions (e.g., obesity, cardiovascular disease, diabetes, and arthritis)?				
22. Do exercise classes have different levels of intensity, duration, and skill level?				
23. Are classes offered:				
a. In a dedicated space?				
b. With participants of different body sizes and shapes?				
c. With participants of similar body sizes and shapes?				
d. To a small number of clients (≤ 5)?				
e. To a moderate number of clients (6 to 15)?				
f. To a large number of clients (≥ 16)?				
24. Is there an adequate screening and assessment process (i.e., medical history, physical activity, nutrition, and health goals)?				
25. Do staff members offer counseling on the following:				
a. Nutrition?				
b. Fitness and physical activity?				
c. Behavioral modification?				
d. Weight management?				
26. Is assessment/monitoring equipment able to accommodate larger-sized individuals? (e.g., scales, blood pressure cuffs, heart rate monitor belts, and skinfold calipers)?				
27. Are assessments conducted in a private area?				
Staff				
28. Do staff members have expertise or specializations in the following areas?				
a. Nutrition?				
b. Fitness and physical activity?				
c. Behavioral modification?				
d. Weight management?				
29. Is the staff polite, friendly, and caring?				

(continued)

30. Is the staff certified by a nationally recognized fitness organization to work with people who have various health issues that may arise with obesity (e.g., osteoarthritis, hypertension, and diabetes)?				
31. Do staff members ask about health history, which movements cause pain, fatigue or discomfort, and which activities or exercises are feasible for each client?				
32. Is the staff properly trained to identify the warning signs of fatigue or distress, and to handle emergencies that may arise?				
33. Is the staff knowledgeable about the impact that obesity can have on exercise ability?				
34. Is the staff knowledgeable about how to modify exercises to accommodate different body sizes and limitations?				
35. Are different body types and sizes represented among staff members and instructors?				
36. Is the staff knowledgeable about the weight restrictions on facility equipment (cardiovascular equipment, resistance balls, etc.)?				
Additional questions and notes				

CHAPTER 19

■ ■ ■

Changing Media Images of Weight

MICHELE WESTON
DIANE BLISS

The media exerts a powerful influence on how we view ourselves. Chapter 3 reviews the literature on how weight is portrayed in the media and concludes that the media presents far more thin people than heavy people, and the heavy people shown are often in stereotypical roles. Media images can both promote and reflect cultural shifts. Positive images of overweight individuals are becoming more commonplace, and the plus-size movement in the fashion industry has gained notoriety; however, it is too early to tell if there will be a genuine media transformation. The aim of the present chapter is to review the past and current ways weight is portrayed in both print and visual media from the perspective of individuals who work inside those industries.

PORTRAYALS OF FAT PEOPLE ON TELEVISION

Fat is funny. So goes the adage in the entertainment world. But fat in and of itself is just fat. Fat people experience the same range of emotions and demonstrate the same variety of personality quirks and foibles as any other human being, yet the vast majority of representations in the entertainment media are one-dimensional, with the person's size being the only characteristic that is shown or highlighted. And Hollywood continues to perpetuate the myth of fat people as dumb, lazy, and slovenly, as if all these characteristics are inherently part of being fat.

These negative and stereotypical portrayals are slowly changing to include positive portrayals and story lines that reflect the larger woman as a complete person. The most common representations of fat women in the entertainment media tend to fall into one of five categories: (1) the clown, (2) the caretaker, (3) the best friend, (4) the shrew, or (5) the punchline.

The Clown

The character Mimi from *The Drew Carey Show*, the chief antagonist of the lead character, is the archetype for a fat woman as clown. Mimi's visual representation alone screamed "I'm a clown," with wildly colorful prints or polka-dotted clothing and garish, over-the-top make-up. For the majority of the run of the show Mimi was portrayed as an asexual person with no love interests and no life outside the job environment she shared with the main character at a department store. In a major departure from tradition, in the show's final season, Mimi was finally given a story line that included dating, marriage, and motherhood, a marked contrast to the previous story lines in which we were led to believe that no one could possibly want Mimi in a romantic way.

The Caretaker

In the 1950s and 1960s, *The Andy Griffith Show* featured Aunt Bea, the fat matriarch taking care of the "boys" in the Griffith household. Aunt Bea was always portrayed as being fulfilled simply by the act of caring for Andy and his son, Opie, and she was seldom featured in a story line that included romance or any interests outside of home and family.

The Best Friend

Among classic sitcoms, the leading lady was most often slender and pretty with a pudgier, less traditionally attractive sidekick/best friend. *I Love Lucy* and *The Lucy Show* featured Lucille Ball as the clown with her straight woman, Vivian Vance. Vance never got to ham it up as much as Lucy, and there was a clause in Vance's contract stating that she would maintain a weight that was more than Lucille Ball. Mary Tyler Moore was the happy-go-lucky girl about town, while her best friend, Rhoda was heavier and appeared more desperate in her search for a man. The spin-off for Rhoda was never as successful as *The Mary Tyler Moore Show*, only lasting for a few seasons.

The Shrew

In the 1980s, women of substantial physical stature were in leading roles in sitcoms for the first time: Bea Arthur in *Maude* and *The Golden Girls* and Nell Carter in *Gimme a Break*. The contrast between the two actors' roles is striking. Maude was portrayed as a strong, independent, feminist woman with no emotional encumbrances or children—the archetype of the shrewish Amazon. In contrast, Nell Carter was portrayed as the traditional "Mammy" caretaker to a white family, reinforcing negative stereotypes of not only size but also socioeconomic status and race.

During the same time period, we finally saw a plus-size woman of means with Isabel Sanford as Weezie on *The Jeffersons*. While Weezie was caretaker to her husband, George, she also had a maid of her own and was not boxed into any of the other stereotypical roles for women of size or color, making this a break-out role on many levels.

Designing Women was another sitcom from the 1980s that featured a plus-size character, with Delta Burke as Suzanne Sugarbaker. While the show never intended to feature a plus-size character, Burke's weight gain during the run of the show made it a fact. While viewers never seemed to mind that Burke gained weight during the show, Burke was repeatedly hounded by the show's producers and network executives to lose the weight, and her struggles with her weight were frequently fodder for the tabloids and entertainment news. Burke eventually embraced her new-found shape and launched a successful clothing line catering to plus-sizes and carried by major department stores across the country.

The Punchline

Shallow Hal, a film by the Farrelly Brothers, is the archetype of fat woman as punchline. The leading man falls madly in love with an obese woman after being shown her "true inner beauty" through hypnosis. He is the only one who sees her as the lovely, and notably *slender*, Gwyneth Paltrow. From broken chairs and tipping canoes, to a rear shot of a fat woman in a too-small bikini, every fat joke in the film used the plus-size woman as the visual punchline. Even the basic premise of the film is insulting, since it implies that no one could possibly fall in love with an obese woman unless he was hypnotized or conned into believing she was thin. Advocates of the film might view it as promoting the positive message of loving the person within rather than the outward appearance, but there are so many fat jokes along the way that it is hard for the film as a whole to convey a positive message about size acceptance.

POSITIVE PORTRAYALS ON TELEVISION

In the fall of 1990, a new sitcom featuring plus-size women debuted called *Babes*. It was the first television show ever to focus on a group of plus-size women as the leading characters. Wendy Jo Sperber, Lesley Boone, and Susan Peretz starred in the sitcom, which was about the three Gilbert sisters (Marlene, Charlene, and Darlene), who happened to be plus-size. Simply featuring plus-size women in leading roles was certainly a step in a positive direction, but the show was chock-full of weight jokes and diatribes about how difficult it is for a woman of size to find a man. While the show made an honest and good-intentioned effort at portraying the three leading characters as fully developed, three-dimensional human beings, the show only lasted one season on the FOX network. Boone has been most recently seen as series regular Molly Hudson on the show *Ed*, a part notable for seldom discussing her size.

Since that initial foray into the world of plus-size women, there have been some positive portrayals of plus-size women, a few of which have barely even acknowledged that the character happens to not be thin. One of the first to break out of the mold was Patrika Darbo in her role of Nancy Miller Wesley on *Days of Our Lives* (1998–2003). The 1990s also brought us Roseanne Arnold as a white-trash version of herself on her self-titled sitcom, and demonstrated that someone of size can be a wife, mother, and business owner, as well as being the clown, the shrew, and the caretaker.

Veronica's Closet featured the voluptuous Kirstie Alley in the lead role with the plus-size Kathy Najimy as a best friend/sidekick. As with Delta Burke, Alley's weight was frequently a topic for discussion behind the scenes, and she was repeatedly told by network executives that her failure to keep her weight at a certain level jeopardized the continuation of the show. Alley stood strong and refused to let her weight be dictated by the powers that be, and rumor has it that Alley's refusal to cave on her weight contributed to the demise of the show. Alley signed with Showtime in 2004 to executive produce and star in a show titled *Fat Actress*, which aired in the new TV season for 2005 (discussed later in the chapter).

In the dramatic arena, the most prominent and recognizable role has been Ellenor Frutt on *The Practice*, an ABC drama created by David E. Kelley. Camryn Manheim won an Emmy and national acclaim as the feisty, determined lawyer who just happened to be a size 22. Manheim's one-woman show, *Wake Up, I'm Fat!,* paired with her incredible talent, opened doors for her in her quest for recognition and roles. In her book of the same name, she describes her meeting with Kelley, where she challenged him to a game of cribbage and won, earning her an audition for the part of Ellenor. While her weight was a sidebar in one or two episodes, for the most part, the character of Ellenor Frutt was portrayed as being a woman of stature for whom size just was not an issue.

In 2003, the ABC sitcom *Less Than Perfect* debuted. Created by Terri Minsky, the show was developed with the intention of showing the life of a woman who is not a perfect size 2. The lead character of Claude is played by size 10 Sara Rue, who is adamant that she is just a regular-size woman, not someone who is plus-sized. The show also features Claude's best friend and cohort in crime, Ramona, played by the very voluptuous Sherri Shepherd.

The Gilmore Girls on the WB network features Melissa McCarthy in the role of best friend, Sookie St. James. She is another actress who chooses not to identify as a plus-size woman, but rather as an actress just doing her job. Yet the portrayal of Sookie's love life has been a groundbreaking and positive representation of a plus-size woman.

There are currently two new TV series that star plus-size women. The HBO series, *Good in Bed*, which is based on the book by the same name by Jennifer Weiner and set to star Tony award-winning actress Marissa Jaret Winokour in the lead role, is still in development. As noted earlier, Showtime's series, *Fat Actress*, a mostly improvised show that stars Kirstie Alley, aired in the 2005 TV season. *Fat Actress* initially had the potential to provide a positive portrayal of a large woman; however, *People* magazine stories report that Kirstie Alley vowed she has not had sex in her "fat body" and she would be thin by the time the show aired in spring 2005. Alley's vow to be thin by the time the show aired, however, was not to be. Her show has been met with lukewarm reception.

THE PORTRAYAL OF WEIGHT IN FASHION AND ENTERTAINMENT PUBLICATIONS

In the mid-1800s, fashion models were voluptuous women. By the mid-1900s, designers felt that ample bodies detracted attention from the clothes, so thinner women were employed because the clothing hung on them as it would a clothes hanger. The "skinny mini" image of women in the fashion media continued for several decades, but as the size-acceptance movement has gained momentum, the fashion industry has begun to change. There were early size-acceptance magazines in the 1980s of titles such as *BBW*, *Dimensions*, and *Radiance*. In 1997, *Mode* magazine opened the doors to beautiful, compelling imagery of full-figured women. The founding team of *Mode* magazine saw the opportunity to "shape shift" and helped lead the industry to see beauty and fashion as an aspirational ideal, not limited by size. While neither *Mode,* nor the subsequent *Grace,* survived, their legacy is greater attention to the issue of diversity among body shapes and sizes in the magazine industry.

At least a decade in the making, a new female image is now coming to mainstream magazines and advertisement billboards. More mass media industries seem to be devouring full, curvy figures and spitting out the bones. By providing positive examples in magazine editorial articles, newspapers, and advertising campaigns in beauty and fashion, there can be a shift in language of how people, especially teens and women, speak about themselves.

Cover Stories

Recent years have seen a huge crossover with Hollywood celebrities and Grammy-winning singers becoming "cover model gurus" for fashion and lifestyle magazines. The cover lines range from "Make Peace with Your Shape" to "Fat Busting Secrets of the Stars." The body-type standards for most magazine covers are still severely limited. Actress Renée Zellweger ended up on the cutting room floor as she launched *Bridget Jones' Diary* because her curvy figure was considered too heavy for the cover of *Harper's Bazaar.* However, for the first time, former editor Kate Betts shared her struggle with the decision. She began an article in the "Style Section" of the *New York Times* with the statement "I owe Renée Zellweger an apology" and went on to say:

> These days, fashion's antifat bias and obsession with thinness, so ingrained among those who make careers in the business, is looking increasingly like a blind spot, one that could ultimately shortchange designers, retailers and even magazine publishers. . . . Over the last century, body types have gone in and out of style like hemlines and haircuts. . . . All of these permutations occurred against a backdrop of larger questions about the role of women and the power of images. Fashion, which can make people feel beautiful and glamorous, can also make people feel worse about themselves if they're not as beautiful, or as thin, or as fabulous as the swans in the pictures. (Betts, 2002, p. 1)

Actress Kate Winslet is another example of a Hollywood actress who is not "fat" but who keeps being dumped in that category. Her already fabulous curvy legs were retouched for a cover of *British GQ,* which stirred up the debate on airbrushing (Davies, 2003). Some editors claim women want to see a fantasy when they turn the pages of a magazine, and insist these technological touch-ups are necessary. Other media outlets and celebrities have spoken out against the blatant physical fabrications of airbrushing photographs and state that these fantasy images are part of the reason why it has been impossible to promote size acceptance in the media.

Some magazine cover lines are promising. In October 2002 *People* magazine had a cover story, "Sexy at Any Size," and in the same season, an article featured on the cover of *Us* magazine stated: "Who's Sexy Now? Short. Tall. Big. Small. What Really Counts Is Attitude, Not Size. And Hollywood May Be Getting the Message."

Editors and Models

In 2000, Liz Jones, editor-in-chief of British *Marie Claire* magazine, attended the Supermodel Summit in England—a body-image symposium in which figures from the worlds of fashion, modeling, and women's media met to discuss how the media pressures young women to be thin rather than feel beautiful in their own skin. As a result, European fashion editors committed to using more 12-plus models in fashion editorials.

Several publications have made a concerted effort to create issues that are more inclusive and less hostile to our frames. Editors-in-chief who have addressed the body-image dilemma include Atoosa Rubenstein, founder of *CosmoGirl!* and now editor of *Seventeen* magazine. She has made it clear that her magazines would be more diversified and inclusive of myriad body shapes. Liz Tilberis, the legendary editor of *Harper's Bazaar* who passed away from ovarian cancer in 1999, was also vocal in her stand on this issue.

Even editor-in-chief Anna Wintour of American *Vogue* dips in halfheartedly once a year with "The Shape Issue." One year we saw the darling of the plus-size world, model Kate Dillon, portrayed in a fashion spread as an "Amazon stature shape" next to a shrunken figure of a man as her partner. The following year featured another plus-size model, Mia Tyler. Ms. Wintour's language in the body-issue's Editor's letter reflects this shift as well. In 2002 she states: "I fully take on board the complex issues of body dysmorphia, isolation, and manipulation that presenting images of idealized women may give rise to," and in 2003 her letter from the editor began with, "I couldn't help but thinking, as we prepared this issue, how confused we all are about matters of size, weight and speech. If it's politically incorrect to call someone fat—in a country where one in three people suffers from (medical) obesity—why is there no prohibition against labeling a skinny person "skeletal" or "anorexic." . . . It's tiresome. Why can't we just accept that people come in different sizes?"

The Beauty Industry

Some beauty companies have started to see the world through a different lens. Celebrities Queen Latifah and plus-size supermodel Emme were seen in beauty campaigns for Cover Girl and Clairol, supporting the message that beauty comes in all sizes. Another example of this message is found in Dove's "Campaign for Real Beauty 2004" (www. campaignforrealbeauty.com). This is the first time a major beauty company has appeared to be truly committed to using real women in their print and television media—going far enough to announce inclusion with a billboard in Times Square that shows women of all body shapes.

Clothing Industry Responses

The power of the media recently led fashion companies such as Ralph Lauren, Tommy Hilfiger, Oscar de la Renta, and Anne Klein to size up in order to include women who wear sizes 14–24W. Chain stores such as Old Navy not only extended their missy line to size 20 but also launched a plus-size line for women's sizes starting at size 16W. Torrid, a division of Hot Topic, was created to offer contemporary junior clothes for plus-size teens. Even well-established chains created exclusively for plus-size women, such as Lane Bryant, Ashley Stewart, and Avenue, have adapted their collections to more contemporary lines and offer a more fitted silhouette instead of a boxy bigger fit. These new designs are finally answering the needs of the younger, hipper, curvy female consumer.

The Role of Teenagers

The new interest in plus-size consumers may not be due entirely to the shifting standards of attractiveness; teen customers also have tremendous spending power. The plus-size business for kids has become critical for the retailers who work with this age group. As kids returned to school in 2004, news stations and local newspaper articles across the country asked how the industry is going to dress these teens. Unfortunately, this media coverage also included destructive articles such as "Do Kids' Plus Sizes Legitimize Obesity?: Teen-Plus Sizes Risk of Accepting Obesity" (Nicita, 2004).

Teenagers are effective spokespeople. Teen readers responded to an article written in 1996 in *People* on the pressures of being thin and wrote, "I'm so much more than my body size, and I don't have time for those who would judge me just on what I look like." Teenagers also need our support. We need to teach our daughters and sons to choose role models for their hearts and minds, as well as looks. We should continue to aim to be the best of *ourselves* due to *their* inspiration—*not aspiration.*

How do we raise self-awareness and self-esteem in the media so that our children learn body self-acceptance? How do we angle and reposition celebrity role models and real role models that have found some sense of peace within their bigger bodies as an example of health and well-being? The media holds so much power to educate and support what was started by *Mode* magazine in 1997. Since that time, *Glamour* has included columns like "So, You're Not a Size 10—What Do You Call Yourself—Shapely? Plus Size? Big Boned?" Today's fashion magazines and entertainment publications can become even more inclusive by using female models and celebrities above a size 12. Cover lines should continue to read like *Glamour* in the December 2004 issue: "Sexy Clothes for Real Bodies: Size 2 or Size 24? Who Cares! Flattery for All!"

There are positive signs. This year, *Allure* has made "Total Makeover" a standing column, following women who learn new diet and exercise programs to become healthy in their bodies over the course of one calendar year. *Marie Claire* has regular articles on body-image and food-issue concerns. *Cosmogirl!* has "Body Beautiful" coverage on a monthly basis and *Seventeen* has added a "Curvy" column to every month's issue. It has also been a record couple of years for magazine coverage about body image and dressing for your body type.

THE FUTURE FOR MEDIA IMAGES

Diane Bliss is a Los Angeles-based actress and comedian and who became disenchanted with the industry due to the dearth of positive roles for plus-size women in film and television, so she founded and now chairs the Plus-Size Task Force of the Screen Actors Guild. The mission of this group is to inform and educate the industry about the negative portrayals of plus-size people, particularly women, and to increase the quantity and quality of available roles.

There are several obstacles to achieving the stated goal; the most important one is that plus-size people are not recognized as a protected class under federal, state or local anti-discrimination laws (see Chapter 14, this volume). This means that even though the director of the office of Affirmative Action and the chair of the Women's Committee of the Screen Actors Guild are sympathetic to the cause, there are so many demands on the limited resources available for the protected classes that plus-size actors are virtually dead last in the priority list for funding. Nevertheless, this group is moving forward with plans to sponsor a career night where members can meet individually with casting directors and agents. A website features the most active members of the Task Force (www.actorsatlarge.com).

While past portrayals of plus-size people have been predominantly negative, there are signs the landscape is slowly changing. NBC's *Jane Pauley Show* had a program on the topic of body image in December 2004. HBO has a new documentary slated on the roster based on Lauren Greenfield's (2002) book *Girl Culture*. HBO has also gotten behind the groundbreaking independent film *Real Women Have Curves* (La Voo & Cardoso, 2002). On stage, activist and award-winning playwright Eve Ensler addresses these issues in the *Vagina Monologues* and her newest play, *Good Body*. Author Jennifer Weiner is currently touring with her new book, *Little Earthquakes*, which has another fabulous plus-size woman as one of the major characters and has been optioned to Universal Pictures. As in her first book, *Good in Bed*, Jennifer mixes women characters of all sizes into her stories, with truth, skill, care, and humor.

Michele Weston is a body-image author (*Learning Curves*) and is currently on the founding magazine team, as Executive Editor, Style and News, for *AmaZe* magazine (www.AmaZemagazine.com) for curvy women. She co-owns the retail consulting firm Selling Style, which helps clothing companies develop their sales strategies to meet the needs of curvy women (www.SellingStyle.com). She believes the impact of plus-size/curvy models and the motto "Style beyond Size" was a turning point in mainstream fashion magazines. The visuals are shifting and the eye is becoming retrained to be more inclusive. What is next and how do we go about this shift? With passion for change, but *slowly* and with purpose. All the outrage, all the publicity has worked, and as a result there is a greater push for acceptance of women of all sizes in fashion magazines and all forms of media—certainly more genuine than ever before.

REFERENCES

Betts, K. (2002, March 31). The tyranny of skinny, fashion insider's secret. *New York Times*, Section 9, p. 1.

Davies, H. (2003, January 10). Why there's more to Slimline Kate than meets the eye; Lads' mag gives star a digital makeover. *Daily Telegraph (London)*, p. 13.

Greenfield, L. (2002). *Girl culture*. San Francisco, CA: Chronicle Books.

La Voo, G. (Producer), & Cardoso, P. (Director). (2002). *Real women have curves* [Motion picture]. United States: HBO Films.

Nicita, L. (2004, June 2). Do kids' plus sizes legitimize obesity?: Teen-plus sizes risk of accepting obesity. *Gannett News Service*.

CHAPTER 20

■ ■ ■

Coping with Weight Stigma

REBECCA M. PUHL

The social consequences of obesity occur in multiple areas affecting the health and well-being of obese individuals. A disquieting number of such consequences have been documented, including disadvantages in employment, health care, education, interpersonal relationships, and overall quality of life (Puhl & Brownell, 2001; Puhl, Henderson, & Brownell, 2005). The impact on individuals is beginning to be studied, but it is probable that stigma results in negative outcomes that compromise well-being and psychosocial functioning. Given that obesity is associated with increased risk for many medical problems and chronic illnesses, it is especially important to prevent additional consequences created by stigma.

Despite the vast numbers of people affected, little work has examined the ways in which obese individuals cope with bias and discrimination. The topic is important given the limited success of existing treatments, leaving millions overweight and exposed to bias, stigma, and discrimination. We believe it is important to identify how people cope with a stigmatizing environment, whether some approaches are more beneficial than others, and how interventions might be developed to assist obese patients in their efforts to cope effectively. Without sufficient examination of coping methods, it will be difficult to assist obese people in managing bias and participating in activities of daily life that most people take for granted. The aim in this chapter is to review what is known about the ways that obese people cope with stigma, and to identify areas that require further study to help the field move forward.

Coping with stigma involves dealing with stress in social interactions, making decisions about whether to avoid or confront the perpetrator of stigma, and deciding to accept, internalize, or reject the content of the stigmatizing message or a discriminatory action. There are different ways that individuals attempt to adapt to or reduce distress in these situations.

CONFIRMATION

Obese persons may cope with stigmatizing situations by confirming negative perceptions attributed to them by others, and behaving or thinking in ways consistent with stereotypes. Confirmation has been demonstrated among obese women in two experimental studies. In one study, male participants were instructed to engage in telephone conversations with female participants, and males were led to believe that their telephone partner was either an obese or normal-weight woman. Obese female participants confirmed males' negative weight-related perceptions during telephone conversations by portraying themselves as being similar to the stereotyped assumptions made by their phone partners. The authors suggested that obese women may have confirmed stereotypes as a way to facilitate social interactions (Snyder & Haugen, 1995).

In a second experiment, obese and nonobese women received either positive or negative feedback from a male confederate who rated their attractiveness as a potential dating partner. Heavier women reacted to negative feedback by attributing this criticism to their weight, and instead of placing blame on the confederate for his response, reacted by accepting negative stereotypes (Crocker, Cornwell, & Major, 1993).

Quinn and Crocker (1998) hypothesize that obese people may confirm negative stereotypes as a way of feeling more similar to members of society who endorse these normative views, and as a means of increasing personal motivation to lose weight. Research suggests that coping strategies of confirming or internalizing obese stereotypes have negative consequences of increasing negative affect, depression, hostility, and vulnerability to low self-esteem (Crocker et al., 1993; Fuller & Groce, 1991; Quinn & Crocker, 1998).

SELF-PROTECTION

Some obese individuals may use self-protective coping strategies to buffer themselves from bias and to preserve their self-esteem (Crocker & Major, 1989). Self-protection can involve ascribing negative feedback to prejudiced attitudes of others, comparing one's outcomes to others in the stigmatized group, or selectively minimizing domains in which one's stigmatized group is perceived as inadequate and instead valuing those traits in which they excel. Studies have not yet examined self-protective strategies of coping among obese persons, although examples can be found in certain obese populations. Members of the National Association to Advance Fat Acceptance (NAAFA), for example, publicly attribute negative stereotypes about obese people to biased societal attitudes and instead embrace positive attributes of being obese.

Research by Crandall, Tsang, Harvey, and Britt (2000) showed that self-protective coping strategies were only correlated with increased self-esteem when stigmatized individuals perceived themselves to be legitimate members of the stigmatized group, but not when they were attributed a stigmatizing label without feeling part of the group. This work did not assess obese individuals, but it can be predicted that self-protective strategies may be most useful if an obese person feels that his or her stigma is part of a larger group identity. However, obese individuals may be reluctant to identify themselves as members of a larger population of "obese people" if they hope to eventually lose weight and escape their stigma. Thus, for those who do not identify with a larger group membership, self-protection strategies may be less effective.

Crocker (1999) proposes that self-esteem among obese people is shaped by attributions about the causes of obesity, and that in situations where uncontrollable causes of obesity are emphasized, stigma is more likely to be attributed to biased attitudes rather than personal traits, thus protecting self-esteem. These views have not yet been tested with obese populations, and more work is needed to know whether self-protective processes are intentional and viable coping responses.

COMPENSATION

Obese people may try to compensate for stigma by focusing on personal skills or traits that can facilitate achievement of desired goals and positive feedback. Limited research has examined this coping strategy, but existing work supports compensation as a tool that some use to deal with weight stigma. In one study, obese and nonobese women participated in telephone conversations with individuals who they believed either could or could not see them (Miller, Rothblum, Felicio, & Brand, 1995). When obese women believed that they were visible to partners, they rated themselves as more likable and socially skilled than nonobese women, who decreased their self-ratings. The authors suggest that obese women presented themselves more positively to compensate for anticipated negative reactions from being visible (Miller et al., 1995).

Research on compensation strategies in obese adults found that involvement in community organizations and engaging in excessive "helping" behaviors increased social acceptance and likability (Hughes & Degher, 1993). Other work suggests that individuals who were obese since childhood may be more likely to use compensation (Degher & Hughes, 1999), presumably because those who confront stigma at a young age learn to achieve success in other areas in order to be accepted (Hughes & Degher, 1993).

Additional research is needed to determine whether compensation strategies produce more favorable perceptions of obese people when faced with stigma, and to determine the criteria used to judge the amount of effort necessary to compensate sufficiently. For example, negative outcomes may be more likely to occur for obese individuals if they compensate inappropriately, which might be the case if weight stigma is perceived to be low, or if an individual tries too hard to compensate, in which excessive emphasis of skills could result in negative reactions (Miller et al., 1995; Miller & Myers, 1998).

CONFRONTATION

Obese individuals may be able to increase feelings of empowerment and prevent further stigmatizing encounters by confronting the "perpetrator" of stigma. Levy (1993) defines confrontation as challenging the reasons for and consequences of another's behavior. In a self-report study of obese adults, verbal assertion and physical aggression were reported as responses to perpetrators of stigma (Joanisse & Synnott, 1999). Verbal assertions included filing formal complaints, responding with witty comebacks or insults, or making verbal threats to end relationships with individuals if negative comments did not cease. Physical aggression was reported less frequently, but included minor acts of aggression. Participants reported that asserting their rights and challenging the perpetrator was their preferred method of coping. Research in this area remains scarce, and studies are needed to identify under what circumstances confrontation is effective in ending additional stigmatization and how useful it is in improving self-esteem or overall well-being.

SOCIAL ACTIVISM

Protesting weight stigma is another possible coping strategy. Social activism has been identified as a common method used by homosexuals to deal with the stigma of AIDS (Siegal, Lune, & Meyer, 1998), and this strategy has also been observed among obese advocacy groups like NAAFA, who promote size acceptance, battle weight discrimination, and challenge stigma in a variety of public domains. Dealing with weight stigma through social activism may provide benefits of communal coping, such as allowing obese individuals to achieve acceptance, support, and meaningful group membership.

It has been suggested that social activism is most likely to be used when individuals believe that their stigmatized status cannot be changed (Deaux & Ethier, 1998). While some obese individuals may believe that their overweight status is temporary and can be altered once weight loss occurs, others may have experienced years of unsuccessful dieting and perceive their obese status to be unalterable. Widespread societal perceptions that obesity is controllable and that people are personally responsible for being overweight are often internalized, leading some people to never cease hoping they will wrestle the situation under control. Under these conditions, social activism may be less likely.

Social action is slowly leading to policy-level changes with the implementation of anti-weight discrimination legislation, but some authors suggest that it may be challenging to eradicate prejudice and discrimination by challenging societal attitudes given the automatic and deep-rooted quality of stereotypes (Major, Quinton, McCoy, & Schmader, 2000). More needs to be known about the types of benefits one might experience from this form of coping, and under what conditions activism can change social attitudes.

AVOIDANCE

Negative outcomes of stigmatizing encounters may lead some obese individuals to avoid social interactions or public situations as a way of coping. Stigmatized individuals who have low confidence in their ability to cope may default to avoidance responses (Swim, Cohen, & Hyers, 1998). Hughes and Degher (1993) found that avoidance strategies were commonly reported by obese individuals in their study who were confronted with stigma. Situations that were avoided included shopping in public places or going to the beach, where they believed that being observed could potentially place them at higher risk for ridicule and stigma.

Research has documented that avoidance is associated with higher levels of distress among obese persons confronted with stigma (Myers & Rosen, 1999). Increased distress may come from diminished social support and few opportunities to express emotions. One form of avoidance is psychological disengagement from stigmatizing areas of life. Disengagement may involve attributing less value to areas that are stigmatized and placing more value in others. A risk is that disengagement may lead to long-term avoidance in multiple areas, therefore compromising skills and further reducing incentives to participate in these areas (Major & Schmader, 1998).

It is not known whether obese individuals are more likely than other stigmatized people to disengage when confronted with bias. Some argue that obese individuals may be less likely to discount negative feedback and more likely to engage in self-blame due to normative perceptions that obesity is under personal control, a belief which would make it more difficult to disengage (Major & Schmader, 1998). Research is needed to explore the frequency and types of avoidance strategies used by obese individuals and whether avoidance is an effective coping strategy.

ATTEMPTING TO LOSE WEIGHT

Individuals who believe that weight is within personal control may attempt to escape stigma by trying to lose weight (even with approaches as dramatic as surgery) and to blame themselves for stigmatizing situations; thus, they may be less likely to try other coping strategies (Miller & Major, 2000). Although very little work has examined the association between gastric bypass surgery and stigma, self-report studies indicate that people's perceptions of stigma change prior to and following surgery. In one study, 87% of presurgical patients reported that their weight prevented them from being hired for a job, 90% reported stigma from coworkers, and 84% avoided being in public places due to their weight (Rand & MacGregor, 1990). Following surgery, all patients reported reduced discrimination (stating that they rarely or never perceived prejudice since the operation), and 90% reported increased cheerfulness and confidence (Rand & MacGregor, 1990).

Another study examining obese patients undergoing gastric restriction surgery documented that 59% of patients requested the surgery for social reasons such as embarrassment, and only 10% emphasized medical reasons (Peace, Dyne, Russell, & Stewart, 1989). Following the operation, patients reported improved interpersonal and occupational outcomes. The self-report nature and self-selected samples of this research are limits to these studies, yet this research suggests that social perceptions may contribute to surgery decisions. An important question is whether surgery is more likely to be sought by individuals without other means of coping.

METHODOLOGICAL CONSIDERATIONS

Because the literature addressing moderating factors of coping has not addressed weight stigma, the individual difference variables influencing how obese persons experience and cope with weight stigma have not been studied. It is likely that gender, age, personality, self-perceived problem-solving abilities, self-esteem, social support, and beliefs about the causes of obesity have some impact on the ways in which obese people might best cope with stigma (Puhl & Brownell, 2003).

Several other methodological issues arise from the existing literature on coping with weight stigma. First, some coping strategies seem theoretically analogous despite distinct labels. As an example, coping methods like compensation, self-protection, and even disengagement strategies may be better categorized as strategies that aim to maintain and buffer self-esteem. It may therefore be useful to identify fewer categories of coping strategies to facilitate comparisons of coping styles.

Second, the measurement of coping must improve for advances to be made. Many self-report measures of coping exist, but they often assess different types of coping, arise from opposing theoretical perspectives, and differ in whether they measure coping dispositions versus strategies used in specific situations. Much more work is needed to determine which approaches of measurement are most appropriate, and to clarify fundamental questions about the structure of coping processes.

Third, attempting to determine the usefulness and effectiveness of coping strategies are challenges. Strategies perceived to be useful in coping with certain situations may be less effective in others, and some methods (e.g., physical aggression) may have short-term adaptiveness but little value in general. This picture is complicated when the meaning of effectiveness is considered. Effectiveness could be defined by reduction of future stigma, psychosocial functioning, motivation for weight loss, decrease in distress, or short-term versus long-term consequences. It may be wise to identify coping strategies that both prevent stigma and improve emotional/physical well-being.

WHICH COPING METHODS ARE BEST?

With scarce research on this topic in general, it is too early to predict which methods of coping are most appropriate for obese individuals. Some cross-sectional data has documented multiple coping strategies reported by obese individuals, including problem solving, confrontation, social support, avoidance, wishful thinking, and thought modification (Myers & Rosen, 1999). Certain types of coping, such as self-blame, isolation, and avoidance were associated with higher distress and mental health symptoms, whereas strategies like self-acceptance and positive self-talk were somewhat related to more positive psychological adjustment. The frequency of coping responses increased in proportion to increased stigmatization, and coping strategies were used more frequently with increasing severity of obesity (Myers & Rosen, 1999). This study does not address whether specific coping methods decrease stigma or whether different coping methods are likely to be effective in certain situations. However, the results suggest that a variety of coping methods are likely being practiced across and within stigmatizing encounters, and point to the need for further work to investigate the relationships among weight stigma and distress, psychological variables, and other indices of well-being in populations of obese persons.

CONCLUSION

Research on coping with weight stigma is just beginning. This chapter has presented information on an array of coping strategies, and although there are significant gaps in knowledge, there is sufficient information to help guide future research.

The visibility and perceived controllability of obesity make weight stigma distinct from many other forms of stigma, but it can be beneficial to learn from research with other stigmatized groups to help identify methods for investigating coping in obese individuals. Other priorities for research include examination of individual differences and situational factors that affect coping by obese people, theoretical consideration of how to conceptualize effectiveness of coping strategies, and implementation of multidimensional assessments of coping responses for stigma experiences.

The implications for advancing the field in this area are potentially far-reaching. With focused efforts to address existing empirical and conceptual questions, we can begin to identify and test clinical tools that will provide health care professionals with strategies to help obese patients manage stigma, and can offer parents and educators ways of helping obese children cope with prejudice. Of course, without changes in societal attitudes toward obesity and significant reformation of larger social systems, the utility of coping strategies may be limited. Eradicating pervasive societal attitudes is a considerable challenge, and should not be a burden for obese individuals to bear alone.

REFERENCES

Crandall, C. S., Tsang, J., Harvey, R. D., & Britt, T. W. (2000). Group identity-based protective strategies: The stigma of race, gender, and garlic. *European Journal of Social Psychology, 30*, 355–381.

Crocker, J. (1999). Social stigma and self-esteem: Situational construction of self-worth. *Journal of Experimental Social Psychology, 35*, 89–107.

Crocker, J., Cornwell, B., & Major, B. (1993). The stigma of overweight: Affective consequences and attributional ambiguity. *Journal of Personality and Social Psychology, 64*, 60–70.

Crocker, J., & Major, B. (1989). Social stigma and self-esteem: The self-protective properties of stigma. *Psychological Review, 96*, 608–630.

Deaux, K., & Ethier, K. A. (1998). Negotiating social identity. In J. K. Swim & C. Stangor (Eds.), *Prejudice: The target's perspective* (pp. 301–323). New York: Academic Press.

Degher, D., & Hughes, G. (1999). The adoption and management of a "fat" identity. In J. Sobal & D. Maurer (Eds.), *Interpreting weight: The social management of fatness and thinness* (pp. 11–27). Hawthorne, NY: Aldine de Gruyter.

Fuller, M. L., & Groce, S. B. (1991). Obese women's responses to appearance norms. *Free Inquiry in Creative Sociology, 19*, 167–174.

Hughes, G., & Degher, D. (1993). Coping with a deviant identity. *Deviant Behavior, 14*, 297–315.

Joanisse, L., & Synnott, A. (1999). Fighting back: Reactions and resistance to the stigma of obesity. In J. Sobal & D. Maurer (Eds.), *Interpreting weight: The social management of fatness and thinness* (pp. 49–70). Hawthorne, NY: Aldine de Gruyter.

Levy, A. J. (1993). Stigma management: A new clinical service. *Families in Society, 74*, 226–231.

Major, B., Quinton, W. J., McCoy, S. K., & Schmader, T. (2000). Reducing prejudice: The target's perspective. In S. Oskamp (Ed.), *Reducing prejudice and discrimination* (pp. 211–237). Mahwah, NJ: Erlbaum.

Major, B., & Schmader, T. (1998). Coping with stigma through psychological disengagement. In J. K. Swim & C. Stangor (Eds.), *Prejudice: The target's perspective* (pp. 219–241). New York: Academic Press.

Miller, C. T., & Major, B. (2000). Coping with stigma and prejudice. In T. F. Heatherton, R. E. Kleck, M. R. Hebl, & J. G. Hull (Eds.), *The social psychology of stigma* (pp. 243–272). New York: Guilford Press.

Miller, C. T., & Myers, A. M. (1998). Compensating for prejudice: How heavyweight people (and others) control outcomes despite prejudice. In J. K. Swim & C. Stangor (Eds.), *Prejudice: The target's perspective* (pp. 191–218). New York: Academic Press.

Miller, C. T., Rothblum, E. D., Felicio, D., & Brand, P. (1995). Compensating for stigma: Obese and nonobese women's reactions to being visible. *Personality and Social Psychology Bulletin, 21*, 1093–1106.

Myers, A., & Rosen, J. C. (1999). Obesity stigmatization and coping: Relation to mental health symptoms, body image, and self-esteem. *International Journal of Obesity, 23,* 221–230.

Peace, K., Dyne, J., Russell, G., & Stewart, R. (1989). Psychological effects of gastric restriction surgery for morbid obesity. *New Zealand Medical Journal, 102*, 76–78.

Puhl, R., & Brownell, K. D. (2001). Obesity, bias, and discrimination. *Obesity Research, 8*, 788–805.

Puhl, R., & Brownell, K. D. (2003). Ways of coping with obesity stigma: Review and conceptual analysis. *Eating Behaviors, 4,* 53–78.

Puhl, R., M., Henderson, K., E., & Brownell, K. D. (2005). Social consequences of obesity. In P. Kopelman, I. Caterson, & W. Dietz (Eds.), *Clinical obesity and related metabolic disease in adults and children* (pp. 29–45). London: Blackwell.

Quinn, D. M., & Crocker, J. (1998). Vulnerability to the affective consequences of the stigma of overweight. In J. K. Swim & C. Stangor (Eds.), *Prejudice: The target's perspective* (pp. 125–143). New York: Academic Press.

Rand, C. S., & MacGregor, A. M. (1990). Morbidly obese patients' perceptions of social discrimination before and after surgery for obesity. *Southern Medical Journal, 83*, 1390–1395.

Siegal, K., Lune, H., & Meyer, I. H. (1998). Stigma management among gay/bisexual men with HIV/AIDS. *Qualitative Sociology, 21*, 3–24.

Snyder, M., & Haugen, J. A. (1995). Why does behavioral confirmation occur? A functional perspective on the role of the target. *Personality and Social Psychology Bulletin, 21*, 963–974.

Swim, J., K., Cohen, L. L., & Hyers, L. L. (1998). Experience everyday prejudice and discrimination. In J. K. Swim & C. Stangor (Eds.), *Prejudice: The target's perspective* (pp. 37–59). New York: Academic Press.

CHAPTER 21

Advocacy

LYNN McAFEE
MIRIAM BERG

In our hearts, we all know prejudice and discrimination when we see it. The false stereotypes about fat people—that they are weak-willed, lazy, stupid, selfish, and ugly—have resulted in rampant discrimination in all areas of life, from employment to health care to family and social interactions. The question is, what can one individual do about it?

Other social change movements have shown us that advocacy is critical in the fight for equality. Imagine being in a room with friends and hearing someone telling a racist joke. How would you handle the situation? Would you find a way to tell the friend that you found the joke offensive? If so, you are an advocate. One of the basic principles of activism is "Think Globally, Act Locally." Being an advocate in one's daily life can make a difference, ultimately, in the world. Advocacy can happen on any scale. You can advocate within your family, your school, your local or state government, your workplace, public places, private places—in short, everywhere.

In order to become advocates, we must first confront the prejudice within ourselves. Even for a plus-size person it is not possible to live in this culture and not be prejudiced against fat people. As we have learned with other prejudices like racism and sexism, prejudice is deeply ingrained and must be confronted by both the individual and society. Confronting your own prejudice is an ongoing process, not a job you can do in an afternoon. Reading books on body image and size acceptance, joining organizations or online discussions, even starting a group, can be steps toward self-acceptance.

Information does not always equal change, but it is a tool that is critical in effecting change. This book is a major resource for anyone who wants to advocate for plus-size people. Advocates need to have a solid foundation of facts and principles. These need to be ideas that most people can understand and relate to. For advocacy against weight discrimination, basic tenets include the following:

1. Diets don't work. There is no successful treatment for individuals that takes off weight and keeps it off.
2. Ideas of attractiveness change through history. Today's cultural obsession with extreme thinness is damaging to people's self-esteem and, indeed, to their physical health.
3. People should be judged on the basis of their actions and their character, not on the basis of their weight.

The debate over whether weight is "voluntary" is meaningless until science discovers a way to allow people to lose weight and keep it off. Once we stop blaming people for being fat, our society will start dealing with the diversity of sizes in a rational way. Public accommodations, including seating, will be made more size-friendly; health care professionals will be educated in how to treat larger patients for their medical conditions just as they would thin patients with the same conditions, instead of automatically prescribing weight loss; job applicants would be chosen on basis of how well they could do the job, and weight prejudice would play no part in the decisions.

The civil rights movement was galvanized in part by the phrase "Black is beautiful." In the same way, we can advocate for fat people's rights by advocating for a new aesthetic. It is important to remember that fat has not always been considered unattractive. In the 1890s, Lillian Russell was considered the most beautiful woman in the world, at over 200 pounds. The women portrayed in Reubens' paintings would today be classified as supersize. "Ideal" body sizes are merely fashions, changing as quickly as clothing styles.

The personal is the political. But for those who want to take advocacy to the next level, one thing to consider is finding your own strengths. Do you feel more comfortable speaking to someone in person, or on the phone? Do you prefer to talk or write? Do you prefer to work alone or with others? Find a way to be an advocate that fits your personal style.

One advocate called the diversity office in her city when she found out they were doing a sign campaign. She had to call back a few times, but she finally succeeded in getting them to include size as one of the characteristics included in diversity. The office printed signs that businesses can post that say: "This space respects all aspects of people, including race, ethnicity, age, sexual orientation, ability, size, and gender expression."

Another advocate went to the hospital and discovered they had no wider wheelchairs. She had to be wheeled through the corridors on a gurney. She asked to speak to an administrator, and explained the problem. Within 2 weeks, the hospital had purchased an extra-wide wheelchair.

WRITING LETTERS

Letters can be very effective in creating change. One advocate learned that her local movie theater was under renovation. She wrote to the owner and suggested that putting in a few of the new "love seats" would make it possible for larger people to attend more movies. The owner wrote back saying he appreciated the suggestion, and the new movie theater has a few double seats that can fit a thin couple or one fat person.

Here is an example of a powerful letter, sent to the Council on Size & Weight Discrimination by someone who said we had inspired her to become an activist, and that this was her first such letter:

Dear Father Smith,

I had the privilege of attending Holy Cross Church on a Sunday in late August with my parents. There was a visiting priest there.

I would like to tell you why I found his homily distasteful and inappropriate. He started out speaking of the Olympic games and how the athletes train for years to condition their bodies, which of course is true and I have no objection to. He then went on to describe how we must do the same for our souls or they will atrophy. I also believe this statement to be true.

Then he went on to describe how so many American are fat. He then went on to speak out about almost every single fat prejudice that people have today. He equated being fat with being lazy and gluttonous. He also implied that fat people are failures and that fat is evil and should be avoided at all costs.

I am a fat woman and although I am a vegetarian, ride my bicycle to work in clement weather and do yoga, obviously, this priest wants parishioners to see me otherwise. Instead of getting to know me they can prejudge me because of the way I look.

I felt like I didn't belong there, like this church did not welcome me, a visiting Catholic, into their fold as Jesus would have, because I am fat.

Our bodies are what they are. God in His infinite and incomprehensible wisdom made us all different and all special, yet in the same image as the Holy One. "Gentile or Jew, servant or free" as the popular hymn goes. We are all a part of God's family and no one should ever feel left out.

If all the priests preach love and acceptance maybe we can help recovering bulimic and anorexic individuals, or, even better, prevent these conditions from occurring altogether. Perhaps the person at the end of his or her rope will find strength to continue because here, amongst God's family, in the Catholic Church, this person has found the love and acceptance that has always eluded her.

Yours in Christ,

Here is a letter to a health food store objecting to an ad campaign. Although it is fairly long, I include it because it contains many arguments that advocates can use in their own letters.

Dear Health Food Store,

I just saw your ad in the newspaper, in which you prominently display the headline:

One in seven children is obese.

I am offended by this ad on so many levels it is difficult to know where to begin.

1. *My first reaction is "So what?" Kids come in all sizes, and weights are distributed in the population in a normal bell curve. But your ad makes the strong implication that we should be very concerned about those kids at the higher end of the range, and that we should try to change their size so that they are "normal."*
2. *Children who are heavier than average deserve to have the opportunity to lead ordinary, happy lives. Why should their size mean they are not well-adjusted, interesting, intelligent, or any number of characteristics that go into making a good life?*
3. *Obese is a medical term with a specific meaning. But when used as it is used in your ad, it becomes a taunt with the power to do serious emotional damage. Giving the word such prominence*

lets bullies know that it is perfectly all right to torment the fat kids.

4. *Since your ad is obviously aimed not at kids but at parents, your purpose is to create guilt about parents' roles in their children's weight. You are in effect advising parents to put their kids on weight-loss diets at a time when the kids need adequate nutrition for growth.*
5. *Despite the mass media hysteria about weight that is going on right now, the scientific facts are far from clear. Body weight is a very complex issue. It has not been proven that higher weights lead to shorter lives. What is clear is that lack of exercise, and poor nutrition, lead to higher risk of chronic diseases such as diabetes.*
6. *Lack of exercise and poor nutrition are behaviors. Body size is a characteristic. The two are not at all the same, and should not be confused or used as substitutes for one another.*
7. *Lack of exercise and poor nutrition are not always behaviors that can be controlled by choice. Much of the disease caused by these factors is really caused by poverty and lack of access to fresh foods. Many children don't have safe places to be active.*
8. *Countless controlled studies have shown that weight-loss diets have an abysmally low long-term success rate. There is currently no known method of weight loss that will take off weight and keep it off for more than 1 or 2 years. Some studies have shown, and many dieters have confirmed, that it becomes harder to lose with each diet, and that yo-yo dieting ultimately results in a higher body weight over time.*
9. *Our culture is obsessed with thinness rather than with healthfulness, and the media supports that obsession. The standard for ideal body size gets progressively smaller. Celebrities who fail to stay thin are ridiculed and kicked out of the spotlight. Thinness is falsely equated with beauty, star quality, acting ability, and virtue.*
10. *Promoting thinness and dieting, as your ad does, is part of the reason eating disorders are epidemic in our country and in Europe. Seventy percent of normal-weight high school girls feel fat and are on a diet. One in ten of those will develop a full-blown eating disorder. Eating disorders have a 5–20% mortality rate, the highest of any psychiatric diagnosis (see enclosed fact sheet with citations).*
11. *Your ad falsely implies that if parents shop in a health food store, their kids won't get fat, or will lose weight if they already are. Are all your customers thin? Have you never seen a fat veg-*

etarian, or a skinny meat-eater? Are you implying that the snacks you sell don't have any calories? don't you sell butter, which is 100% fat—mostly artery-clogging saturated fat?

12. *Assuming that the foods you carry promote health, why does your ad target only the obese? If children are average weight or thin, does that mean their parents should not worry about the quality of their nutrition?*

In populations where the standard of living is fairly high, both children and adults can be healthy at whatever size they are naturally. Physical activity, fresh whole foods, and healthy lifestyle behaviors can improve health for people of every size.

This is what your ads should be promoting: Health for all people, no matter what their size. Improving one's health by eating better, whether or not that causes you to lose weight. Letting your children be who they are, feeding them well, and honoring their body sizes.

don't use the scare tactics of the weight-loss industry. Tell parents to make a commitment to health for themselves and their children.

I hope you will change your ads and make no references to obesity, overweight, or weight loss in future ads. Please let me know your position on this issue. If you wish to discuss this further, please call me.

Sincerely,

LETTERS TO THE EDITOR

One of the most widely read section of the newspaper is the letters to the editor. Advocates should consider this a form of free publicity for the cause. Some suggestions for writing letters to the editor: Keep it short; read other letters to that publication and match their style; don't use irony or sarcasm; refer to an article or letter, and briefly summarize the content of that piece; include a cover letter and documentation of any statistics (this is for the editor's information, not to be published); and end with a dramatic statement. Here are some examples:

Letter in response to an article on dangerous fad diets, fasting, and weight-loss surgery:

To the Editor:

Your article "Dying to be Thin" told the story of a few desperate people who went to extreme measures to lose weight, but this problem affects all of us, everyday. Fear of being fat permeates our culture and distorts our perceptions. Every time we compliment someone for losing weight we are contributing to this distorted standard of what is attractive. Beauty—like health, strength, character, and happiness—comes in all shapes and sizes.

Letter in response to a letter to the editor on the effectiveness of dieting:

To the Editor:

In a letter to the editor, dietitian Jane Doe says that "simply" buying less, practicing portion control, and staying active are "tried and true methods to fight fat." If losing weight were as easy as she makes it sound, everyone who wanted to be thin would be thin. Instead, the long-term success rate for all methods of weight loss is abysmally low.

Our genes have prepared us for lives of physical labor. Instead, we spend our workdays in front of computers. The human metabolism is set up to withstand famine, but we live in a nation where quick and easy food is a major industry. These trends will not likely be reversed.

Poor nutrition and lack of exercise have dangerous health consequences for all people, regardless of weight. Rather than blame individuals for their weight or for their health condition, we need to acknowledge these cultural changes and take appropriate steps.

Instead of allowing fast-food companies to run lunch programs, schools should be given the funding to provide nutritious and appealing choices. Opportunities for safe and pleasurable physical activity should be made available to people of all sizes in schools, workplaces, and communities. And health practitioners should, without judgment, help their patients be as healthy as they can be no matter what their size.

Changes such as these would be much more effective at promoting health than stern lectures on "self-control," which have so far proven to be useless.

Letter in response to an op-ed piece that denounced the San Francisco law against weight discrimination:

To the Editor:

The author of this op-ed betrays his own bigoted attitudes at the end of his article. After claiming to use purely scientific research and legal opinion to denounce San Francisco's ordinance against weight discrimination, he ends his column with the sarcastic suggestion that a ballet school, to satisfy the new ordinance, might want to put in "disability handrails that heavy people could use while climbing the building's long flight of steep stairs." He then adds: "Oh. An elevator might be nice, too."

He is trying to create a mental image of fat people struggling with stairs to show that it would be absurd for heavy people to learn to dance. Yet earlier in the piece, he takes fat people to task for failing to exercise. Apparently he feels that dance is not a proper type of exercise for people who do not meet his stringent requirements of body size, shape, and weight.

Whether the cause is social, environmental, behavioral, or genetic, the fact is that many Americans are fat. We can continue to make life difficult for them, in the misguided belief that teasing, rejection, and discriminatory treatment will make them lose weight. Or we can change our attitudes and accommodate people of all sizes in our lives.

One way to change cultural attitudes is by changing laws. I applaud San Francisco for taking a stand against weight discrimination.

ACTIONS IN DAILY LIFE

Effective advocacy may involve writing letters or making phone calls to protest unfair treatment or portrayal of fat people. But advocacy can also mean taking simple action in daily life on behalf of oneself or a friend. One of the more important things fat advocates can do for themselves is to insist on respectful health care. Fat people need to talk to their doctors, and to ask them for advice on how to be as healthy as possible whether or not they lose weight. They need to ask for specific changes if necessary, such as not being given lectures on weight loss or dieting, and moving the scale to a more private area or not being weighed at all. This is an area where thin allies can play an important part by going along with a friend and helping to facilitate the discussion. Another benefit of this kind of advocacy is that the physician is introduced to the concept of health at every size.

Media messages and images can be very damaging, especially to young minds. Children are the most susceptible to the hurtful messages they see and hear every day from the media, their peers, and even the adults in their lives. People of all sizes should learn to be critical of these messages, to recognize their subtle manipulations, and to educate others about them. Testimonials are compelling, but it must be pointed out that they are not the same as scientific proof. Diet ads that show before-and-after pictures need to be countered with the correct information: The people in those ads probably regained all the weight they lost within a year or two. Portrayals of fat people stuffing themselves, or breathing heavily, or acting in malicious ways need to be identified as degrading and insulting. As mentioned earlier, humor that makes fun of people for their weight has to be interrupted.

In any kind of advocacy, follow-up is very important. The issue is not as important to the other person as it is to you. It is also essential to meet hidden objections. In the case of health care professionals, that might mean taking along some information from medical journals on the ineffectiveness of dieting. Finally, advocates need to pick their battles. It is not worth trying to change the mind of someone who is a hard-liner on the issue of weight. There are so many people who would be open to these ideas if they had the opportunity to hear them.

Advocacy is about the personal and the political, about passion, commitment, and personal growth. Those who confront their own prejudices will feel better about themselves, no matter what their size. There is no better feeling than knowing that you expressed the truth, argued for fairness and tolerance, and took action toward making the world a safer place for people of all sizes. Perhaps the most useful thing an advocate can do is to advocate for young people: Compliment plus-size kids, give them positive messages, let them know they are OK just the way they are, and encourage them to stand up for themselves. In that way, the advocacy can be passed on to the next generation.

AUTHORS' NOTE

For further information about advocacy against weight bias, see www.cswd.org.

CHAPTER 22

■ ■ ■

Expression of Bias against Obesity in Public Policy and Its Remedies

MORGAN DOWNEY

Bias may be expressed in many ways. Individuals can express bias by overt actions and statements as well as by inactions or departures from normative behavior, such as not helping someone who has fallen down or had an accident. Institutions can also express bias by their actions and by their omissions. The determinants of institutional action are multifactorial and open to debate. Nevertheless, such actions or omissions are available to discernment and evaluation. To this end, obesity can be viewed through the prism of what institutions do or fail to do regarding obesity. We can compare their actions and policies with those for other diseases of a comparable nature. The most obvious place to start is with governmental and nongovernmental health care institutions, not only because they literally make life and death decisions but also because obesity is a physiological condition and the decisions or omissions they make regarding obesity are, to a large extent, more transparent than with other institutions.

Let us begin by looking at a hypothetical condition. This condition is a fatal, disabling, and relapsing chronic disease. While it has been in existence for a very long time, it quickly increases in prevalence across every age, gender, racial, and socioeconomic group (Flegal, Carroll, Odgen, & Johnson, 2002). Children and adolescents are affected, implying ever increasing generations of very sick individuals continuing into the future (Hedley et al., 2004). The condition becomes a major cause of preventable death in the society (Olshansky et al., 2005). It also is recognized as a major cause of other long-term chronic diseases that affect every organ system in the body (Bray, 2003). The costs associated with treating this condition are very high and lead to increases in the overall costs of health care in the society (Thrope, Florence, Howard, & Joski, 2004). Many individuals become disabled, usually by a combination of diseases caused by this condition, and are unable to work, becoming dependent on governmental assistance (Strum, Ringel, & Andreyeva, 2004). Now imagine that this society has evolved a highly sophisticated science-based response for dealing with similar conditions. Its response typically involves a combination of basic science, clinical or applied research, prevention efforts, treatments for the afflicted, and education for providers, patients, and the public.

We can uncloak this hypothetical condition and the affected society. The condition, of course, is obesity and the society is the United States at the outset of the 21st century. We can ask, therefore, does the U.S. health care system deal with obesity in the same way that it has dealt with similar threats to public health? How would the U.S. health care system respond to our hypothetical disease if it weren't obesity?

Over previous decades, the United States has suffered through several major public health challenges. These include tuberculosis, influenza, polio, cancer, smoking, and HIV/AIDS. Each disease had its own unique aspects in terms of scientific understanding, public attitudes, and models of intervention. Yet, the governmental responses all share a similar pattern, which include:

1. Expansion of research to understand the basic physiology of the condition.
2. Treatment of the afflicted population.
3. Prevention to halt spread of the disease.
4. Educational efforts for the public and health professionals.
5. Efforts to combat discrimination, which interferes with prevention, treatment, or control over the disease.

However, the federal government's response to the obesity epidemic has fallen far short of this historical expectation. The obesity paradigm currently in place is basically this: We know what causes obesity and what to do about it so research is relatively unimportant. The critical step is preventing future cases of persons who are at normal weight from becoming overweight. Therefore, prevention is to be preferred to treatment. Obesity is overwhelmingly a failure of personal protective actions, so the appropriate role is for the government to tell people how they should act to avoid obesity in the future. Stigma and discrimination are unfortunate but do not rise to the level of significance of other criteria, such as race, gender, and religion. Some stigma may actually be helpful, as in the case of stigmatizing smokers to make smoking less socially desirable.

Examples of this paradigm can be found in Healthy People 2010 (U.S. Department of Health and Human Services, 2000), which establishes goals for reduction in obesity rates, and in the Surgeon General's Call to Action to Prevent and Decrease Overweight and Obesity (U.S. Department of Health and Human Services, 2001), which make almost no reference to treatment of obesity and little to research. Let us now look at the various aspects of the federal government's response to elucidate this paradigm.

RESEARCH

The National Institutes of Health (NIH) is the major biomedical research organization both in the United States and the world. Its current budget is over $28 billion. Operationally, NIH is divided into some 27 institutes and centers. The institutes are the major budgetary sources of funding and include the National Cancer Institute, the National Institute on Aging, the National Institute of Child Health and Human Development, the National Institute of Neurological Disorders and Stroke, the National Institute of Mental Health, the National Heart, Lung and Blood Institute, the National Institute on Deafness and Other Communication Disorders, the National Institute on Nursing Research, the National Institute on Diabetes and Digestive and Kidney Diseases, the National Institute on Arthritis, Musculoskeletal Disorders and Skin Diseases, the National Eye Institute, the National Institute of Allergy and Infectious Diseases, the National Institute on Alcohol Abuse and Alcoholism, the National Institute of Dental and Craniofacial Research, and the National Institute on Drug Abuse. Institutes receive a line-item appropriation from the U.S. Congress and engage in a host of activities, including funding extramural research grants, some intramural programs, research training, translation of research into clinical practice, conferences, and other forms of education for health care professionals and the public. Institutes rely heavily on outside experts for advice and review of research proposals. Institute leaders play major roles in explaining to Congress and the public important health developments, as was the case with the HIV/AIDS epidemic and the anthrax outbreak. They also have many consultative roles with other federal agencies.

Obesity does not have an institute of its own, although arguably it is at least as important a health concern as eye diseases, allergies, skin diseases, and deafness. The lead institute for obesity research is the

National Institute on Diabetes and Digestive and Kidney Diseases (NIDDK), although other institutes, such as the National Heart, Lung and Blood Institute (NHLBI), play significant roles. There are five major divisions within NIDDK. Obesity is not one of them; it is organized as a separate office.

The lack of a significant role for obesity research has major implications for the efforts to prevent and treat obesity. Obesity research funding is far below what is needed. Many other disorders of similar magnitude or diseases that are significantly attributable to obesity receive far greater funding. In fiscal year 2004, obesity research funding was just $422 million, or about 1.5% of the total NIH budget, while substance abuse was funded $1.5 billion; cancer, $5.6 billion; heart disease, $2.1 billion; diabetes, $996 million; and HIV/AIDS, $2.8 billion. Alzheimer's disease, which affects about 4 million Americans, received 150% of the obesity funding, although obesity affects over 15 times as many people (National Institutes of Health, 2005a).

The low organizational status of obesity research may mean that there are missed opportunities for important collaborations. One such opportunity was missed in 2002 when one NIH Center, the Fogarty International Center held a conference on the global effects on health of stigma. The NIDDK declined to participate, and so obesity was not included in the agenda (National Institutes of Health, 2001) or in subsequent requests for research proposals (National Institutes of Health, 2005b).

In recent years, the NIH has increased its obesity activities. Funding has increased from $97 million in 1997 to $420 million in 2004. In 1997, the NHLBI published the Guidance for the Treatment of Adult Obesity (National Heart, Lung and Blood Institute, 1998). In 2001, the director of the NIH created an internal "Task Force on Obesity," which created an NIH Strategic Plan on Obesity Research (Strategic Plan for NIH Obesity Research, 2004). However, the previous "Task Force on the Prevention and Treatment of Obesity," composed of outside experts, was downgraded at the same time. Although this NIH Strategic Plan was generally well-regarded in the field, it carried no additional funding commitment.

EDUCATION

Understanding the nature and extent of a major threat to public health is an essential component of any effective strategy. During such crises, emotional responses can run high, interfering with sound public health strategies and impeding access to treatment by affected individuals. The federal government's efforts in promoting improved awareness of obesity have been substantial—a large number of websites have been developed. The former Secretary of Health and Human Services and the Surgeon General have addressed the issue in numerous public statements. Major components of the federal government, including the Centers for Disease Control and Prevention (CDC), the National Institutes of Health (NIH), and the Food and Drug Administration (FDA) and Federal Trade Commission have all instituted some efforts at public education about obesity.

Yet, in most instances, important opportunities have been missed. For example, there has been little effort to educate health care providers and the public on the meaning and use of the Body Mass Index (BMI), resulting in public confusion over the "obesity epidemic." Little information has been conveyed about the influences of genetics and the environment on obesity compared with personal "lifestyle" aspects. Almost no attention has been focused on morbid or severe obesity (BMI ≥ 40), compared with a BMI of 30 or more. This is a major omission since the mortality, morbidity, health care utilization, and health care costs increase dramatically at higher body weights. The population with morbid obesity has increased at a faster rate than the population at a BMI of 30 (Must et al., 1999).

Furthermore, major efforts to aid consumers seeking nutrition information have been uncoordinated. Until the announcement of the new Food Guide Pyramid on April 19, 2005, the pyramid used different portion sizes than the FDA-regulated food label provided. For example, the pyramid serving size for pasta is a half cup while on the nutrition label it is a full cup (U.S. Department of Agriculture Center for Nutrition Policy and Promotion, 2000). Additionally, many Americans view obesity as just a U.S. issue and do not appreciate its global dimension (Monteiro, Moura, Conde, & Popkin, 2004). This view can have two effects. First, to the extent that obesity is only characterized as poor behavior, it is a challenge to perceive a worldwide epidemic of sloth and overeating. Second, it causes us to miss important research opportunities as different societies have different experiences with putative causes, such as transportation, breastfeeding of infants, childhood physical activity, television viewing, fast-food access, and vending machines.

TREATMENT

Federal health programs generally exclude coverage of obesity treatments. Medicare, the largest federal health program, had a policy until July 2004, which held that obesity was not an illness or disease and therefore no program payment could be made (U.S. Department of Health and Human Services, 2004).For some time, Medicare has had limited coverage of gastric bypass surgery when used to treat other conditions, such as cardiovascular disease or diabetes. The Medicare policy change in July 2004 eliminated the language that obesity is not an illness and began a process of evaluation of different therapies. Medicare does not cover physician and dietician counseling on obesity, however, and drugs for treatment of obesity were excluded from the new Medicare drug benefit.

Likewise Medicaid, the federal–state program for low-income individuals, generally has little to no coverage of drugs for the treatment of obesity or for physician or dietician counseling. Surgery is apparently covered in some states, but often the patient must have multiple obesity-related problems (making them very high-risk patients). Or the reimbursement rate is so low as to deter surgeons and hospitals from providing the service to patients. It is reasonable to assume, although no hard figures exist, that obesity is highly prevalent in the Medicaid population. This has created an analomous situation wherein the Department of Health and Human Services ordered state Medicaid programs to pay for Viagra even when they did not cover treatments for obesity (Associated Press, 1998).

Other federal health programs, such as the Veteran's Administration health care services, the Indian Health Service, and the Department of Defense program for military personnel and their dependents likewise have limited to nonexistent coverage. The picture on the private insurance side is hardly more hopeful. Most commercial insurance programs have little to no coverage for treatment of obesity. Drugs for weight loss are generally not covered; if they are covered, it is usually for only a short duration. Counseling is almost never covered. Bariatric surgery had modest insurance coverage until 2004 (Stein, 2004) when several large national insurance companies and many local ones announced that they were dropping coverage from their standard benefits. In some cases, employers could purchase coverage for an additional premium. Some plans have increased demands for documentation of prior failed weight loss attempts. For some patients, this is a "catch-22." If they do not lose weight during a year before surgery, they are deemed noncompliant and the surgery coverage is denied. If they do lose weight, the surgery is regarded as unnecessary. In some states, if an obese individual loses group health insurance coverage, they cannot purchase individual coverage because of their weight. Even in cases where the policy provides coverage of items such as bariatric surgery, denials necessitating appeals over a long period of time are common. On the positive side, Blue Cross and Blue Shield of North Carolina announced in 2004 that it would begin offering a package of obesity treatments, which included physician and dietician counseling, FDA-approved medications for weight loss, and bariatric surgery at selected centers of excellence (BCBS, 2004).

As mentioned above, the existing paradigm for obesity stresses prevention virtually to the exclusion of treatment. It is almost a mantra of policymakers to state that they do not want to treat obesity; they want to prevent it. This binary choice exists nowhere else in the health care system. It would be unheard of for a policymaker to say, "I don't want to treat breast cancer (or HIV/AIDS); I want to prevent it." The apparent reasons—that treatments are not effective or costly—may not be the real reasons. After all, studies to prevent obesity have not shown much effectiveness, and preventive interventions can be expensive as well.

The situation of bariatric surgery is especially informative. As discussed above, the population with morbid obesity is where most of the mortality, morbidity, disability, suffering, and discrimination are found. Bariatric surgery has long-term studies showing effective weight loss. In fact, bariatric surgery is one of the most powerful interventions in all of modern medicine. According to a meta-analysis (Buchwald et al., 2004), surgery not only results in long-term weight loss, but it also resolves or eliminates several long-term chronic diseases, including type 2 diabetes, obstructive sleep apnea, hypertension, and hyperlipidemia. Furthermore, a recent Canadian study showed that patients who had the surgery survived markedly longer than those who did not (Flum & Dellinger, 2004).

It strains credulity to imagine a surgical procedure with this profile, including a mortality rate of less than 2% (Christou et al., 2004), being eliminated from coverage for any other disease state.

REMEDIES

From this brief survey, it should be clear that the United States has a serious disconnect between the impact of the rising tide of obesity and the responses of policymakers to this problem. In fact, it may be observed that the principal policy outcome in Congress and in many states since the Surgeon General's report is to consider legislation to insulate the food and restaurant industries from any possible civil injury claims. Furthermore, in spite of abundant information on the obesity crisis, little attention has been paid to the millions of dollars of subsidies at the federal and state level for agriculture and programs to increase food consumption.

The American Obesity Association (AOA) has decided to focus advocacy efforts to affect the direction of federal health care policies related to obesity. At the heart of these efforts is advancing the concept of obesity as a disease rather than an unwanted personal behavior. Under this paradigm, obesity is seen as a complex, multifactorial disease in its own right; a fatal, relapsing chronic disease due to a combination (or interaction) of genetic, environmental, and behavioral factors that we do not fully understand. Research is at the core of these advocacy efforts. It provides the science base for prevention strategies and can lead to more effective interventions than are currently available. Likewise, the obese person is not seen as a failure but as a patient trying to manage a lifelong complex disease. We look at obesity like skin cancer. Skin cancer is a result of a genetic predisposition to fair skin, environmental exposure to the sun, and the failure to take personal protective steps. In fact, there are numerous other diseases that share a similar profile of genetic, environmental, and behavioral interaction. Advocating this view, the AOA has been successful in having obesity recognized as a disease by the Social Security Administration in its revision of regulations for when persons with morbid obesity can qualify for disability (Federal Register, 1998).

A major step was taken when, after urging from AOA, the Internal Revenue Service reversed its policy and recognized obesity as a disease whose costs were eligible for the medical deduction from individual taxes (IRS Revenue Ruling 2002-19). This step led to the change in Medicare policy discussed earlier.

AOA's advocacy goals are straightforward. It seeks:

1. The creation of a National Institute of Obesity Research at the National Institutes of Health to expand, focus, and broaden basic and clinical research on obesity and to speed the development of new therapies. In addition, this institute could initiate much needed health policy and economics research to evaluate policy recommendations.
2. Coverage of obesity treatments in federal health plans, such as Medicare and Medicaid.
3. Modernizing guidances of the Food and Drug Administration for the development of a new generation of drugs to treat obesity.
4. A federal "human activity impact statement," similar to the environmental impact statement, which would require federal construction projects to evaluate the effect of physical activity on a community's patterns and, if necessary, take remedial steps to maintain or expand physical activity.
5. Review of federal and state legislation, such as the No Child Left Behind Act, which appear to inhibit programs of physical activity in the nation's schools.
6. Bans on discrimination against persons with obesity in health care, education, and employment.
7. Creation of an Office of Obesity Policy in the Secretary of

Health and Human Services Office charged with coordination of agencies within Health and Human Services and among other federal agencies.

AOA believes that such steps are needed to create an infrastructure to deal with the multiple aspects of obesity.

The questions raised at the outset of the chapter, "Does the U.S. health care system deal with obesity in the same way that it has dealt with similar threats to public health? How would the U.S. health care system respond to our hypothetical disease if it weren't obesity?" can be answered in the negative. It is clear, however, that we have the tools to affect the course of this epidemic if we choose to use them. By attacking obesity and not the obese we may be able to promote public health, reduce suffering, and alleviate the stigma associated with obesity.

REFERENCES

Associated Press. (1998, July 2). *Medicaid must cover Viagra.*

BCBS. (2004, October 12). *Blue Cross and Blue Shield of North Carolina expands coverage to treat obesity.* Available on-line at: www.bcbsnc.com/news/press-releases/PR2004-1012.cfm

Bray, G. (2003). Risks of obesity. *Endocrinology Metabolism Clinics of North America, 32*, 787–804.

Buchwald, H., Avidor, Y., Braunwald, E., Jensen, M.D., Poires, W., Fahrbach, K., et al. (2004). Bariatric surgery: A systematic review and meta-analysis. *Journal of the American Medical Association, 292*, 1724–1737.

Christou, N. V., Sampalis, J. S., Liberman, M., Look, D., Auger, S., McLean, A. P., et al. (2004). Surgery decreases long-term mortality, morbidity, and health care use in morbidly obese patients. *Annals of Surgery, 240*, 416–423.

Federal Register 63, 11854. (1998, March 11). Available on-line at: www.obesity.org/subs/disability/

Flegal, K. M., Carroll, M. D., Odgen, C. L., & Johnson, C. L. (2002). Prevalence and trends in obesity among U.S. adults, 1999–2000. *Journal of the American Medical Association, 288*, 1723–1727.

Flum, D. R., & Dellinger, E. P. (2004). Impact of gastric bypass operation on survival: A population-based analysis. *Journal of the American College of Surgeons, 199*, 543–551.

Hedley, A. A., Ogden, C. L., Johnson, C. L., Carroll, M. D., Curtin, L. R., & Flegal, K. M. (2004). Prevalence of overweight and obesity among U.S. children, adolescents and adults, 1999–2002. *Journal of the American Medical Association, 291*, 2847–2850.

IRS Revenue Ruling (2002-19). Available on-line at: www.obesity.org/subs/tax/taxbreak.shtml

Monteiro, C. A., Moura, E. C., Conde, W. L., & Popkin, B. M. (2004). Socioeconomic status and obesity in adult populations of developing countries: A review. *Bulletin of the World Health Organization, 82*, 940–946.

Must, A., Spandano, J., Coakley, E. H., Field, A. E., Colditz, G., & Dietz, W. (1999). The disease burden associated with overweight and obesity. *Journal of the American Medical Association, 282*, 1523–1529.

National Heart, Lung and Blood Institute. (1998). *Clinical guidelines on the identification, evaluation, and treatment of overweight and obesity in adults: The evidence report.* Available on-line at: www.nhlbi.nih.gov/guidelines/obesity/e_txtbk/intro/intro.htm

National Institutes of Health. (2001). Available on-line at: www. stigmaconference.nih.gov/

National Institutes of Health. (2005a). *Estimates of funding for various diseases, condition, research areas.* Available on-line at: www.nih.gov/news/fundingresearchareas.htm

National Institutes of Health. (2005b). Available on-line at: www.grants.nih.gov/grants/guide/rfa-files/RFA-TW-03-001.html

Olshansky, S. J., Passaro, D. J., Hershow, R. C., Layden, J., Carnes, B. A., Brody, J., et al. (2005). A potential decline in life expectancy in the United States in the 21st century. *New England Journal of Medicine, 352,* 1138–1145.

Stein, R. (2004, April 11). As obesity surgeries soar, so do safety, cost concerns. *Washington Post.*

Strategic Plan for NIH Obesity Research. (2004). Available on-line at: www.obesityresearch.nih.gov/About/strategic-plan.htm

Strum, R., Ringel, J. S., & Andreyeva, T. (2004). Increasing obesity rates and disability trends. *Health Affairs, 23,* 199–205.

Thrope, K. E., Florence, C. S., Howard, D. H., & Joski, P. (2004, October 20). Trends: The impact of obesity on rising medical spending. *Health Affairs, W4*, 480–486.

U.S. Department of Agriculture Center for Nutrition Policy and Promotion. (2000, December). *Serving sizes in the food guide pyramid and on the nutrition facts label: What's different and why?* Available on-line at: www.usda.gov/cnpp/Insight22.PDF

U.S. Department of Health and Human Services. (2000). *Healthy people 2010 (2nd ed.): With understanding and improving health and objectives for improving health* (2 vols.). Washington, DC: U.S. Government Printing Office.

U.S. Department of Health and Human Services. (2001). *The Surgeon General's call to action to prevent and decrease overweight and obesity.* Rockville, MD: U.S. Department of Health and Human Services, Public Health Service, Office of the Surgeon General.

U.S. Department of Health and Human Services. (2004, July 15). *HHS announces revised medicare obesity coverage policy.* Press Release.

Summary and Concluding Remarks

MARLENE B. SCHWARTZ
REBECCA M. PUHL

There is clear evidence of stigmatization of obese people in multiple domains of living, including education, employment, and health care. Bias places numerous obstacles in everyday life and threatens the emotional and physical health of obese individuals. There is also a growing literature documenting the extent to which obese children and adolescents are targets of stigmatization from both peers and adults, resulting in impaired social functioning, increased psychological distress, and greater vulnerability to eating disordered behavior and other self-harming behaviors. Taken together, existing research documents widely held perceptions that obese people have multiple negative characteristics, ranging from flaws in personal effort (such as lack of willpower or laziness), to central attributes of competence, attractiveness, and even morality. With increasing rates of obesity among adults and children, and evidence that the stigma is intensifying, the situation may worsen if steps are not taken to alleviate negative attitudes.

AREAS IN NEED OF FURTHER RESEARCH

The chapters in this book demonstrate that weight stigma is pervasive and difficult to change. Many key research questions remain unanswered. To address the gaps that exist in knowledge about weight stigma, several methodological advances are needed. As a first step, some experimental studies (such as those testing interventions) should be replicated with larger samples, and those with cross-sectional designs (such as the studies that link teasing to psychological distress) should be tested with longitudinal research. Because the ecological validity of the laboratory experiments on employment discrimination has been questioned, it will be especially important to test for discrimination in real world settings such as schools and workplaces, to examine whether the severity and frequency of discriminatory behaviors match those reported in the laboratory.

Second, the psychosocial and health consequences of weight stigma must be clarified. Some research suggests that negative psychological consequences of obesity are more a function of the bias experienced by the individual than the obesity itself. Assessing the direct impact of weight stigma will be important in understanding the range of adverse outcomes of obesity on health and well-being. It is possible that the impact of bias and discrimination on public health is significant.

Third, the etiology of weight bias needs to be better understood. While research has documented the presence of bias toward obese people in numerous settings, less work has examined why this population has become increasingly derogated, and why it is socially acceptable to hold these attitudes.

Theory-driven research on the psychological origins of weight bias is necessary to guide stigma-reduction efforts. Attribution theories have identified the components of causality, stability, and controllability in forming weight bias, suggesting that these be targeted in efforts to help individuals recognize how their attributions lead to stigma. A truly comprehensive theory of obesity stigma must identify the origins of weight bias and explain the association between certain negative traits and obesity and why stigma is elicited by obese body types. The ultimate goal is to develop methods to reduce bias.

Finally, the chapters in this book highlight the need for additional research to identify and test stigma-reduction interventions. Lack of research and mixed findings indicate the need to integrate theories and to find new stigma prevention methods. The social consensus framework may be one potential method, but is not yet adequately tested. The potential to alter negative attitudes by changing perceptions about the normative acceptability of beliefs is encouraging. It may be especially useful to determine how to utilize and disseminate perceived social consensus approaches in real-world settings.

LEVELS OF INTERVENTION

Given the pervasiveness of negative attitudes toward obese people, multiple intervention strategies are likely needed. Efforts to train employers, educators, and health care professionals to advocate weight tolerance requires recognition of both the physical and interpersonal environment in which weight stigma occurs. Physical barriers in classrooms, medical settings, and places of employment must be considered in addition to subtle and overt forms of communication that stigmatize obese individuals. Honest self-examination of one's own attitudes may be critical to fostering effective and empathic interactions with obese individuals.

Changing social conditions sometimes requires legal interventions. The absence of federal law specifically prohibiting weight discrimination illustrates bias itself. The legal remedies currently available to individuals who believe they have been discriminated against are limited. In order to seek protection under the Americans with Disabilities Act or Rehabilitation Act, plaintiffs must argue that their weight is a disability, which can be difficult to do and conflicts with the mission of those promoting fat acceptance. Title VII of the Civil Rights Act of 1964 does not provide protection because it specifically prohibits employment discrimination based on race, color, religion, sex, or national origin; weight is not included on this list. At the present time, only Michigan, the District of Columbia, San Francisco, and Santa Cruz have laws prohibiting discrimination on the basis of weight.

While the complex medical problems associated with obesity must be addressed, efforts to improve the experiences of patients using the health care system are also worthwhile. Understanding the complex etiology of obesity and learning how to work with obese patients in kind ways should be included in standard training for medicine, psychology, nursing, nutrition and other health-related fields. Health care professionals and those who educate them can play a vital role in stigma reduction by advocating weight tolerance and communicating positive attributes of obese people. Concrete strategies for health care settings are discussed in Chapters 2, 16, and 17.

The collective attitude about the controllability of weight must be challenged. We live in a society where the body is seen as infinitely malleable. Educating people about the genetic, biological, and environmental contributors to body weight may be helpful as a means of reducing anti-fat attitudes. Existing work using education about etiology to change attitudes has found mixed results, but the strong link between the concept of personal responsibility and obesity stigma suggests it is an important area for intervention research. One possible strategy is to provide accurate information about the complex etiology of obesity by admired individuals, peer leaders, or through written materials as part of course curricula.

The portrayal of obese individuals in various media, including the entertainment and fashion industries, requires ongoing attention. While there have been a handful of positive portrayals of overweight people on television, there is a disturbing trend of engaging people in weight loss efforts as a form of entertainment.

We also must identify and question the subtle messages conveyed to children through movies, television, and books about the relationship between body weight and personal characteristics such as intelligence and generosity. The fact that even very small children exhibit weight bias suggests we must challenge the avenues through which children are learning these negative attitudes.

Health professionals, educators, and parents need strategies to help obese children and adults cope with adverse experiences. We need a better understanding of which coping methods can improve daily functioning in stigmatizing environments, protect psychological health, and reduce the negative consequences of future prejudiced encounters. Coping effectively with weight stigma may require a range of strategies, including those that help individuals feel less isolated in their experiences of stigma, reduce feelings of self-blame, lift self-imposed restrictions in living, remove barriers to coping, and encourage individuals to become advocates for themselves.

CONCLUSION

The longer prejudice against obese individuals remains widespread, the more likely that negative attitudes will become institutionalized. In the words of Albert Einstein, "problems cannot be solved at the same level of awareness that created them." It is critical to find ways to address the epidemic of obesity without further stigmatizing individuals. This will involve integrating physical, psychological, and social functioning into measures of health. Reliance on the concept of personal responsibility for weight has not only contributed to stigma, but has dangerously delayed viewing obesity as a public health issue and prevented the needed shift to public health strategies for obesity intervention and prevention. Clinicians, educators, legal advocates, obesity researchers, and health care professionals have a responsibility to improve the well-being of obese adults and children. Our success with this challenge depends on focused research efforts, intensified legal and legislative action, and increased acceptance that weight prejudice must be reduced.

Index

"f" following a page number indicates a figure;
"t" following a page number indicates a table.